Pathology of Granulomas and Neoplasms of the Nose and Paranasal Sinuses

Pathology of Granulomas and Neoplasms of the Nose and Paranasal Sinuses

Imrich Friedmann
MD, DSc, FRCS, FRCPath, DCP

Emeritus Professor of Pathology in the University of London;
Consulting Pathologist, Royal National Throat, Nose and Ear
Hospital, London; Honorary Consultant Pathologist,
Northwick Park Hospital, Harrow; Research Fellow,
Imperial Cancer Research Fund, London; Consultant in
Electron Microscopy, House Ear Institute, Los Angeles;
Formerly Director of the Department of Pathology and
Bacteriology, Institute of Laryngology and Otology,
University of London

The late
Denis A. Osborn
MD, FRCPath

Formerly, Reader in Pathology and Deputy Director
Department of Pathology, The Institute of Laryngology and
Otology, British Postgraduate Medical Federation, University
of London
and
Consultant Pathologist, Royal National Throat, Nose and Ear
Hospital, London

CHURCHILL LIVINGSTONE
EDINBURGH LONDON MELBOURNE AND NEW YORK 1982

CHURCHILL LIVINGSTONE
Medical Division of Longman Group Limited

Distributed in the United States of America by Churchill
Livingstone Inc., 19 West 44th Street, New York, N.Y.
10036, and by associated companies, branches and
representatives throughout the world.

First published 1982

ISBN 0 443 01410 8

British Library Cataloguing in Publication Data
  Friedmann, Imrich
    Pathology of granulomas and neoplasms of the nose and
    paranasal sinuses.
    1. Nose—Tumours
    2. Nose, Accessory sinuses of Tumors
    I. Title   II. Osborn, Denis A.
    616.99'286   RC280.N6

Library of Congress Catalog Card Number 81–68398

Printed and bound in Great Britain by
William Clowes (Beccles) Limited, Beccles and London

Preface

Granulomas and neoplasms of the nose and paranasal sinuses are of great interest to surgeon and pathologist alike and their correct interpretation, often difficult, can influence treatment and prognosis. Semantic and terminological intricacies abound and have defied the imagination of many a lesser and greater authority. We have been aware of these practical and theoretical problems and the presented opinions and conclusions reflect our personal experience and interest in this field over a period of thirty years.

It is with great regret that the writer of these introductory remarks has to announce the untimely loss of his friend and colleague of so many years, Denis Allan Osborn, Reader in Pathology, University of London. He died on the 21st February, 1981 having finished the manuscript but alas could not live to see it in print. A pathologist of great experience has been lost and it is hoped that this book, with his historical reviews, will serve as a monument *aere perennius*, to his scholarship and be of value to the postgraduate and to the practising pathologist and otolaryngologist.

Our thanks are due to our former surgical colleagues at the Royal National Throat, Nose and Ear Hospital, at the Institute of Laryngology and Otology and at the Royal Marsden Hospital. We are also grateful to other pathologists, in particular, the members of the ENT Tumour Panel whose discussions have assisted us in the preparation of this book. Sincerest thanks are due to those colleagues whose photographs and specimens have enhanced the quality of the relevant chapters. To our wives go our thanks for their tacit patience. To our publishers, Churchill Livingstone, go my sincerest thanks for all their help, encouragement and equally tacit patience.

1982   I.F.

To
JOAN and ROSE,
our wives

Contents

Anatomical considerations

ANATOMICAL CONSIDERATIONS

The anatomy of the external nose has hitherto been poorly defined. Dion, Jafek and Tobin (1978) referred to this discrepancy and have described more accurately the cartilages, bone and supporting tissues. They emphasized the variable relations between the upper and lower lateral nasal cartilages that determine the configuration of the external nose which is a matter of considerable interest to the plastic surgeon.

The anatomy of the paranasal sinuses has been known for several centuries and Highmore (1651) defined the maxillary antrum (rightly bearing his name) and described the anatomy of the maxillary and frontal sinuses. The gross anatomical relations of the paranasal sinuses are indicated in Figures 1.1, 1.2, 1.3 and 1.4.

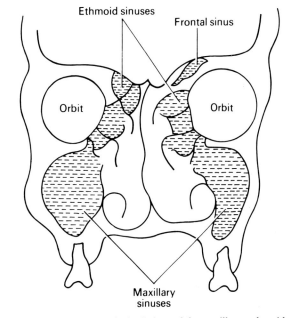

Fig. 1.2 Gross anatomical relations of the maxillary, ethmoid and frontal sinuses.

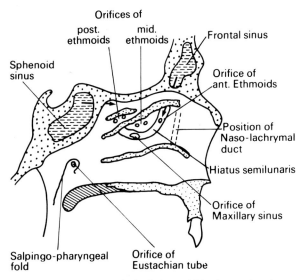

Fig. 1.1 Gross anatomical relations within the nasal cavity.

Normal histology

The anterior part of the vestibule is lined by keratinizing squamous epithelium which is a continuation of the skin covering the external nose. Further back in the vestibule, the squamous cells are no longer keratinized and occasionally they present short knob-like microvilli. As the lining is traced backwards into the nasal fossa, the epithelium undergoes a marked change, becoming a pseudostratified, ciliated, columnar type characterizing the respiratory type epithelium. However, squamous epithelium may be found on the anterior ends of the middle and inferior turbinates, as a result of metaplasia due to exposure to the drying effect of inspired air. It may be of interest to recall that the nasal mucous membrane was first described by Schneider (1660) who

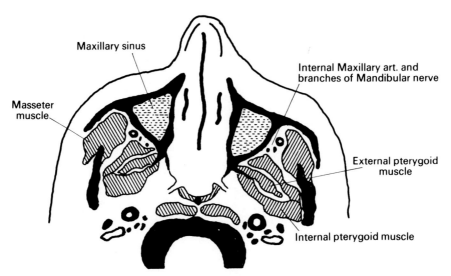

Fig. 1.3 Gross anatomical relations of the maxillary sinus.

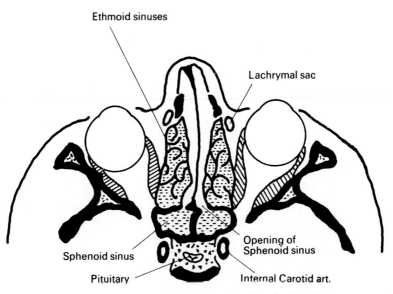

Fig. 1.4 Gross anatomical relations of the ethmoid and sphenoid sinuses.

disproved the theory that mucus originated in the pituitary gland. The lining of the nasal cavity subsequently became known as the Schneiderian membrane. Interspersed amongst the ciliated cells in the respiratory type epithelium are varying numbers of mucus-producing goblet cells. The secretion from these cells supplemented by the product of the mucosal glands, forms a 'mucous blanket' on the surface of the epithelium (Proetz, 1941) which is in constant motion due to the action of the cilia, operating like a conveyor belt. Particles deposited on the anterior aspect of the nasal respiratory mucosa appear in the nasopharynx in about three minutes under normal conditions (Hilding, 1932). Ciliated cells bear a large number of cilia projecting from their free surface. It has been estimated that such cells in the trachea carry nearly 300 cilia. The ultrastructure of cilia was first described by Fawcett and Porter (1954). The cilia are normally endowed with nine peripheral, double microtubules which surround a central pair forming the basic $9+2$ pattern of the axoneme (Figs. 1.5, 1.6 & 1.6a). The microtubules terminate in a basal body or plate by which the cilium is anchored within the cell (Figs. 1.7 & 1.8). Rootlets extend from the basal body deep into the cell, composed of longitudinally arranged fibres, interdigitating with transverse bands (Fig. 1.9) or striations (Anderson, 1971). There are important links between the peripheral and central microtubules (Hilding and Heywood, 1971) and there are two arms attached to one of the outer microtubules which are referred to as 'dynein arms' (Figs. 1.6a and 1.6b). The absence of these structures has been associated with the 'immotile ciliary phenomenon' in Kartagener's syndrome (mucoviscidosis) and also in Retinitis Pig-

mentosa (Arden and Fox, 1979). The last mentioned authors showed that nasal cilia in Retinitis Pigmentosa and congenital deafness (Usher's syndrome) exhibited a high incidence of compound cilia with deviation from the $9+2$ pattern of microtubules and a relative absence of dynein arms. Atypical or giant cilia are a variation of the normal structure (Figs. 1.10 & 1.11), probably due to the precocious regeneration of the true cilia. Kawabata and Paparella (1969) have described atypical cilia in the normal human and guineapig middle ear mucosa and anomalies have also been observed in tissue cultures of the embryonic chick otocyst and also in the antral, laryngeal and postnasal mucosa (Friedmann and Bird, 1971). Such atypical cilia are usually multiple so that several true cilia form a complex enveloped by the bulging outer membrane of the cell. Atypical cilia appear to be more frequent in inflamed or otherwise diseased mucosa and it seems likely that they might impede the regular rhythmic action of the muco-ciliary apparatus.

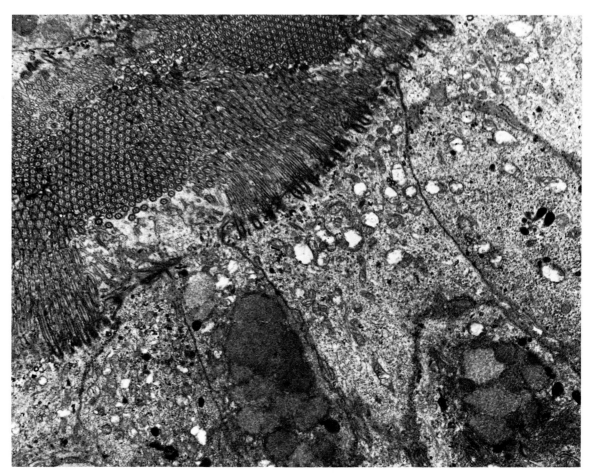

Fig. 1.5 Ciliated epithelium with dense ciliary carpet. M $\times 5950$ By courtesy of the Journal of Laryngology and Otology.

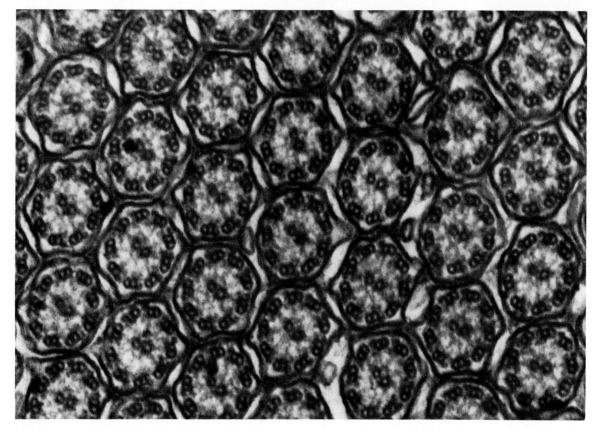

Fig. 1.6 Cilia in transverse section showing the 9 + 2 axoneme pattern of microtubules. Note also connections between peripheral and central structures. M × 111 560.

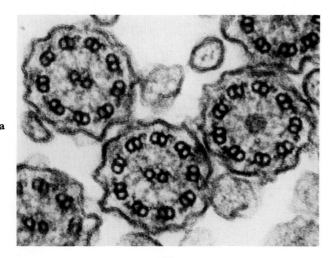

a

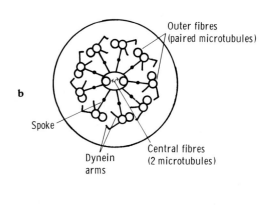

b

Transverse sections of nasal cilia (By courtesy of B. Fox, 1980).

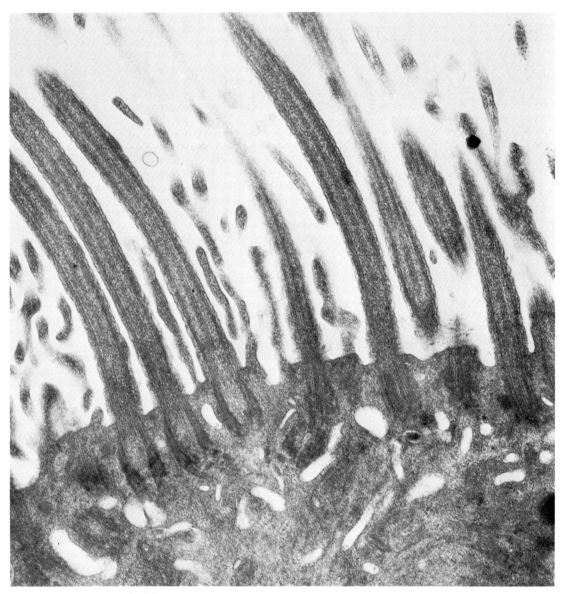

Fig. 1.7 Cilia in longitudinal section showing microtubules and basal bodies. M ×45 500.

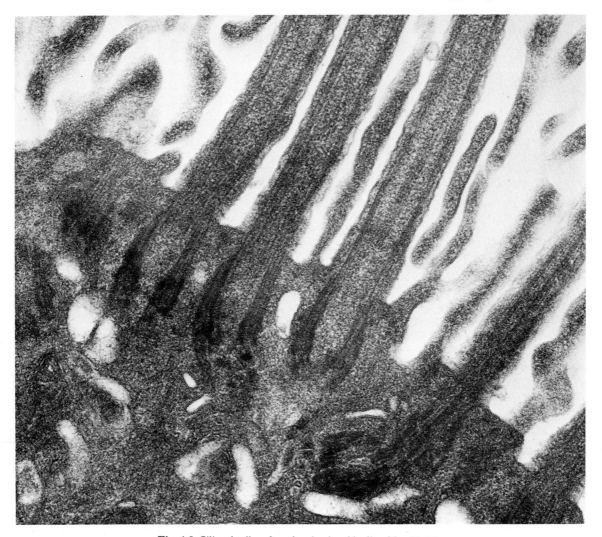

Fig. 1.8 Ciliated cell surface showing basal bodies. M ×98 000.

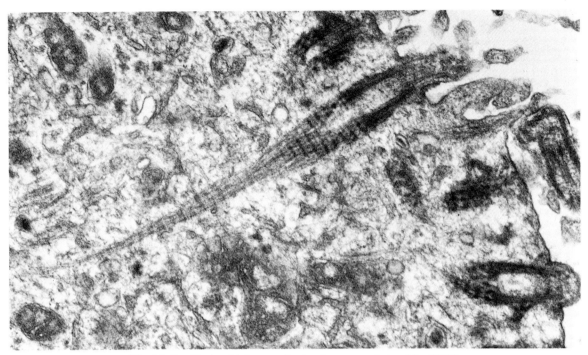

Fig. 1.9 Basal body with long rootlet showing cross striation. M ×56 700.

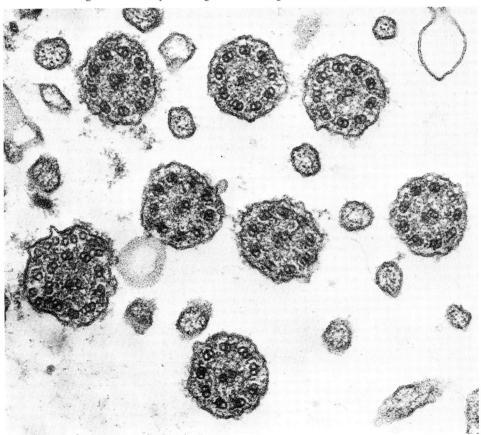

Fig. 1.10 Cross sections of cilia. Note atypical axoneme with supernumerary microtubules (lower left). M ×108 000.

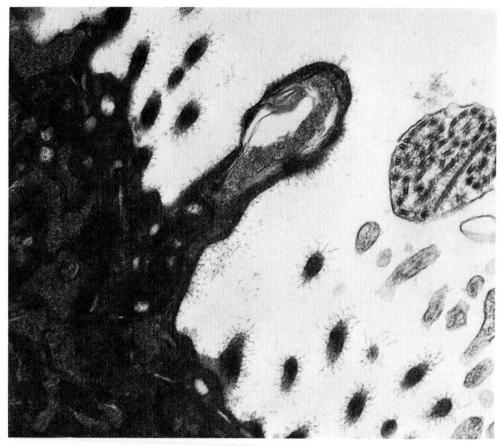

Fig. 1.11 Oblique section of atypical compound cilium (upper right) and abnormal bulbous microvillus. M × 54 000.

Goblet cells vary in number and it has been claimed that there are fewer in the paranasal mucosa. This may be debatable since one of the present authors has examined postmortem paranasal mucosa from apparently normal sinuses and noted a large number of goblet cells. Poulsen and Tos (1975) studied the distribution of goblet cells in the developing human nose. These cells appeared between the 13th and 30th week, commencing anteriorly and were preceded by the establishment of ciliated cells. There has been no supporting evidence for the former view that ciliated cells were capable of transmutation to goblet cells. The modern view is that the latter cells are derived from the basal cells which are to be found in respiratory type epithelium. Under light microscopy with routine haematoxylin and eosin staining, goblet cells are usually identified as unstained areas. Under the electron microscope, the cells are seen to contain numerous membrane-bound mucous granules, usually only moderately electron-dense (Fig. 1.12) but occasionally containing circumscribed denser material. The free border exhibits microvilli which are often coated by mucopolysaccharides (Fig. 1.13) forming a glycocalyx (Friedmann and Bird, 1971).

There are numerous mucosal glands lying deep in the lamina propria. These glands are mixed (Fig. 1.14), comprising mucus-secreting cells and two types of serous secretory units. The ductular systems are not as formalistic as those in the major salivary glands and sometimes ducts may be difficult to identify. The serous elements show two features. Some of the secretory acini contain well defined basophilic granules comparable with those seen in the major salivary glands whilst other acini contain eosinophilic granules resembling those seen in the lachrymal gland. Random analysis of nasal secretions has revealed the presence of amylase-like activity, hence it is a reasonable assumption that the basophilic granules are comparable with the zymogen granules in the salivary glands. It has long been known that tears and nasal secretion contain lysozyme (muramidase). This was established by Fleming (1922) and it is likely that cells containing eosinophilic granules are lysozyme producers.

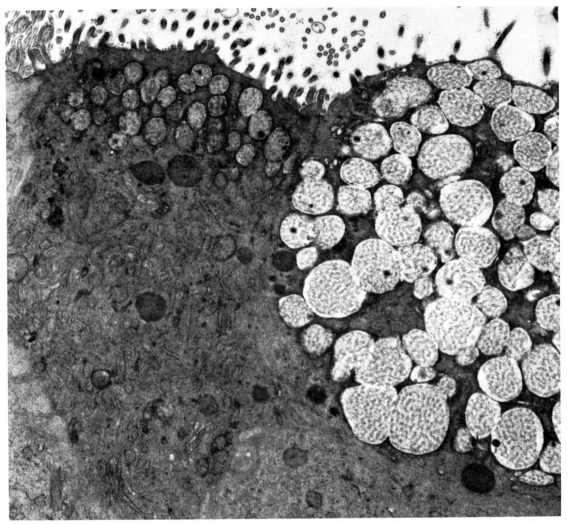

Fig. 1.12 Two goblet cells showing variable content of mucous product. Note microvilli on the free surface and variable electron density of the mucous granules. M × 5400.

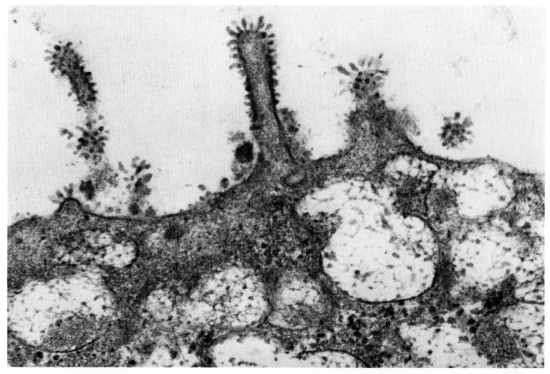

Fig. 1.13 Microvilli on goblet cell showing coating by mucopolysaccharide. M × 63 000.

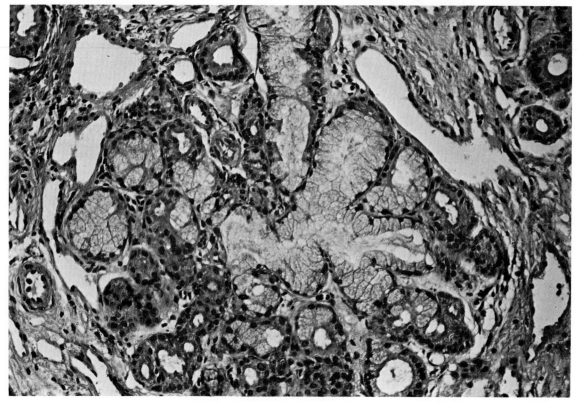

Fig. 1.14 Nasal mucosal gland showing mixed mucous and serous secretory units. M × 223.

On the periphery of both mucous and serous secretory units are located the myo-epithelial cells. These are important since they have relevance to the pathogenesis of certain mucosal gland tumours. In human material, light microscopy is not always successful in demonstrating adequately these cells though occasionally the phosphotungstic acid haematoxylin stain will show up the so-called myofibrils. In human glands, the myo-epithelial cells contain a high concentration of alkaline phosphatase which can be used to delineate the multiple processes of these cells (Fig. 1.15). Electron microscopy reveals the myofilaments with their aggregation zones, resembling smooth muscle (Figs. 1.16a & b).

The mucus-producing cells package their product in the Golgi apparatus forming membrane-bound granules, some of which later become confluent. Electron microscopy also reveals an interesting mechanism of discharge (Osborn, 1974); the apical membrane appears to rupture followed by the release of the cell contents (Figs. 1.17a, b, & c). To what extent this is a holocrine type of discharge is not clear and even if the cell survives there must be an inevitable loss of some of its basic content. The mechanism occurs both in goblet cells and cells of mucosal glands. Under the scanning electron microscope, crater-like traces mark the sites of recent apocrine secretion of the goblet cells (Andrews, 1979).

The mucous product contains two main types of mucopolysaccharide. Neutral mucopolysaccharide exhibits a positive periodic acid Schiff reaction which characterizes the epithelial type mucin whilst acid mucopolysaccharide often differs from that in connective tissue mucin inasmuch as it produces a hyaluronidase-fast metachromasia with Toluidine Blue.

The paranasal mucosa is essentially similar to that of the nasal fossa, though there are slight differences. The columnar cells tend to be shorter resulting in a somewhat thinner epithelium. Columnar cells bear cilia and there are large numbers of microvilli (Figs. 1.18 & 1.19). The lamina propria also tends to be thinner and usually bears fewer mucosal glands. The lamina propria of the nasal and paranasal mucosa often contains a sprinkling of assorted inflammatory cells, including plasmacytes, lymphocytes, macrophages and occasional polymorphonuclear leucocytes and eosinophils, even when the mucosa is apparently healthy. Control of nasal secretion is believed to be under the influence of the parasympathetic system, fibres reaching the mucosa via the sphenopalatine ganglion.

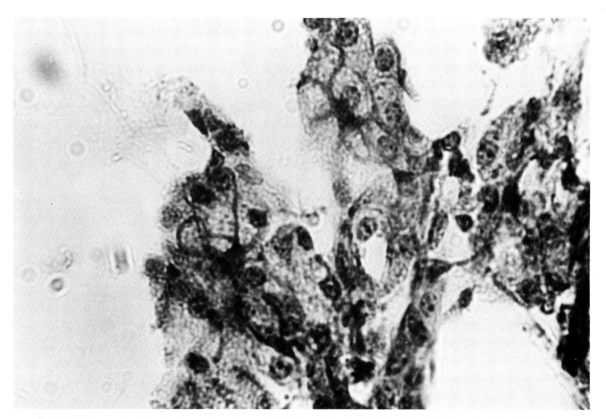

Fig. 1.15 Myo-epithelial cells, in a guineapig parotid gland, outlined by the histochemical demonstration of alkaline phosphatase. M × 600.

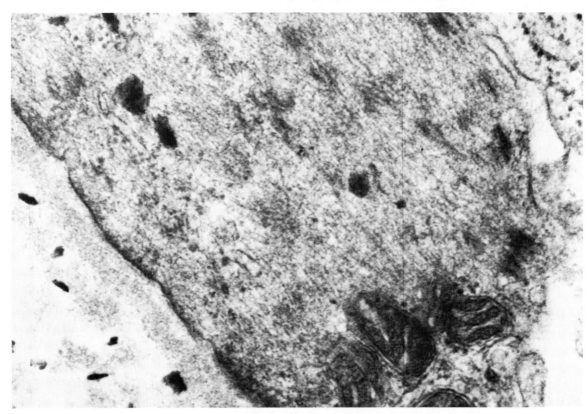

Fig. 1.16a Myo-epithelial cell in nasal mucosal gland showing filamentous cytoplasm with aggregation zones. M ×75 000.

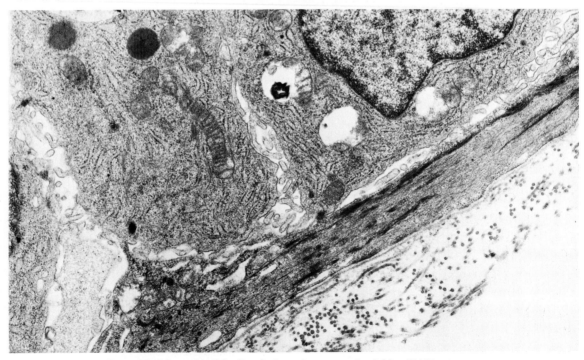

Fig. 1.16b Myo-epithelial cell at the base of a mucous gland. M ×23 170.

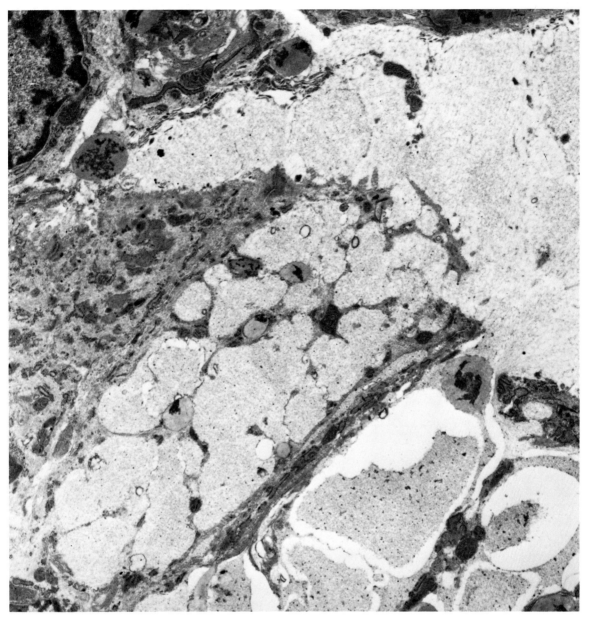

Fig. 1.17a Mucous gland in nasal mucosa showing rupture of the luminal cell surface, leading to liberation of the mucous product. M × 12 000.

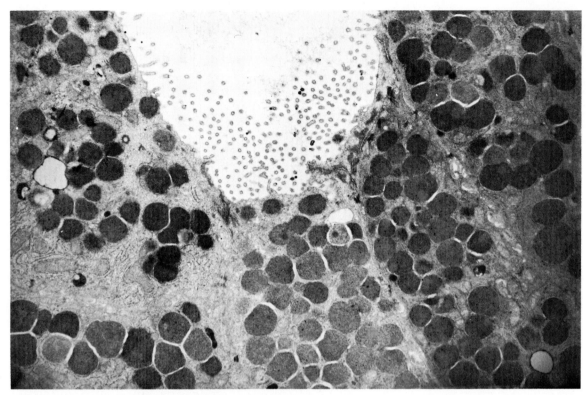

Fig. 1.17b Lumen of gland surrounded by secretory cells. M × 8890.

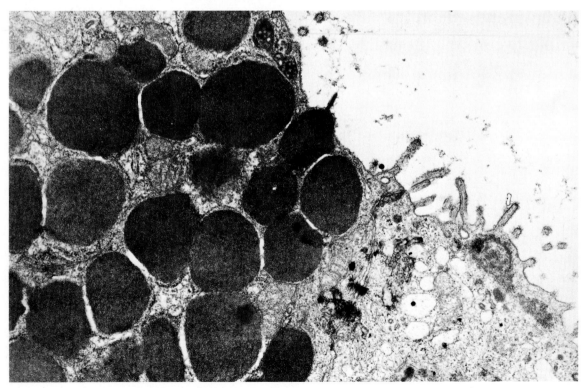

Fig. 1.17c Detail showing secretory granules and microvilli. M × 11 830.

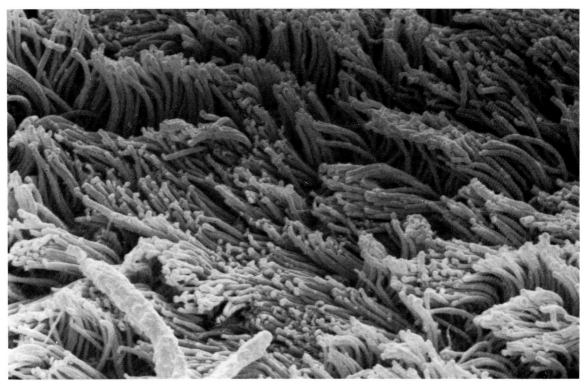

Fig. 1.18 Scanning electronmicrograph of paranasal epithelium, showing mainly long microvilli. Note two cilia (bottom left). By courtesy of Mr R Gray.

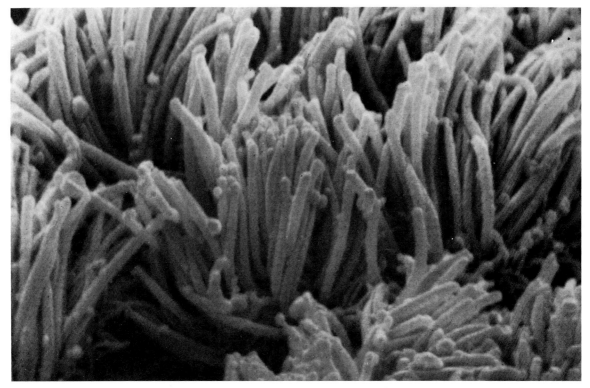

Fig. 1.19 Scanning electronmicrograph of paranasal epithelium, showing detail of Fig. 1.18. By courtesy of Mr R Gray.

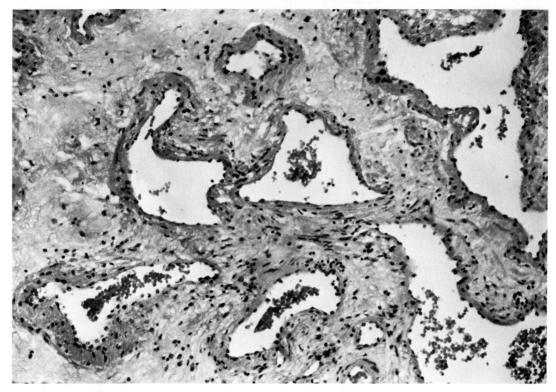

Fig. 1.20 Nasal erectile tissue showing the irregular muscular wall due to the spiral arrangement of the fibres. M ×135.

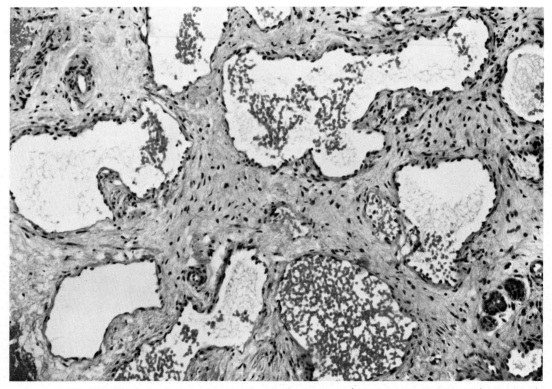

Fig. 1.21 Nasal erectile tissue showing distension and engorgement of the vessels. M ×135.

Nasal erectile tissue

An interesting feature in the lamina propria of the nasal mucosa is the presence of complex blood vessels which are designated 'erectile tissue'. This vascular component is found on the side of walls and also on the septum, concentrated posteriorly around the choanal orifices, whence it may extend into the postnasal space. The same tissue is also found occasionally in the paranasal mucosa, especially in the antrum and there are clinical reasons for believing that heterotopic representation may be found, very occasionally in the pterygoid fossa.

The vessels in this system contain a substantial amount of smooth muscle which is not arranged in the conventional pattern of ordinary arteries and veins. The muscle fibres are orientated in a spiral fashion, thus giving rise to an irregular arrangement in cross section (Figs. 1.20 & 1.21). Studies of the development of this tissue in animals have shown it to be very complex (Swindle, 1935 and 1937). The vessels develop in three strata, connected by arterial, venous and arterio-venous anastomoses. Swindle (1935) noted the existence of shunts which he called arterio-capillary anastomoses and, in 1937, he showed that, at or shortly after birth, the deepest stratum undergoes atrophy leaving the more superficial strata which gradually lose their identity as distinguishable layers. The musculature of this tissue is under the influence of the autonomic nervous system and it also reacts to chemical reagents, including some hormones. The main purpose of this tissue is to effect changes in local blood flow, causing rapid mucosal congestion. A link has been observed between the nasal and genital erectile tissue, nasal congestion sometimes accompanying sexual excitement (Mackenzie, 1898; Watson-Williams, 1952). It has been suggested that this association is a vestigial reflection of the role of smell in the mating activity of animals.

Melanin-producing cells

Another interesting aspect of the nasal cavity is the existence of melanocytes. These cells have been readily demonstrated in the skin of the vestibule (Szabo, 1959) but, in white races, melanocytes have not been demonstrated satisfactorily in the nasal fossa although they undoubtedly exist in the epithelial lining. Zak and Lawson (1974) claimed to have identified melanocytes in the nasal cavity on the basis of finding pigmented cells. Unfortunately, melanocytes have long been recognized as having the capacity to inject their pigment into adjacent epithelial cells, hence pigmented cells are not necessarily melanocytes. Attempts to demonstrate these cells by the D.O.P.A. oxidase technique are liable to be confusing due to the inevitable infiltration of the

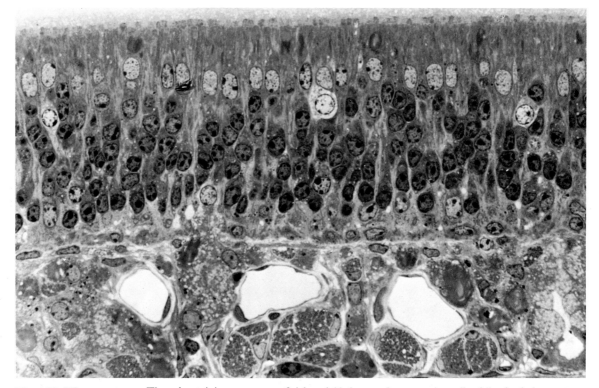

Fig. 1.22 Olfactory mucosa. The paler staining, more superficial nuclei belong to the supporting cells whilst the darker more rounded nuclei lie in the receptor cells. Note the element of Bowman's gland (lower right). M × 1000. By courtesy of P P C Graziadei.

epithelium by polymorphonuclear leucocytes containing an oxidase which will act upon the substrate. However, an interesting observation was made by one of the present authors on the nasal mucosa of a coloured patient from North Africa; dendritic cells were seen, outlined by melanin pigment and the morphology of these cells suggested that they were melanocytes rather than pigmented epithelial cells. It is probable that nasal melanocytes in white skinned subjects are comparable with the 'white dendritic cells' found in unpigmented skin (Billingham, 1948).

The olfactory mucosa
Topographically, the human olfactory area extends from the roof of the nasal cavity about one centimetre downwards on either side of the nasal septum and on the medial surface of the superior turbinate. In the recent state, the area appears slightly yellowish as compared with the pink colour of the respiratory mucosa. In contrast with the extensive studies carried out on other sensory organs, the ultrastructure of the olfactory system has received comparatively less attention. However, following the pioneering work of De Lorenzo (1957, 1960 and 1963), there has been enhanced interest in this field and Graziadei and his team (1966, 1971 and 1973) have contributed greatly to our knowledge of the olfactory epithelium and nerve.

The development of the olfactory mucosa has been studied in mice by Cuschier and Bannister (1975). The essential features of the tissue are established by the 13th day of gestation but their functional capability may be achieved sometime later. Bowman's glands develop about the 17th of gestation but certain histochemical and cytological manifestations appear only shortly before birth. We possess little information regarding the development of human olfactory mucosa.

Normal histology
The light microscopical features of the olfactory mucosa of lower animals have been described by Allison and

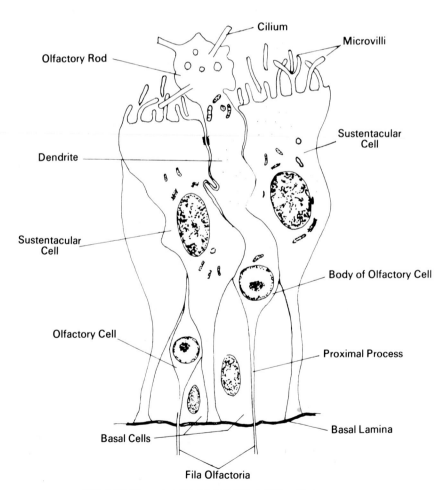

Fig. 1.23 Diagrammatic representation of the olfactory mucosa.

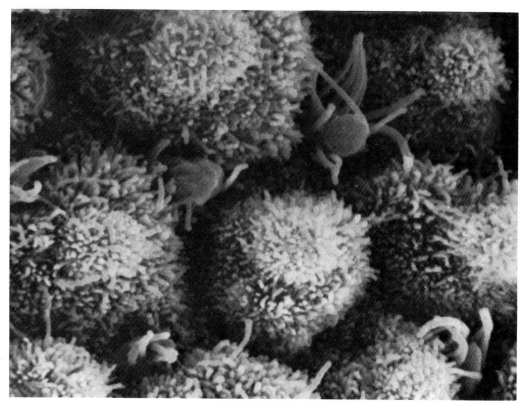

Fig. 1.24 Scanning electronmicrograph of the olfactory mucosa. Note ciliated olfactory rods surrounded by microvillus-bearing supporting cells. By courtesy of K H Andres.

Warwick (1949) and by Allison (1953). The olfactory area is covered by a pseudostratified epithelium which tends to be not only more extensive but thicker in lower animals as compared with Man. In reptiles and rabbits the olfactory epithelium was found to be of the order of 65 microns in thickness (Allison, 1953; De Lorenzo, 1960). Three layers of nuclei can be recognized (Fig. 1.22). The nuclei of the supporting cells lie nearest to the epithelial surface whilst the middle layer of nuclei belong to the olfactory receptor cells and the deepest layer is formed by the nuclei of the basal cells. In the recent state there is a fluid layer covering the epithelial surface, in which the projections from the cells are embedded (Fig. 1.23). There are three types of cell in the olfactory epithelium.

The supporting or sustentacular cells are cylindrical in their distal portions, extending from the surface to the basement membrane. The nuclei are oval and lie more or less in one plane and, proximal to the nucleus, the body of the cell narrows to accomodate the receptor and basal cells. Under the electron microscope, these cells bear a large number of microvilli on their free surface, projecting into the fluid layer and forming a

close meshwork (Graziadei, 1973). In addition to mitochondria and flattened profiles of rough endoplasmic reticulum, the supporting cells also contain yellowish-brown pigment which accounts for the gross appearance.

The basal cells are roughly conical in shape and lie between the basal portions of the supporting cells. They may also envelope the proximal parts of the receptor cells and Graziadei (1973) believes that they might function as Schwann cells.

The olfactory cells are essentially bipolar receptor neurones. The slender, flask-like cells contain rounded nuclei and are provided with distal and proximal processes. The distal process, known as the dendrite, passes towards the surface between the supporting cells. Under the electron microscope, it is seen to contain microtubules and mitochondria. When the dendrite reaches the surface it expands slightly to form the olfactory rod or olfactory vesicle (Figs. 1.24, 1.25 & 1.26) of Van der Stricht (1909). This structure contains a number of small vesicular structures but projecting from its surface are several cilia which lie in the fluid layer in association with the microvilli of the supporting cells.

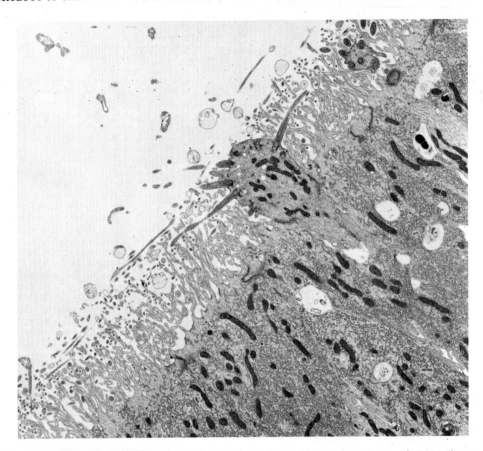

Fig. 1.25 Olfactory mucosa. Olfactory vesicle bearing several cilia. M × 8000. By courtesy of P P C Graziadei.

The olfactory cilia have a short proximal segment containing the 9+2 pattern of microtubules typical of kinocilia and a longer distal portion with two sub-fibres. Within the olfactory rod, the cilia terminate in basal bodies. The number of cilia varies and their length varies in different species. In rabbits, the length ranges from 0.3 to 3.0 microns (De Lorenzo, 1960). Lenz (1977), with the aid of the scanning electron microscope, studied the surface of the olfactory mucosa of a 25 year-old man who was killed in an accident. Several fairly uniform planes could be distinguished; uppermost there was a layer of fluid of varying thickness into which dipped the long, closely packed olfactory cilia. The proximal process of the olfactory cell is essentially an axon which passes between the basal cells to penetrate the basal lamina where it comes into association with many similar, non-myelinated axons known as the fila olfactoria. They ultimately form synaptic connections with neurones of the second order in the olfactory bulb. De Lorenzo observed that the terminations of the fila olfactoria pushed themselves into the dendrites of mitral cells.

The lamina propria contains the exocrine glands of Bowman which supply the fluid layer covering the epithelial surface. This layer is believed to entrap the molecules of odorous substances. The ultrastructure of these glands is somewhat variable, possessing a profuse rough and smooth endoplasmic reticulum and containing secretory granules which exhibit a positive periodic acid Schiff reaction, implying the presence of muco-polysaccharides (Graziadei, 1973).

Function

'Even the most learned of men is guided by his sense of smell at least in matters of love' (Groddeck, 1925). The molecular structure of various odorous substances plays an important role in relationship to smelling and taste (Ohloff and Thomas, 1971). Lenz (1977) noted the uniformity of the distal ends of the olfactory receptors and concluded that active molecules would need to be of varied shape. Sex hormones are odorous (resembling musk) and are believed to stimulate the olfactory mucosa. Getchell and Getchell (1974) believe that odorant molecules react with specific receptor proteins located in the receptor cell membrane. They also thought that receptor cells might have varying thresholds to different stimuli.

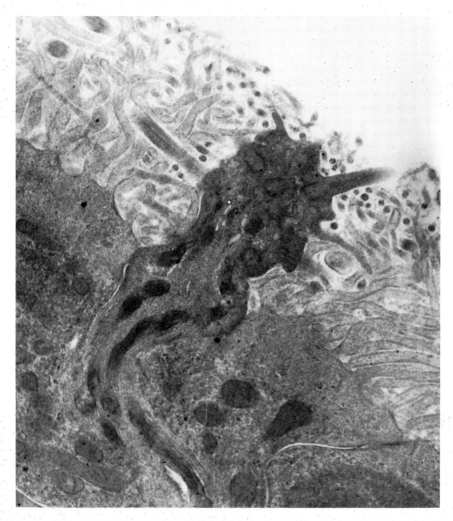

Fig. 1.26 Olfactory rod or vesicle in the nose of a guineapig. Note the supporting cells surrounding the dendrite and the large number of microvilli enmeshed with the olfactory cilia. M × 24 000.

Regeneration

There is general acceptance that many highly specialized cells in the body cannot be replaced during adult life. However, the concept of neuronal permanency has been doubted and the tendency of the olfactory epithelium to undergo regeneration has been put forward by many workers in this field (Mulvaney and Heist, 1971; Graziadei, 1973; Matulionis, 1975; Andres, 1975). Certainly, in lower animals there is clear evidence that development of olfactory receptor cells continues during adult life. The underlying mechanism of regeneration of the olfactory epithelium has been investigated by exposing it to the action of toxic agents such as zinc sulphate (Matulionis, 1975) or antbiotics (Arstila and Wersäll, 1967). The centrioles play an important part in the regeneration of olfactory epithelium. There are large numbers of centrioles in the olfactory neurone in the early stage of development, the number declining as the centrioles reach the surface to form basal bodies and generate cilia. Regeneration of the epithelium is thought to derive from the basal cells.

BIBLIOGRAPHY

Allison A C 1953 The morphology of the olfactory system in the vertebrates. Biological Reviews 28 : 195–244

Allison A C, Warwick R T 1949 Quantitative observations on the olfactory system of the rabbit. Brain 72 : 186–197

Anderson R G W 1971 Structure of cilia. Primate News 9 : 5 ff

Andres K H 1975 Neue morphologische Grundlagen zur Physiologie des Riechens und Schmeckens. Archiv für Ohren-, Nasen und Kehlkopfheilkunde 210 : 1–41

Andrews P M 1979 In : Hodges G and Hallowes R C (eds) The respiratory system in biomedical research applications of scanning electron microscopy. Academic Press, New York, vol 1, ch 3

Arden G B, Fox B 1979 Increased incidence of abnormal nasal cilia in patients with retinitis pigmentosa. Nature 279 : 534–536

Arstila A, Wersäll J 1967 Neomycin-induced changes in the ultra-structure of the olfactory epithelium of the guinea-pig. Acta Otolaryngologica 64 : 298–312

Billingham R E 1948 Dendritic cells. Journal of Anatomy 82 : 93–109

Brokaw C J, Gibbons J R 1975 Mechanisms of Movement in Flagella and Cilia. In Wu T, Brokaw C J, Brennan C (eds) Swimming and Flying in Nature. Plenum Publ Co, New York, 1 : 89–125

Cuschier I A, Bannister L H 1975 The development of the olfactory mucosa of the mouse. Journal of Anatomy 119 : 277–286

De Lorenzo A J 1957 Electron microscopic observations of the olfactory mucosa and olfactory nerve. Journal of Biophysical and Biochemical cytology 3 : 839–850

De Lorenzo A J 1960 Electron microscopy of the olfactory and gustatory pathways. Annals of Otology, Rhinology and Laryngology 69 : 410–419

De Lorenzo A J 1963 In : Zetterman Y (ed) Studies on the ultrastructure and histopathology of cell membranes, nerve fibres and synaptic junctions in chemo-receptors in olfaction and taste. Pergamon Press

Dion M C, Jafek B W, Tobin C E 1978 The anatomy of the nose. Archives of Otolaryngology 104 : 145–150

Fawcett D V, Porter K R 1954 Study of fine structure of ciliated epithelium. Journal of Morphology 94 : 221–281

Fleming A 1922 On a remarkable bacteriolytic element found in tissues and secretions. Proceedings of the Royal Society (London) Section B, 93 : 306–317

Fox B. Bull T B, Arden G B 1980 Variations in the ultrastructure of human nasal cilia including abnormalities found in Retinitis Pigmentosa. Journal of Clinical Pathology 33 : 327–335

Friedmann I, Bird E S 1971 Ciliary structure, ciliogenesis and microvilli. Laryngoscope 81 : 1852–1868

Getchell T V, Getchell M L 1974 Signal-detecting mechanisms in the olfactory epithelium : molecular discrimination. Annals of the New York Academy of Sciences 237 : 62–75

Graziadei P P C 1966 Comparative study of the vertebrate olfactory receptors. Journal of Anatomy 100 : 700–

Graziadei P P C, Metcalf J F 1971 Autoradiographic and ultra-structural observations on the frog's olfactory mucosa. Zeitschrift für Zellforschung 116 : 305–318

Graziadei P P C 1973 In : Friedmann I (ed) The ultrastructure of vertebrates' olfactory mucosa in Ultrastructure of Sensory Organs. Elsevier, Amsterdam

Graziadei P P C 1973 Cell dynamics in the olfactory mucosa. Tissue and Cell 5 : 113–131

Groddeck G 1925 The unknown self. London

Highmore N 1651 Corporis humani disquisito anatomica. Hagae Comitis, S Broun

Hilding A 1932 The physiology of drainage of mucus. Archives of Otolaryngology 15 : 92–100

Hilding D A, Heywood P 1971 Ultrastructure of middle ear mucosa and organization of ciliary matrix. Annals of Otology, Rhinology and Laryngology 80 : 306–312

Kawabaa I, Paparella M 1969 A typical cilia in normal human and guinea-pig middle ear mucosa. Acta Otolaryngologica 67 : 511–515

Lenz H 1977 Die Oberfläche der regio olfactoria des Menschen im Rasterelektronenmikroskop. Acta Otolaryngologica 84 : 145–154

Mackenzie J N 1898 The physiological and pathological relations between the nose and the sexual apparatus of Man. Journal of Laryngology and Otology 13 : 109–123

Matulionis D H 1975 Ultrastructural study of mouse olfactory epithelium following destruction by $ZnSO_4$ and its subsequent regeneration. American Journal of Anatomy 142 : 67–90

Mulvaney B D, Heist H E 1971 Centriole migration during regeneration and normal development of olfactory epithelium. Journal of Ultrastructure Research 35 : 274–281

Ohloff G, Thomas A F 1971 Gustation and olfaction. Academic Press, New York

Osborn D A 1974 The tumours of subsidiary or mucosal glands. M D Thesis, University of London

Poulsen J, Tos M 1975 Goblet cells in the developing human nose. Acta Otolaryngologica 80 : 434–442

Proetz A W 1941 Essays on the applied physiology of the nose. Annals publishing Company (St. Louis), ch 13, p 201

Schneider C V 1660 De Catarrho sorum diaeta et de Speciebus Catarrhorum, Wittebergae

Swindle P F 1935 The architecture of the blood vascular networks in the erectile tissue and secretory lining of the nasal passages. Annals of Otology, Rhinology and Laryngology 44 : 913–932

Swindle P F 1937 Nasal blood vessels which serve as arteries in some mammals and as veins in others. Annals of Otology, Rhinology and Laryngology 46 : 600–628

Szabo G 1959 Pigment cell biology. Editor : Gordon M Proceedings of the 4th conference on Biology and atypical pigment cell growth, p 99

Van der Stricht O 1909 Le neuro-épithélium olfactif et sa membrane limitante interne. Mémoires Courannés et autres mémoires. Publié par l'Acadamie royale de médecine de Belgique, 20, fascicule 2, 1–45

Watson-Williams E 1952 Endocrines and the nose. Journal of Laryngology and Otology 66 : 29–38

Zak F G, Lawson W 1974 The presence of melanocytes in the nasal cavity. Annals of Otology, Rhinology and Laryngology 83 : 515–519

2

Miscellaneous granulomas and nasal polyposis

GENERAL COMMENTS ON GRANULOMAS

Granulomatous inflammatory reaction has attracted a great deal of attention in so far as it exhibits considerable variations both clinically and histologically. Turk (1971) defined a granuloma as a collection of cells of the macrophage-histiocyte series with or without the admixture of other inflammatory cells. The principal elements of the granulomas are macrophages, epithelioid cells and giant cells primarily derived from monocytes formed in the bone marrow. Necrosis is not a constant component but in more complex granulomas this change may be observed. Differentiation of the mononuclear phagocytes into epithelioid or giant cells may be enhanced by delayed hypersensitivity reaction. Thus epithelioid and giant cell granulomas are formed.

Spector (1969 and 1971) has studied granulomas on a general basis. This author has pointed out that histological study gives no indication of the great variation in cellular dynamics that exists between one granuloma and another. The dynamic behaviour of granulomas varies greatly according to the nature of the granuloma-forming agent and Spector has drawn attention to the crucial role of persistence of the irritant within the mononuclear phagocytes. Two broad types (high and low turnover) of granulomatous reaction have been recognized by this author on the basis of the rate of replacement of cells either by mitosis or from the circulation. In the low turnover type, virtually all participating cells are laden with the irritant; cell turnover is slow and many of the macrophages are very long-lived. In the high turnover variety, only a small proportion of the cells contain the irritant and the bulk of the reaction is composed of cells with a high turnover rate, many corresponding to epithelioid or lymphoid cells. The constituent macrophages and giant cells contain lysosomes and potent enzymes capable of extensive tissue destruction when released by various mechanisms such as delayed hypersensitivity (Friedmann, 1971). Vascular spasm and vasculitis might ensue with subsequent ischaemia and necrosis. The release of soluble mediators from the macrophages may in turn cause delayed hypersensitivity reactions enhancing the differentiation of macrophages.

Granulomas of the nose and sinuses may be caused by specific or non-specific agents. Specific causes are largely infections which will be dealt with individually but certain non-specific or unknown agents produce characteristic clinical and histopathological patterns, such as sarcoidosis and the midfacial granuloma syndrome. These also merit separate consideration. In the general context, one of the commonest non-specific granulomas is caused by reaction to foreign bodies but these are not commonly encountered in pathological material from the nose and sinuses although reaction to foreign material, probably introduced by a nasal spray is sometimes seen. A variety of miscellaneous granulomas is encountered in the nasal and paranasal region though the incidence is variable and not very high. Three separate lesions are about to be described, namely eosinophilic granuloma, cholesterol granuloma and 'myospherulosis'.

Pregnancy granuloma may occur during pregnancy forming a vascular tumour-like lesion arising from the mucosa at the mucocutaneous junction. The usual location is in the upper gum, but, although rarely, it may present in the nose (Bicknell, 1971). Usually unilateral it resolves spontaneously, but may recur at subsequent pregnancies. Microscopically it resembles the features of a pyogenic granuloma or haemangioma.

EOSINOPHILIC GRANULOMA OF THE NOSE AND SINUSES

Introduction

In 1929, Finzi described a lesion in the frontal bone of a 15 year-old boy in which he noted the presence of many eosinophils but concluded that it was a form of myeloma. Lichtenstein and Jaffe (1940) published a case of a femoral lesion in a four year-old girl under the title of 'eosinophilic granuloma of bone'. Perusal of the literature showed that, in addition to Finzi's case, another frontal bone lesion was reported by Mignon (1930) and two cases involving the parietal bones

(Schairer, 1938). All these cases appeared to resemble each other microscopically and, on the basis of further histological resemblance, Farber (1941) suggested that there was a link between the eosinophilic granuloma, Schüller-Christian syndrome and Letterer-Siwe disease. In 1953, Lichtenstein embraced this concept, designating the three conditions as 'Histiocytosis X'. This view, however, was not universally accepted and eosinophilic granuloma is now regarded as a separate entity.

Incidence
Eosinophilic granuloma is uncommon in the general context and, although there is a particular tendency for the lesions to occur in the skull, involvement of the nose and sinuses is extremely rare. In the ILO material one case (involving the frontal sinus) has been encountered over a period of 30 years whilst one of us has seen material from an antro-nasal lesion.

Clinical features
Predominantly a disease of very young subjects, more than 60 per cent of cases are encountered during the first decade of life. However, in the series reported by Lieberman, Jones, Dargeon and Begg (1969), a number of cases occurred in older subjects including one in the seventh decade. Most series have recorded a predominance of males though no particular significance has been attached to the observation. The common form of presentation is that of painful swelling, usually of not more than a few weeks' duration.

Anatomical site of origin
Most eosinophilic granulomas have their origin in bone though lesions in soft tissues (skin, alimentary tract and lungs) have also been reported. About 40 per cent of published cases have involved the head region (Ochsner, 1966), particularly the frontal, parietal and temporal bones. In the ILO case the lesion occurred in the frontal bone of a 19 year-old male and had invaded the frontal sinus. In the antro-nasal lesion, referred to one of the present authors, the granuloma appeared to have arisen in the lateral nasal wall, involving both the nasal and antral cavities.

Gross appearances
To the naked eye, the lesion is usually a circumscribed, soft, yellowish brown mass, thus accounting for the punched out appearance on X-ray.

Histopathology
The microscopical picture shows characteristic features in varying proportions. Eosinophils are always present either as a diffuse infiltration or as more localized masses and noteworthy is the relative maturity of these cells.

Interspersed are larger cells with large palely staining, ovoid or indented nuclei whilst cytoplasmic boundaries show variable definition, some cells being sharply delineated whilst other present a syncytial appearance. These larger cells, which are either diffusely scattered or concentrated in small groups, have the appearance of histiocytes (Figs. 2.1, 2.2) and a variable number may show evidence of phagocytosis, including complete cells such as eosinophils. The cytoplasm varies from being amphophilic to eosinophilic and occasionally presents a foamy appearance, though intracellular lipid is not a prominent feature. Many of the histiocytic cells are binucleate and varying numbers of multinucleated giant cells may be present. Polymorphonuclear leucocytes and small numbers of plasmacytes and lymphocytes may also be found. Small areas of haemorrhage and focal necrosis have been observed in some cases. Although the principal features of eosinophilic and histiocytic infiltration are always present, the histological picture is likely to vary in the relative proportions of the different types of cell and the degree of phagocytosis exhibited by the histiocytes.

Aetiology and pathogenesis
The cause of the condition is completely unknown and attempts to link it with Schüller-Christian syndrome and Letterer-Siwe disease has confused rather than elucidated the problem. The common feature of histiocytic infiltration hardly justifies the concept of a unified pathology. Eosinophilic infiltration is a more prominent feature in the granuloma but it also represents a reaction to a variety of aetiological agents and is, therefore, somewhat lacking in specificity. Its presence in Letterer-Siwe disease (Lichtenstein, 1953) or in Schüller-Christian disease (Sissons, 1966) is, consequently, open to alternative interpretations. In a reappraisal of the concept of Histiocytosis X, Lieberman et al (1969) could find no support for the view that these three conditions had a common pathogenesis. They stressed the benign behaviour of the eosinophilic granuloma, the lack of specificity in the Schüller-Christian triad and the probable relationship of Letterer-Siwe disease to malignant lymphoma.

Behaviour
A large proportion of eosinophilic granulomas are and remain solitary. They may cause local bone destruction, giving rise to a clinical and radiological impression of a malignant tumour. Treatment by local surgery or irradiation usually results in non-recurrence (McGavran and Spady, 1960) whilst some lesions undergo spontaneous resolution (Platt and Eisenberg, 1948). Multiple lesions may cause considerable morbidity but are not malignant in a pathological sense.

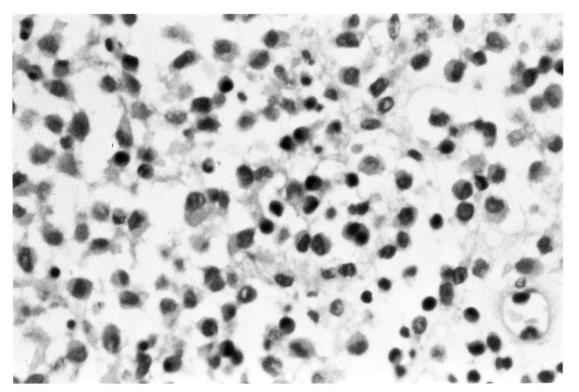

Fig. 2.1 Eosinophilic granuloma of the frontal sinus in a 19-year-old male. M ×640

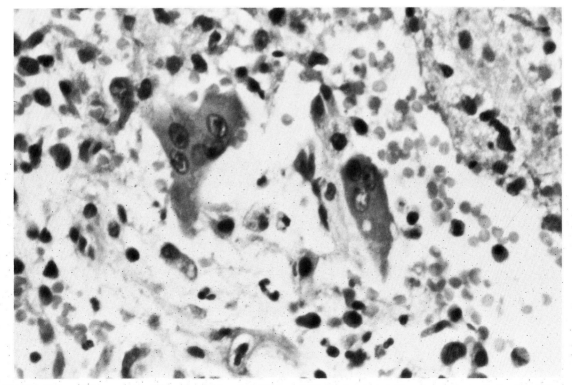

Fig. 2.2 Eosinophilic granuloma of the frontal sinus in a 19-year-old male, showing multinucleated giant cells (see Fig. 2.1). M ×640

CHOLESTEROL GRANULOMA OF THE SINUSES

This lesion is somewhat more common though in the ILO material the order of frequency was approximately one case every two to three years. In former times there was confusion between cholesterol granuloma and 'Cholesteatoma' and a proportion of cases reported under the latter title were clearly cholesterol granulomas (Osborn and Wallace, 1967). Furthermore, the lesion reported under the label of 'rhinitis caseosa' also proved to be cholesterol granuloma.

Although cholesterol granulomas have been reported in the frontal sinus, the ILO material was confined to maxillary sinus origin and the patients were almost invariably very young, the lesion occurring during the first two decades of life. Clinical presentation takes the form of nasal discharge, local discomfort and nasal obstruction, especially when the granuloma is found in an antrochoanal polyp.

Microscopically, the lesion is indistinguishable from that seen in the middle ear. Chronic inflammatory granulation tissue contains numerous foreign body type giant cells which surround and even engulf the cholesterol crystals, marked by empty needle-shaped spaces in paraffin-embedded material (Fig. 2.3). Recent haemorrhage or iron pigment indicating previous haemorrhage may also be seen.

As in all cholesterol granulomas, the basic cause is believed to be haemorrhage though the cause of this in the maxillary lesions has not been defined. However, it is believed that upper dental extraction probably accounts for a proportion of cases. Removal of the granuloma is not usually followed by recurrence.

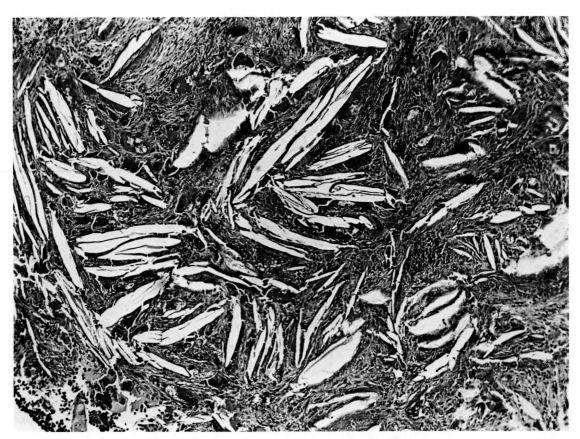

Fig. 2.3 Cholesterol granuloma of the maxillary sinus. M × 95

MYOSPHERULOSIS OF THE NOSE AND SINUSES Figs. 2.4 and 2.5

McClatchie, Warambo and Bremner (1969) described nodular swellings, often painful and apparently related to skeletal muscle, in six Africans. The lesions which were often excised from upper or lower limbs, often appeared to contain creamy purulent material. Histologically, the lesion consisted of fibrosis with inflammatory infiltration and degenerate muscle fibres. Scattered throughout the lesion were numerous cyst-like spaces lined by flattened foam cells, presumed to be histiocytes. Many of these spaces were empty but some contained clusters of rounded bodies, slightly larger than red blood corpuscles and surrounded by a thin refractile membrane. The authors described them as 'partly filled bags of marbles'. There was no obvious internal structure and the spherular bodies did not take up the conventional stains. Histiocytes were seen surrounding these clumps of spherules which they sometimes engulfed. The authors considered the possibility of fungal spores though no organism could be isolated on culture. Hutt, Fernandes and Templeton (1971) reported a further five cases, also in Africans, noting that skeletal muscle was not always involved.

In 1977, Kyriakos reported 16 cases involving the nose, paranasal sinuses and the ear of patients in Missouri. The ages ranged from 15 to 86 years and the sexes were equally divided. Over 50 per cent involved the maxillary sinus with or without other cavities being affected. All cases had had operative procedures prior to the first histological identification of the lesion and about one third had been operated upon for neoplasms of the region. Examination of the initial biopsy was carried out in the majority of cases and revealed no evidence of 'myospherulosis'. A common feature in these cases was the use of gauze packing with petrolatum based ointments and the author considered the possibility that the lesion represented an unusual reaction to this material.

De Schryver-Kecskemeti and Kyriakos (1978) induced the lesion in experimental animals using antibiotic ointments which were petrolatum based. Rosai (1978) encountered the same lesion in the maxillary sinus of an eight year-old boy. A previous biopsy revealed fibromatosis and the site was packed with tetracycline ointment. A subsequent maxillectomy specimen showed, in addition to fibromatosis, the lesion of 'myospherulosis'. This author incubated red cells in test tubes internally smeared with tetracycline ointment and, after five days, smears showed appearances identical with the clumps of spherules in the lesions. The conclusion was that the spherules were red cells modified by the petrolatum based ointment.

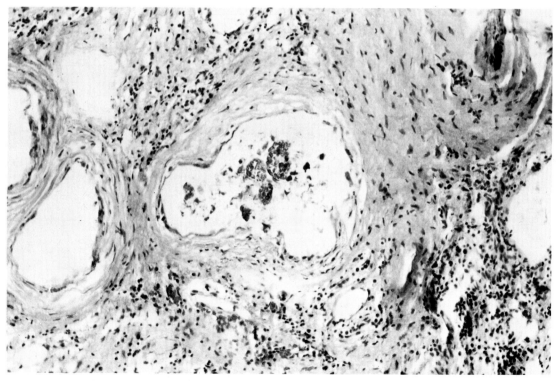

Fig. 2.4 Nasal biopsy showing distended spaces containing microspherules. M × 180

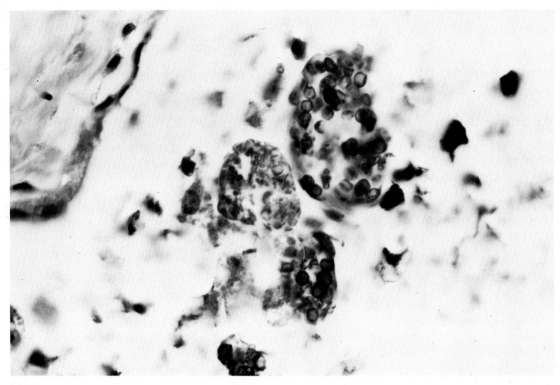

Fig. 2.5 Detail of microspherule formed by a sac-like structure which may be membrane-bound containing collection of erythrocytes altered by foreign substance such as petrolatum-based antibiotic ointment. M ×742 (Section kindly supplied by Professor M H McGavran Houston, Texas.)

POLYPOSIS OF THE NOSE AND SINUSES

The existence of nasal polypi was noted over 100 years ago and, initially, there were differences of opinion as regards their nature. Many believed them to be neoplasms but others maintained that they represented the consequences of chronic infection and this latter view was ultimately established. Subsequently, they were recognized as projections of mucous membrane developing in association with chronic rhinitis and sinusitis but more especially with allergic disease of the upper respiratory tract.

Incidence
In terms of material submitted for histopathology, nasal polyposis represented about four per cent of patients registered with the Royal National Throat, Nose and Ear Hospital over a period of 27 years.

Clinical features
Nasal polypi tend to occur most frequently in middle-aged males. In one year's material, 75 per cent of polypi were removed from patients between 40 and 70 years of age whilst the sex ratio was 3:1 in favour of males. Nevertheless, the age distribution is broadly based and

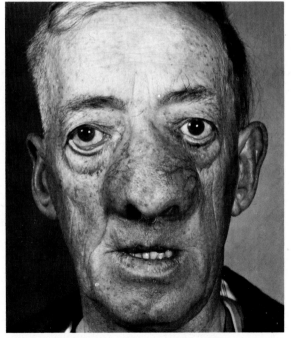

Fig. 2.6a Illustration shows gross enlargement of the left side of the nose by a clinically suspect tumour.

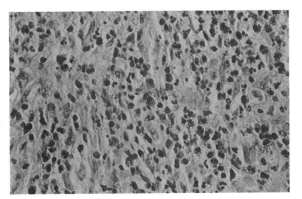

Plate 1 Eosinophilic granuloma'of the maxillary antrum showing diffuse infiltration by eosinophilic cells (19 year-old male) M ×640

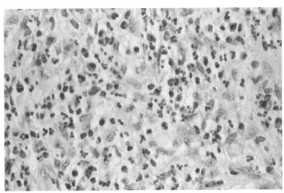

Plate 2. Eosinophilic granuloma of the maxillary antrum showing the histriocytic stroma with interspersed eosinophils (see also Fig 2.1)

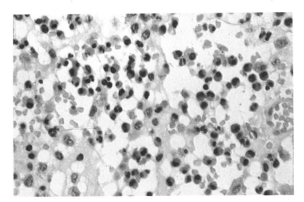

Plate 3. Eosinophilic granuloma of the maxillary antrum showing syncitial histiocytes with interspersed eosinophils (77 year-old male)

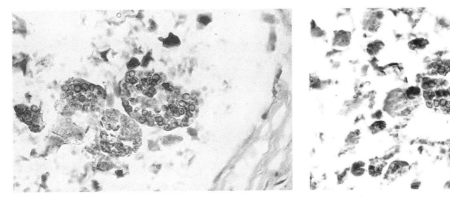

Plates 4 and 5 Myospheruilosis illustrate the red blood cells in the spherules (see also Fig. 2.5)

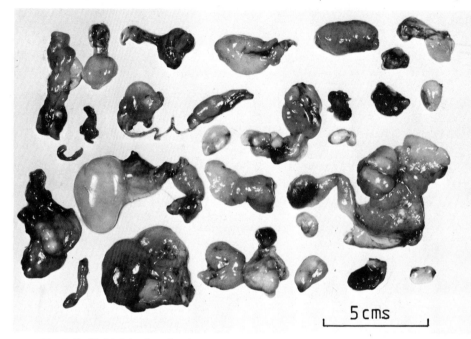

5 cms

Fig. 2.6b Multiple benign allergic type nasal polyps removed from the nose of the old man in Fig. 2.6a.

polypi may be encountered in young patients. Clinical presentation is characterized by nasal obstruction, nasal discharge, sneezing and the lesion may appear at the anterior nares. They are often multiple and bilateral and the filling of the nasal cavity may lead to visible broadening of the external nose. (Fig. 2.6a)

Anatomical site of origin

The common sites of origin are the middle turbinate, middle meatus and especially the hiatus semilunaris. The ethmoid air cells may be filled with sessile polypi and polypoid mucosa may also be found in the maxillary sinus.

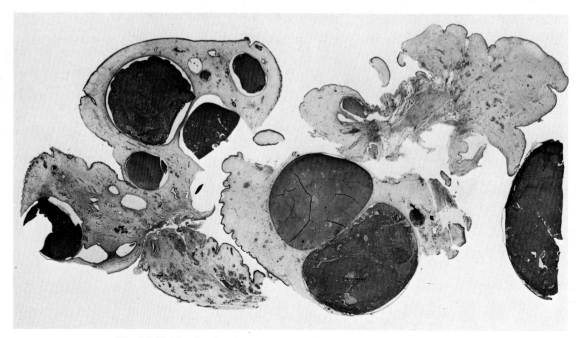

Fig. 2.7 Nasal polyp showing cystic seromucinous distension of glands. M ×4

Gross appearances

They present as smooth shiny swellings, varying in colour from bluish grey to deep pink (Fig. 2.6b). Polypi in the nasal cavity tend to be pedunculated, soft and mobile. Antro-choanal polypi differ from the common variety in being solitary. They arise in the maxillary sinus (Killian, 1906) and occur predominantly in children or young adults. The polyps project through the ostium of the sinus into the middle meatus from whence they enlarge to occupy the nasal cavity, usually being directed backwards towards the choanae.

Histopathology

Nasal polypi consist essentially of an oedematous stroma covered by epithelium which may be respiratory type or metaplastic squamous variety. Ulceration of the epithelium is occasionally encountered, usually with secondary inflammatory infiltration. The respiratory type epithelium contains a fair number of goblet cells whilst the oedematous stroma may contain seromucinous glands with or without cystic distension (Fig. 2.7) due to obstruction of their outlets by kinking or oedema. Large polypi may exhibit a vascular component, particularly elements of the nasal erectile tissue. Infoldings of the epithelium may be seen into which mucosal glands may open. Varying degrees of cellular infiltration may be seen according to the type of polyp.

The greater proportion of polypi appear to be associated with an allergic aetiology and often exhibit a characteristic histological picture. In nearly 700 polypi examined over a period of one year, more than 600 were classified as of allergic type, amounting to nearly 90 per cent.

The common allergic type polyp is characterized by a hyaline thickening in the region of the basement membrane of the surface epithelium (Fig. 2.8), marked mucous secretory activity (involving both goblet cells and mucosal glands) and a predominance of eosinophilic and plasmacytic infiltration. The hyaline thickening does not involve the basement membrane which appears of normal thickness both by silver staining and the periodic acid Schiff reaction and also under the electron microscope which reveals the laying down of collagen beneath the basal lamina. Under the light microscope, this produces a largely clear zone between the epithelium and the infiltrated stroma. The eosinophilic infiltration varies in intensity and may be diffuse or aggregated in masses. Fewer eosinophils may be associated with greater plasmacytic infiltration. The surface epithelium may show extensive replacement of the ciliated component by goblet cells whilst the mucous glands in the stroma may show hyperplasia. In about 40 per cent of allergic

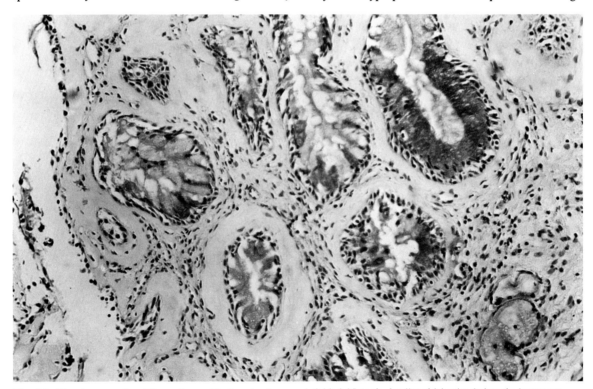

Fig. 2.8 Allergic type polyp. The surface epithelium has become infolded. Note the hyaline thickening below the basement membrane. M × 190

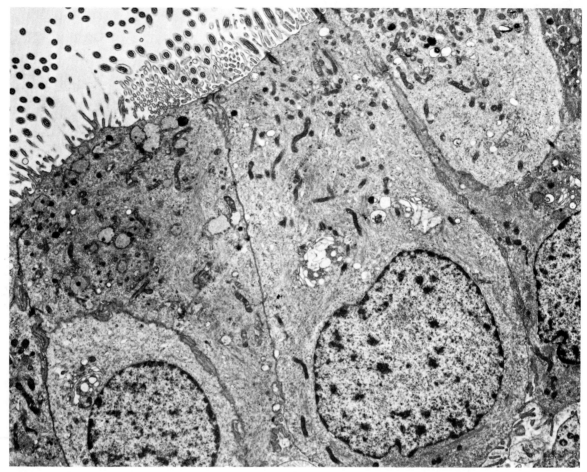

Fig. 2.9 Surface epithelium of a nasal polyp showing cilia and numerous microvilli, some of which appear atypical. M × 6000
By courtesy of Dr A Busuttil.

type polypi there is another characteristic feature consisting of focal granulomas in the stroma, containing eosinophils, plasmacytes and histiocytes.

In non-allergic polypi, there is often a more intense, diffuse cellular infiltration consisting of lymphocytes, plasmacytes, polymorphonuclear leucocytes and histiocytes with a notable absence of eosinophils and the hyaline thickening below the basement membrane. Fibroblasts are often present producing collagen which may be dispersed oedema fluid and lymphoid follicles may be present.

The histological picture of the antro-choanal polyp is usually more akin to that of the non-allergic polyp. The stroma is highly oedematous with scanty cellular infiltration. The accumulation of proteinaceous fluid may impart a degenerative appearance on which may be superimposed haemorrhage and, occasionally as a consequence, the development of a cholesterol granuloma.

Busuttil, More and McSeveney (1977 and 1978) studied the ultrastructure of the respiratory type epithelium covering nasal polypi. There were large numbers of goblet cells and the pseudostratified epithelium ranged from 40 to 100 microns in thickness. Microvilli, with or without complex branching, were abundant near the edge of the free border of the ciliated cells, the cilia being closely packed in the central area. (Figs. 2.9 & 2.10).

Aetiology and pathogenesis

The essential prerequisite for the development of polypi is the occurrence of oedema. In so far as the formation of oedema is a particular feature of acute allergic reactions, this would explain why the majority of polypi are of allergic origin. Furthermore, the more firm attachment of the septal mucosa to underlying structures accounts for the lack of origin of polypi from this location in the nose. Initially, polypi appear simply as bags of oedema fluid covered by the surface epithelium but as they increase in size they tend to take the lamina

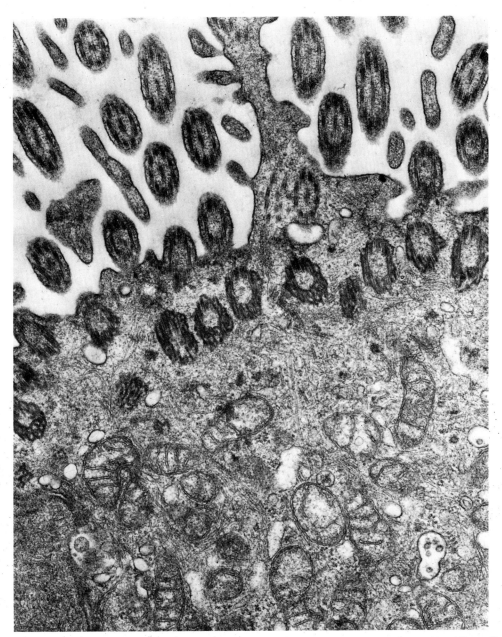

Fig. 2.10 Ciliated cell in nasal polyp with atypical ciliary structure. M × 40 000 By courtesy of Dr A Busuttil.

propria and its contents into the body of the polyp. Tos and Mogensen (1977) put forward a theory that nasal polypi develop as a result of rupture of the surface epithelium and prolapse of the lamina propria. These authors maintained that the prolapsed lamina propria subsequently became covered by psuedostratified epithelium and that the glands found in the polyp were not the original mucosal glands but developed in situ as the polyp increased in size. The present authors cannot accept this view for the following reasons. Long

experience of the histology of nasal polypi has revealed no evidence of rupture of the surface epithelium except due to ulceration at a later stage. This event is caused by trauma or is due to pressure of the enlarging polyp against rigid structures, causing devitalization. The prolapse of the lamina propria must inevitably take its contained structures with it. It is a matter of common observation that the stroma of nasal polypi not infrequently contains seromucinous glands and even nasal erectile tissue. It is unlikely that nasal polypi would exhibit new formation of serous secreting units let alone nasal erectile tissue.

The occurrence of focal granulomas in allergic type polypi suggest the possibility of reaction to an allergen and raises the question of local antibody production. Berdal (1954), using the Prausnitz-Kustner technique on human volunteers, demonstrated increased titres of reaginic antibodies in the oedema fluid of allergic type polypi as compared with those found simultaneously in the sera from the same patients. This technique is no longer used since the dangers are well appreciated. Donovan, Johansson, Bennich and Soothill (1970) studied the concentrations of various immunoglobulin components in both serum and polyp fluid. They noted that the IgE fraction, believed to be responsible for the reaginic activity, was present in the polyp fluid in higher concentration than could be accounted for by simple filtration. Thus they confirmed local antibody production.

Jahnke and Theopold (1977) studied the ultrastructure of nasal polypi in mucoviscidosis. The epithelium showed both intra- and extra-cellular oedema with damage to the cilia. Goblet cells and mucosal glands showed increased activity though the nature of the secretion was normal.

Behaviour

Nasal polypi are liable to recur after removal if the underlying disease persists. Antrochoanal polypi are less likely to recur. The simple nature of nasal polypi cannot always be determined by naked eye examination and the presence of a neoplasm can only be excluded by histological examination. The present authors have frequently observed abnormal connective tissue cells in the stroma of polypi, raising speculations as to their nature but the ultimate conclusion was that they only rarely had pathological significance. Smith, Echevarria and McLelland (1974) reported two cases with pseudo-sarcomatous changes in antrochoanal polypi and warned against a mistaken diagnosis of malignancy in an otherwise benign lesion. Recently, Klenoff and Goodman (1977) also drew attention to the importance of recognizing atypical mesenchymal cells in the stroma of simple nasal polypi. Occasionally, new bone formation is found in nasal polypi (Fig. 2.11).

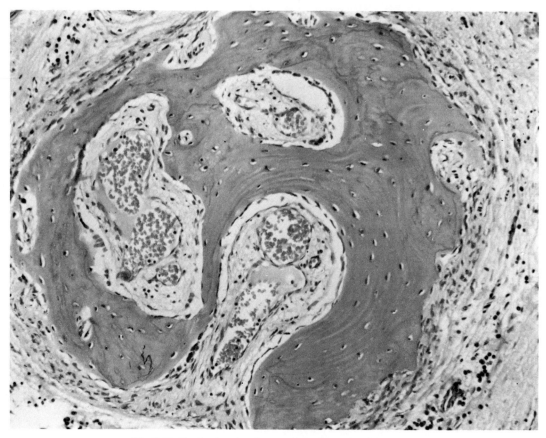

Fig. 2.11 Nasal polyp showing new bone formation. M × 110

BIBLIOGRAPHY

Berdal P 1954 Serological examinations of nasal polyp fluid. Acta Otolaryngologica, Supplementum 115

Busuttil A, More I A R, McSeveney D 1977 A reappraisal of the ultrastructure of the human respiratory nasal mucosa. Journal of Anatomy 124: 445–458

Busuttil A, More I A R, McSeveney D 1978 Branching microvilli in the nasal respiratory epithelium. Archives of Otolaryngology 104: 260–261

De Schryver-Kecskemeti K, Kyriakos M 1978 The induction of human myospherulosis in experimental animals. American Journal of Pathology 87: 33–40

Donovan R, Johansson S G O, Bennich H, Soothill J F 1970 Immunoglobulins in nasal polyp fluid. International Archives of Allergy and Applied Immunology 37: 154–166

Farber S 1941 The nature of solitary or eosinophilic granuloma of bone. American Journal of Pathology 17: 625–626

Finzi O 1929 Mieloma con prevalenza delle cellule eosinofile circoscritto all osso frontale in un giovane di 15 anni. Minerva Medica 91: 239–241

Friedmann I 1971 The changing pattern of granulomas of the upper respiratory tract. Journal of Laryngology and Otology 85: 631–682

Hutt M S R, Fernandes B J J, Templeton A C 1971 Myospherulosis (Subcutaneous spherulocystic disease). Transactions of the Royal Society of Tropical Medicine and Hygiene 65: 182–188

Jahnke V, Theopold H M 1977 Feinstruktur der Nasenschleimhaut bei Mukoviszidose unter besonderer Berucksichtigung der Polyposis. Laryngologie und Otologie (Stuttgart) 56: 773–781

Killian G 1906 The origin of choanal polyp. Lancet 2: 81–82

Klenoff B H, Goodman M L 1977 Mesenchymal cell atypicality in inflammatory polyps. Journal of Laryngology and Otology 91: 751–756

Kyriakos M 1977 Myospherulosis of the paranasal sinuses, nose and ear. American Journal of Clinical Pathology 67: 118–130

Lichtenstein L 1953 Histiocytosis X. Archives of Pathology 56: 84–102

Lichtenstein L, Jaffe H L 1940 Eosinophilic granuloma of bone. American Journal of Pathology 16: 595–604

Lieberman P H, Jones C R, Dargeon H W K, Begg C F 1969 A reappraisal of eosinophilic granuloma of bone, Hand-Schuller-Christian syndrome and Letterer-Siwe syndrome. Medicine (Baltimore) 48: 375–400

McClatchie S, Warambo M W, Bremner A D 1969 Myospherulosis. A previously unreported disease? American Journal of Clinical Pathology 51: 699–704

McGavran M H, Spady H A 1960 Eosinophilic granuloma of bone. Journal of Bone and Joint Surgery 42A: 979–992

Mignon F 1930 Ein Granulationstumor des Stirnbeins. Fortschritte auf dem Gebiete der Röntgenstrahlen 42: 749–751

Ochsner S F 1966 Eosinophilic granuloma of bone. American Journal of Roentgenology 97: 719–726

Osborn D A, Wallace M 1967 Carcinoma of the frontal sinus associated with epidermoid cholesteatoma. Journal of Laryngology and Otology 81: 1021–1032

Platt J L, Eisenberg R B 1948 Eosinophilic granuloma of bone. Journal of Bone and Joint Surgery 30A: 761–768

Rosai J 1978 The nature of myospherulosis in the upper respiratory tract. American Journal of Clinical Pathology 69: 475–481

Schairer E 1938 Über eine eigenartige Erkrankung des kindlichen Schädels (Osteomyelitis mit eosinophiler Reaktion). Zentralblatt für allgemeine Pathologie und pathologische Anatomie 71: 113–117

Sissons H A 1966 Lipidoses involving bone in systemic pathology. In: Systemic Pathology. W St C Symmers (ed) 1st ed. Longmans, ch 37, p 1396

Smith C J, Echevarria R, McLelland C A 1974 Pseudosarcomatous changes in antrochoanal polyps. Archives of Otolaryngology 99: 228–230

Spector W G 1969 Granulomas inflammatory exudate. In: Richter R W, Epstein M A (eds) International Review of Experimental Pathology. Academic Press, New York, 8: 1–53

Spector W G 1971 The cellular dynamics of granulomas. Proceedings of the Royal Society of Medicine 64: 941–942

Tos M, Mogensen C 1977 Mucous glands in nasal polyps. Archives of Otolaryngology 103: 407–413

Turk J L 1971 Granuloma formation in lymphnodes. Proceedings of the Royal Society of Medicine 64: 942–944

Additional References

Burton P A, Dixon M F 1969 A comparison of changes in the mucous glands and goblet cells of nasal, sinus and bronchial mucosa. Thorax 24: 180–185

Michel J 1977 Recherches historiques sur la découverte des maladies des sinus. Annales d'Oto-Laryngologie 94: 753–760

Wheeler T M, Sessions R B, McGavran M H 1980 A preventable iatrogenic nasal and paranasal entity. Archives of Otolaryngology 106: 272–274

3

Tuberculosis of the nose and sinuses

TUBERCULOSIS OF THE NOSE AND SINUSES

Introduction

Although tuberculous infection of this region was never very common, it is even more rare to-day than it was at the beginning of the present century. In 1907 Gleitsmann reviewed 20 published cases of tuberculous maxillary sinusitis. Most of the patients had pulmonary tuberculosis and in 12 cases there was tuberculous disease of the adjacent bones which he regarded as precedent to the sinus infection.

Incidence

Although nearly 50 cases have been published in the English language literature during the present century, the incidence of the disease is difficult to assess. The largest series (five cases) was reported by Havens (1931) but in none was there bacteriological confirmation. The undoubted fall in frequency has resulted in tuberculosis of this region becoming a rare event. In the I.L.O. material, there have been several suspected cases but in only one was Mycobacrerium tuberculosis isolated from the lesion.

Clinical features

Tuberculosis in this region is liable to be encountered at any stage in adult life and it would appear that females are predominantly affected. There seems to have occurred a shift in the age distribution of tuberculosis generally. The normal expectation of life has increased and, with decreasing resistance, re-infection may occur, particularly as a result of increasing travel and immigration which has been rightly emphasized.

Early symptoms consist of nasal discharge with subsequent crusting, foetor and nasal obstruction whilst epistaxis is sometimes encountered. The intranasal lesion commonly appears as a smooth lobulated mass with an unbroken surface but it may sometimes present as a granulation with a tendency to bleed. Some patients may exhibit evidence of pulmonary infection.

Anatomical site of origin

Tuberculosis of the nose may be cutaneous or mucosal. The former type represents *Lupus Vulgaris*, a tuberculous infection of the skin which may extend into the vestibule but the slowly destructive lesions with secondary inflammatory reaction are seen much less frequently today. In the present context, interest is centred on the mucosal form. Ingberg (1958) suggested that involvement was much more commonly nasal than paranasal but published reports present a marked predominance of paranasal lesions, being almost exclusively involvement of the maxillary sinus. When the nose is affected, the site of predilection is the mucosa covering the cartilaginous portion of the nasal septum whence it spreads to the floor and the anterior part of the inferior turbinate and the disease is usually bilateral.

Histopathology

The microscopical picture is essentially that of a tuberculous lesion in any location, characterized by tubercles composed of epithelioid cells, Langhans type giant cells, plasmacytes and lymphocytes (Figs. 3.1, 3.2 & 3.3). Caseating necrosis is not a marked feature but secondary infection may obscure the primary lesion. Acid-fast bacilli may or may not be demonstrable.

The diagnosis depends not only on the classical histological picture but, more important, on the isolation of the causal organism by culture and guineapig inoculation. Frequently, bacteriological investigations have not been carried out in published cases, thus casting doubt on the diagnosis. The characteristic tubercle, first recognized by the Dutch physician Sylvius in the seventeenth century, came to be regarded as pathognomonic of tuberculosis but this is no longer true since the pattern of interpretation has undergone a profound change. There has been an increasing awareness of other 'tuberculoid' lesions, especially in the upper respiratory tract, with the result that pathologists have become reluctant to diagnose tuberculosis solely on histopathological grounds. A variety of conditions may give rise to a 'tuberculoid granuloma', the commonest being sarcoidosis but fungal or nocardial infection may occasion-

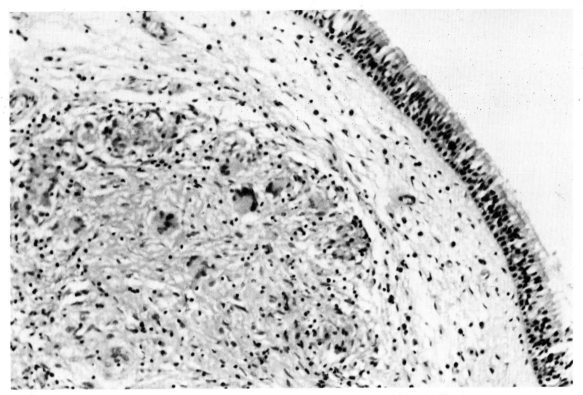

Fig. 3.1 Tuberculoid nodule in the nasal mucosa of a 45 year-old female. M ×225

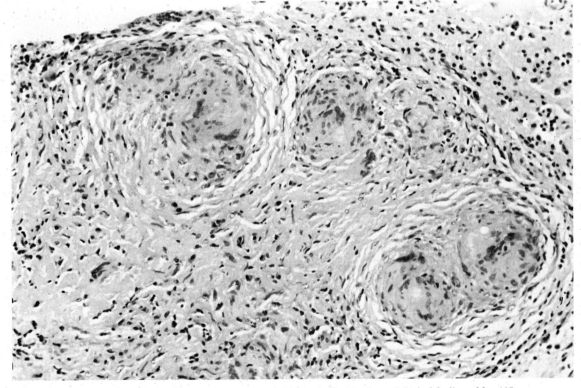

Fig. 3.2 Tuberculosis of the nose in a 32 year-old female. Positive bacteriological findings. M ×225

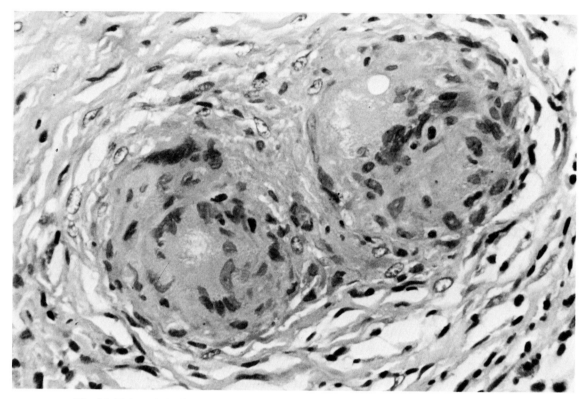

Fig. 3.3 Tuberculosis of the nose in a 32 year-old female. Higher magnification of Fig. 3.2. M × 595

ally be involved. *Beryllium* is also known to induce the same histological pattern though nasal lesions due to this cause have not yet been identified. Nevertheless, the possibility of inhalation of other, at present unidentified, agents has to be considered. Against this background, it must be emphasized that the finding of tuberculoid lesions calls for extensive investigation, including clinical, radiological and bacteriological examinations. The value of microbiological procedures in eliminating an alternative diagnosis was well demonstrated by Messervy (1971) in a case which was initially suspected of being Wegener's Granulomatosis.

Aetiology and pathogenesis

Tuberculosis of the respiratory tract may be encountered at almost any age and, in the present context, radiological evidence suggesting inactive or healed pulmonary infection is not uncommon. Occasionally, active pulmonary lesions are found but in many cases there is no such evidence. It would appear that the relationship of nasal to pulmonary infection is an inconstant one, raising the question of primary or secondary status in the nasal region. Negative bacteriological results on nasal material does not necessarily exclude tuberculous infection;

antral washouts, sputum and urine should also be examined.

Two cases from the I.L.O. material illustrate the diagnostic problems. A 78 year-old woman had nasal obstruction of one month's duration. The chest X-ray was normal but the left antrum was opaque and polypoid mucosa removed from the nasal cavity contained tuberculoid lesions (Fig. 3.4). No acid-fast organisms were found in the tissue and cultures from the nose and sputum were negative but *Myco-bacterium tuberculosis* was isolated from an antral washout. A 49 year-old woman had apical pulmonary fibrosis whilst three biopsies from nasal granulations over a period of several years all showed tuberculoid lesions. Subsequently, a pulmonary relapse occurred, in spite of chemotherapy, producing a positive sputum.

Three out of the five cases reported by Havens (1931) exhibited what were believed to be inactive pulmonary lesions. Nevertheless, even in the presence of active pulmonary tuberculosis, a non-specific purulent sinusitis is not uncommon (Oppenheim, 1955; Page and Jash, 1974). Antral infection may result from direct extension from the nose, teeth or eye or from bloodstream spread from a remote focus in the body.

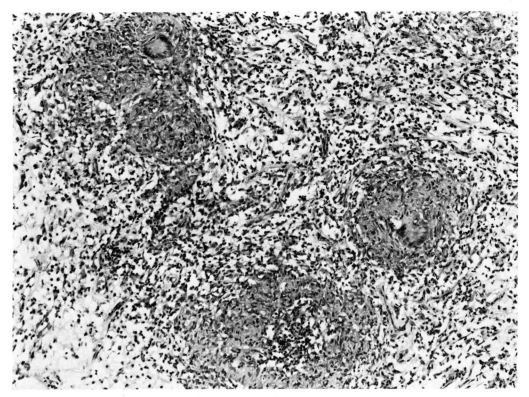

Fig. 3.4 Tuberculosis of the nasal region in a 78 year-old female. Positive bacteriological findings. M × 130

The fall in incidence of tuberculous bone disease (Sissons, 1966) has led to a diminution in the frequency of nasal or paranasal infection whilst control of tuberculous infection generally by antibiotic and chemotherapy has resulted in a marked reduction in the disease with probable influence on nasal and paranasal involvement. Marks (1969) pointed out that the declining tuberculous infection has resulted in a relative increase in importance of diseases caused by 'opportunistic' mycobacteria. These include *M. kansasii, M. avium, M. xenopei* and the Scrofulaceum group. These organisms are capable of producing diseases which are clinically, radiologically and histopathologically identical with tuberculosis. Furthermore, the last mentioned author presented evidence that infections by these organisms had shown an absolute increase in Wales. Stanford and Jeanes (1970) found that nearly nine per cent of mycobacterial infections were caused by the opportunistic group but so far the latter have not been related to nasal or paranasal lesions. However, in so far as many

such cases have not been adequately investigated, the possibility of opportunistic infection remains. It is interesting to note that some of these organisms have been isolated from the soil. Furthermore, another organism, *M. marinum* may contaminate swimming pools and tropical fish aquaria.

Behaviour

Tuberculous granuloma of the nasal septum may lead to perforation (Havens, 1931; Thomas and Gaillard, 1951). Involvement of the maxillary sinus, presumably by direct spread, may also occur (Ingberg, 1958; Page and Jash, 1974) but involvement of bone is uncommon today. Herard (1960) reported a case in which a fistula developed in the scar of a previous Caldwell-Luc operation. Although biopsy from the antrum revealed tuberculoid granulations, culture was negative but the lesion responded to streptomycin. Many cases undergo resolution following antibiotic and chemotherapy but healing with extensive fibrosis is liable to occur.

BIBLIOGRAPHY

Gleitsmann J W 1907 Tuberculosis of the accessory sinuses of the nose. Laryngoscope 17: 445–450

Havens F Z 1931 Primary tuberculosis of the nasal mucous membrane. Archives of Otolaryngology 14: 181–185

Herard M J 1960 Un cas de sinusite maxillaire tuberculeuse. Annales d'Oto-Laryngologie 77: 955–957

Ingberg B 1958 Tuberculous sinusitis. Acta Otolaryngologica Supplement 140: 163–166

Marks J 1969 'Opportunistic' mycobacteria in England and Wales. Tubercle 50 (supplement): 78–80

Messervy M 1971 Primary tuberculosis of the nose with presenting symptoms and lesions resembling a malignant granuloma. Journal of Laryngology and Otology 85: 177–184

Oppenheim H 1955 Rare tuberculous lesions treated with streptomycin. Archives of Otolaryngology 62: 119–129

Page J R, Jash D K 1974 Tuberculosis of the nose and paranasal sinuses. Journal of Laryngology and Otology 88: 579–583

Sissons H A 1966 Tuberculosis of bone. In: Systematic Pathology Wright G P and Symmers W St C (eds) 1st edn. Longmans, ch 37, p 1370

Stanford J L, Jeanes A L 1970 A three-year laboratory survey of bacteriologically confirmed mycobacterial infections. Guy's Hospital Reports 119: 101–110

Thomas R, Gaillard 1951 Un cas de tuberculose isolée du sinus maxillaire et de la fosse nasale gauche à forme tumorale. Annales d'Oto-Laryngologie 68: 863–864

Additional references

Freer O T 1909 Nasal tuberculosis; two cases involving right ethmoid bone with recovery after operation. Transactions of the American Laryngological Association 31: 103–119

Jones E H 1928 Tuberculosis of the maxillary sinus. Laryngoscope 38: 398–401

Juselius H 1961 Tuberculosis of the maxillary sinus. Acta Otolaryngologica 53: 424–428

Kistner F B 1928 Primary tuberculoma of the nasal mucosa. Transactions of the American Laryngological, Rhinological and Otological Society 34: 461–462

Waldman S R, Levine H L, Sebek B A, Parker W, Tucker H M 1981 Nasal Tuberculosis: A Forgotten Entity Laryngoscope 91: 11–16

4

Sarcoidosis of the nose and sinuses

SARCOIDOSIS OF THE NOSE AND SINUSES

Introduction

Sarcoidosis is a generalized disease of protean manifestations, affecting many organs. Although the integument is one of the less frequently involved tissues, the disease was first reported in terms of skin lesions. Besnier (1889) described cutaneous lesions of the face and upper extremities to which he gave the name 'lupus pernio', whilst Hutchinson (1898) referred to similar manifestations as 'Mortimer's malady', named after one of his patients. Boeck (1899) first recognized the generalized nature of the disease which he called 'multiple benign sarcoid' and, in 1905, he noted that four out of nine cases has nasal lesions which had preceded those in the skin whilst, in two other cases, the relationship was coincidental. Since that time it has become evident that the upper respiratory tract is frequently affected and some later workers have supported Boeck's suggestion of primary nasal disease (Ulrich, 1918; Willie, 1946).

Incidence

In the general context, adult coloured people living in rural areas of the south eastern region of the United States and the Scandinavians appear to be the most susceptible. Robinson and Pound (1950) reviewed 30 cases of generalized sarcoidosis and noted nasal or paranasal lesions in six. Lindsay and Perlman (1951) emphasized upper respiratory involvement in their report of nine cases. Later, Scadding (1967) reviewed 47 cases of generalized disease with nasal lesions. Gordon, Cohn, Greenberg and Komorn (1976) found 64 cases of nasal sarcoidosis in the English literature and added three cases of their own. In the I.L.O. material, there were five cases encountered between 1948 and 1974.

Clinical features

The age distribution covers largely the third to the fifth decades, a pattern which coincides with that of the more generalized disease (Keller, 1973). In the present context, there is a female predominance of more than 2:1. The common form of presentation is nasal discharge, nasal obstruction and occasionally epistaxis whilst patients may or may not exhibit signs and symptoms of generalized disease. The septal and turbinal mucosa

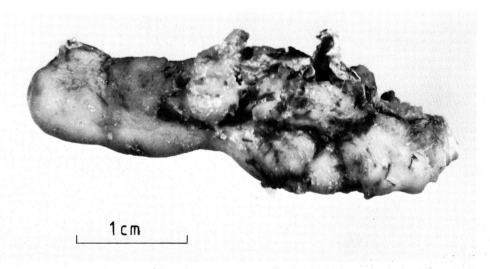

1 cm

Fig. 4.1 Nasal sarcoidosis in a 30 year-old male showing gross involvement of the turbinate.

becomes hypertrophied and granular (Fig. 4.1). It may
be pale or congested but often shows fine greyish-yellow
nodules no larger than a pinhead.

Anatomical site of origin

In the generalized disease, the lungs and lymphnodes
are involved in over 80 per cent of cases, followed by
liver, spleen, heart, kidney, bone, pancreas, skin, salivary
glands and uveal tract. The frequency of involvement of
the upper respiratory tract has not been adequately
assessed but from reports in the literature it would
appear to be a significant proportion. In this context, the
nasal cavity is usually affected but the paranasal region
may also be involved (Lindsay and Perlman, 1951;
Livingstone, 1956; Trachtenberg, Wilkinson and Jacobson, 1974). The nasal septum and the anterior end of the
inferior turbinate are the most commonly affected sites.

Histopathology

The microscopical picture is that of non-caseating
epithelioid tubercles. These so-called hard tubercles
often show a tendency to remain discrete even though
they may be closely packed (Fig. 4.2). A minute amount
of central necrosis is occasionally present. Multinucleated giant cells may be present, often of the

Langhans variety (Figs. 4.3 & 4.4) but sometimes
resembling the foreign body type. Reticulin stain usually
shows fine fibrils penetrating to the centre of the
tubercle. Schaumann bodies are relatively infrequent in
upper respiratory tract lesions. They consist of
concentrically arranged lamellated membranes often
enclosing mitochondria and other organelles (Judd,
Finnegan and Curran, 1975) and have been shown to be
rich in mucopolysaccharides, phospholipids and lipo-
proteins (Jones-Williams and Williams, (1968). Ultrastructural studies of sarcoid granulomas have been
carried out by Greenberg, Györkey and Weg (1970) and
also by Judd et al. (1975). The concensus of opinion is
that the epithelioid cells are derived from macrophages
and the last mentioned authors noted a large variety of
cytoplasmic organelles including rough endoplasmic
reticulum, many mitochondria, large numbers of lysosomes and numerous pinocytic vesicles and they suggested that such cells might be specific.

The microscopical picture is such that the lesion can
only be suspected on histological grounds alone. The
diagnosis will depend ultimately on the supporting
evidence, e.g. signs of generalized disease, negative
bacteriological findings, negative tuberculin test and a
positive Kveim-Siltzbach test (Kveim, 1941; Siltzbach,
1961) (Fig. 4.5)

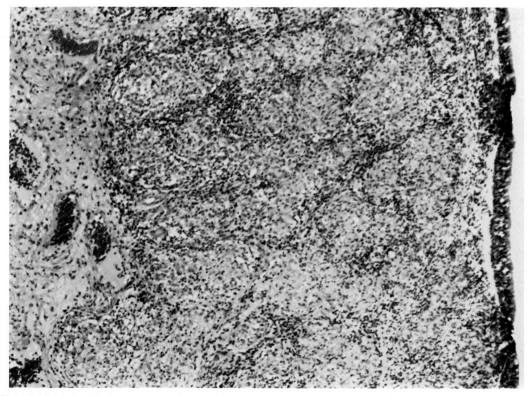

Fig. 4.2 Nasal sarcoidosis in a 30 year-old male (see Fig. 4.1), showing closely packed, discrete 'hard' tubercles. M × 87

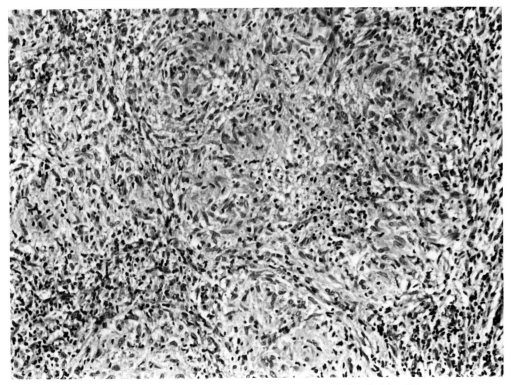

Fig. 4.3 Sarcoidosis of the nasal cavity in a 24 year-old female. M ×208

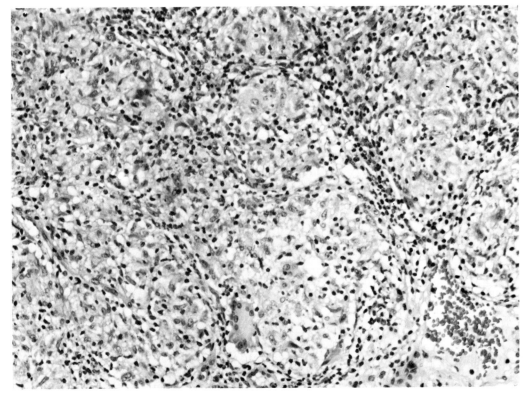

Fig. 4.4 Sarcoidosis of the nose in a 30 year-old male (see Fig. 4.1), showing Langhans type of giant cell. M ×208

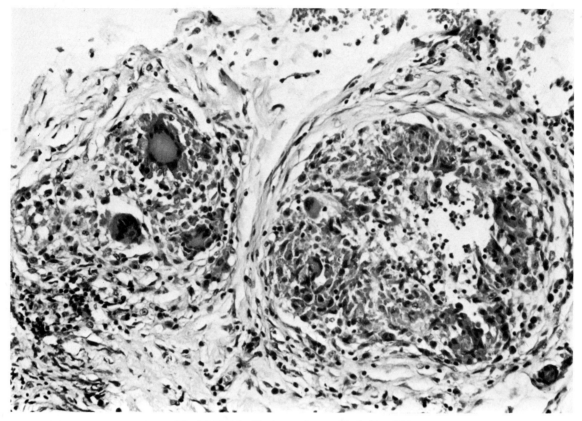

Fig. 4.5 Positive Kveim test in sarcoidosis. M ×225

Aetiology and pathogenesis

The chronological relationship of nasal and paranasal sarcoidosis to the manifestations of systemic disease is ill-defined. In many cases the presence of generalized sarcoidosis has already been established and recognition of upper respiratory involvement follows as a result of investigation of nasal symptoms, though Wille (1946) maintains that these may be minimal and, in one of the cases reported by Lindsay and Perlman (1951), the nasal lesion was an incidental finding in a patient with generalized disease. On the other hand, some cases present with nasal symptoms (Gordon et al., 1976). Clearly, the possibility that nasal sarcoidosis might be a primary manifestation of the disease cannot be excluded and this should be borne in mind in the event of sarcoid-like nasal lesions without supporting evidence of more generalized disease. The five cases in the I.L.O. material all had evidence of generalized disease which in four patients had been previously established.

The aetiology of this condition is still obscure and many of the theories have been examined by Scadding (1967) but, whether the agent is primarily infective or chemical, this pattern of nasal involvement would be consistent with the concept of assault by some extraneous, probably air-borne, antigen (James, 1973). In this context, it should be noted that the common sites of involvement within the nasal cavity are those which are particularly exposed to the inspired air.

It has been suggested that atypical mycobacteria or other organisms might be involved. Acid-fast bacilli may be found in some cases within the lesions but their aetiological role has not been confirmed by bacteriological cultivation. Inoculation of homogenates from human sarcoid lesions into mice by various routes, including the footpads, provided strong evidence that transmissible agents were present and were able to produce local and disseminated epithelioid and giant cell granulomas (Mitchell and Rees, 1969; Mitchell, Rees and Goswami, 1976). It is recognized that not all cases of sarcoidosis are associated with the same infective agent (Mitchell and Scadding, 1974). It was suggested by Burnet (1959) that a protoplast form of the tubercle bacillus might persist as an intracellular parasite of mesenchymal cells and be active in subjects with abnormally efficient production of humoral antibody and poor development of delayed hyper-sensitivity. James (1973) pointed out that cases of sarcoidosis may exhibit raised immunoglobulin levels of various specificities. The possibility of a virus infection has also been suggested.

Behaviour

There is clear evidence that this disease may spread both locally and systematically. Bronson and Fisher (1976) reported extension from the paranasal region into the orbit whilst Gordon et al. (1976) described subsequent remote involvement in two cases. Disturbance of olfaction due not only to involvement of the mucosa but also of the olfactory tract has been emphasized by Delaney, Henkin, Manz, Satterly and Bauer (1977). These authors suggested that deterioration in olfactory and gustatory function may indicate irreversible damage to the nervous system.

Spontaneous remission has been observed in sarcoid lesions though not specifically reported in the nasal region. Variable degrees of regression may be induced by steroid therapy but healing may be associated with fibrosis and structural distortion.

BIBLIOGRAPHY

Besnier E 1889 Lupus pernio de la face; synovites fongueuses (scrofulo-tuberculeuses) symétrique des extremités supérieures. Annales de Demratologie et de Syphiligraphie 2ᵉ série 10: 333–336

Boeck C 1899 Multiple benign sarcoid of the skin. Journal of Cutaneous and Genito-Urinary Diseases 17: 543–550

Boeck C 1905 Fortgesetzte Untersuchungen über des multiple Sarcoid. Archiv für Dermatologie und Syphilis 73: 71–86

Bronson L J, Fisher Y L 1976 Sarcoidosis of the paranasal sinuses with orbital extension. Archives of Ophthalmology 94: 243–244

Burnett F M 1959 The clonal selection of acquired immunity. Vanderbilt Press, Cambridge, p 160

Delaney P, Henkin R I, Manz H, Satterly R A, Bauer H 1977 Olfactory sarcoidosis. Archives of Otolaryngology 103: 717–724

Gordon W N, Cohn A M, Greenberg S D, Komorn R M 1976 Nasal sarcoidosis. Archives of Otolaryngology 102: 11–14

Greenberg S D, Györkey F, Jenkins D E, Györkey P, Weg J 1970 The ultrastructure of the pulmonary granuloma in 'sarcoidosis'. American Review of Respiratory Diseases 102: 648–652

Hutchinson J 1898 Cases of Mortimer's malady. Archives of Surgery 9: 307–314. Hutchinson, London

James G D 1973 Modern concepts of sarcoidosis (Editorial) Chest 64: 675–677

Jones Williams W, Williams D 1968 The properties and development of conchoidal bodies in sarcoid and sarcoid-like granulomas. Journal of Pathology and Bacteriology 96: 491–496

Judd P A, Finnegan P, Curran R C 1975 Pulmonary sarcoidosis: a clinicopathological study. Journal of Pathology 115: 191–198

Keller A Z 1973 Anatomic sites, age attributes and rates of sarcoidosis in US veterans. American Review of Respiratory Diseases 107: 615–620

Kveim A 1941 En ny og spesifik kutan-reackjon ved Boecks sarcoid. Nordisk Medicin 9: 169–172

Lindsay J R, Perlman H B 1951 Sarcoidosis of the upper respiratory tract. Annals of Otology, Rhinology and Laryngology 60: 549–566

Livingstone G 1956 Sarcoidosis of the maxillary antrum. Journal of Laryngology and Otology 75: 426–427

Mitchell D N, Rees R J W 1969 A transmissible agent from sarcoid tissue. Lancet 2: 81–84

Mitchell D N, Rees R J W, Goswami K K A 1976 Transmissible agents from human sarcoid and Crohn's disease tissues. Lancet 2: 761–765

Mitchell D N, Scadding J G 1974 Sarcoidosis. American Review of Respiratory Diseases 110: 774–802

Robinson B, Pound A W 1950 Sarcoidosis: a survey with report of thirty cases. Medical Journal of Australia 2: 568–582

Scadding J G 1967 Sarcoidosis. Eyre and Spottiswoode, London

Siltzbach L E 1961 The Kveim test in sarcoidosis. American Journal of Medicine 30: 495–501

Trachtenberg S B, Wilkinson E E, Jacobson G 1974 Sarcoidosis of the nose and paranasal sinuses. Radiology 113: 619–620

Ulrich K 1918 Die Schleimhautveränderungen der oberen Luftwege beim Boeck'schen Sarcoid und ihre Stellung zum Lupus pernio. Archiv für Laryngologie und Rhinologie 31: 506–534

Wille C 1946 Boeck's Disease on the mucosa. Acta Otolaryngologica 34: 182–191

5

Leprosy of the nose

NASAL LEPROSY

Introduction

Over 25 million people in the World suffer from leprosy (Barton, 1976). Although endemic leprosy is said to have disappeared from the United Kingdom after 1798, large scale immigration in recent times has accentuated the problem and, in 1969, there were over 350 registered cases in England and Wales (Editorial, *British Medical Journal*, 1969). Nasal involvement in leprosy has long been recognized and, even before the turn of the century, the concept of the nose as a portal of entry of the causal organism had been put forward by several observers (Davey, 1974). However, as the last mentioned author pointed out, interest in this site of involvement waned and was overshadowed by the many practical problems relating to the management of leprous patients. As a result, the nasal region tended to be neglected and rhinoscopy was not a routine examination. During the past two decades, increasing attention has been paid to the nasal aspects of the disease, consequently with greater emphasis on its diagnostic and epidemiological significance. Barton (1976) has drawn renewed attention to the importance of nasal involvement in diagnosis, treatment and control.

Incidence

The frequency of the disease is largely related to the endemic regions, particularly, Asia, Central Africa and South America but southern Europe is regarded as lying within the endemic zone. Incidence within the United Kingdom is low in spite of immigration. Amongst the I.L.O. material there has been one case which was reported by Stanton (1964).

Clinical features

Susceptibility to this disease covers a wide age range but those most at risk are children exposed to open cases (Jopling, 1974). There is no sex difference. The presenting symptoms in nasal leprosy consist of discharge (which may be highly infective), obstruction and epistaxis. The mucosa may be oedematous in the early stages and later exhibit grey or pink nodules which are visible on the surface. Ulceration follows and perforation of the septum with destruction of the cartilage is not uncommon. With progression of the disease, complete destruction of the septum may lead to a characteristic flattening of the nose. Not infrequently, at the time of presentation, there may be macular cutaneous lesions and even intra-oral manifestations.

Anatomical site of origin

The nasal mucosa is affected in 95 per cent of cases of early disease (Barton, 1976). The principal sites of election within the nasal cavity are the inferior turbinate and the septum. According to Barton, the anterior end of the inferior turbinate is involved in 97 per cent of cases and the anterior part of the septum in 85 per cent, whilst the posterior aspects of these structures are less frequently affected. Davey (1974) has emphasized the early changes in the inferior turbinate, in which swelling due to lepromatous granulations may be followed by destruction and disappearance before septal lesions are observed.

Histopathology

In the general context it is now accepted that there are two principal microscopical types of leprosy, the lepromatous and the tuberculoid, with an intermediate or borderline pattern. Job, Karat and Karat (1966) pointed out that the intermediate and tuberculoid varieties are rarely seen in the nasal cavity in the absence of adjacent skin lesions. These authors have described four stages of lepromatous rhinitis which they designated (i) invasion, (ii) proliferation, (iii) destruction and ulceration and (iv) resolution and fibrosis. In the invasive stage the mucosa is oedematous with many goblet cells whilst there is an infiltration by lymphocytes, plasmacytes and small numbers of macrophages which contain acid-fast bacilli. Haematoxylin and eosin stained sections at this stage would appear essentially non-specific. Marked proliferation of macrophages may constitute circum-scribed masses which relate to the nodules observed

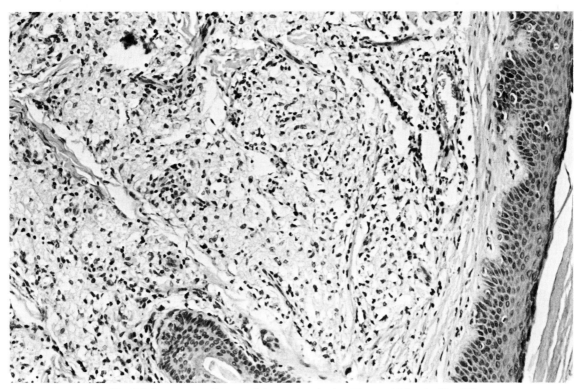

Fig. 5.1 Lepromatous leprosy of the nasal cavity in a 26 year-old female. M × 180

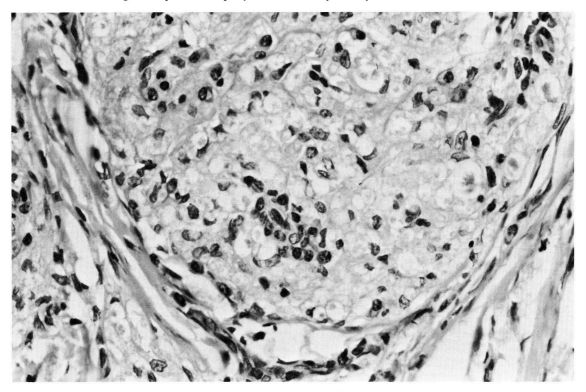

Fig. 5.2 Lepromatous leprosy of the nasal cavity in a 26 year-old female. Higher magnification of Fig. 5.1, showing 'lepra' cells. M × 480

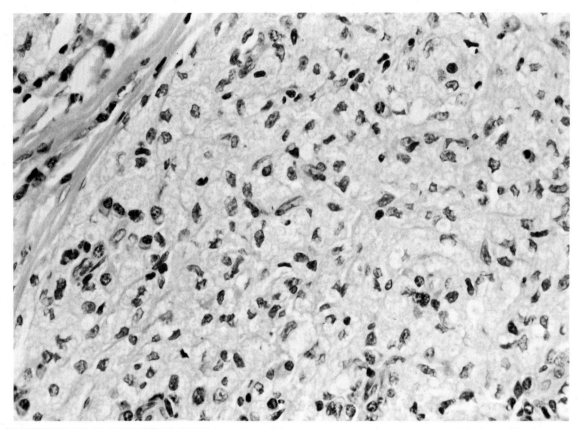

Fig. 5.3 Lepromatous leprosy in the nasal cavity of a 26 year-old female. A further area of 'lepra' cells in the previously illustrated case. M × 480

clinically. The macrophages are loaded with acid-fast bacilli and many assume a foamy appearance characterizing the so-called 'lepra cell' (Figs. 5.1, 5.2 & 5.3). Infiltration of the septum and turbinal bone by lepromatous granulations follows, leading to extensive destruction and in the last phase fibrosis is associated with structural alterations whilst chronic inflammatory infiltration persists with relatively few acid-fast organisms.

Mycobacterium leprae shows a tendency to be decolourized during the routine Ziehl-Neelsen staining technique as applied to tubercle bacilli. Modifications of the technique, involving pre-treatment with a vegetable oil, have been introduced (Fite, Cambre, Turner and Corville, 1947; Wheeler, Hamilton, Harman, 1965). These techniques produce solid staining of viable leprosy bacilli but when the organisms have degenerated, staining is less intense.

McDougall, Rees, Weddell and Wajdi-Kanan (1975) reported histological studies on the nasal mucosa in early cases with particular reference to the distribution of the causal organism in the tissues. In 31 cases of lepromatous leprosy, they noted the presence of viable (solid staining) *Myco. leprae* in macrophages, polymorphonuclear leucocytes, endothelial cells, Schwann cells, mucosal gland elements and even in the cells of the respiratory type epithelium. On the other hand, in four cases of intermediate type, they found no organisms and no specific inflammatory changes.

Following the acceptance of lepromatous, tuberculoid (Fig. 5.4) and intermediate or borderline varieties, a classification with immunological implications was introduced by Ridley and Jopling (1966) which is summarized in Table 5.1.

Table 5.1

Type	Lepromatous (LL)		Borderline (BB)		Tuberculoid (TT)
Subgroup	LL	BL	BB	BT	TT
Resistance of patient	Nil		Moderate		High
No. of *Myco. leprae*	High		Moderate		Low

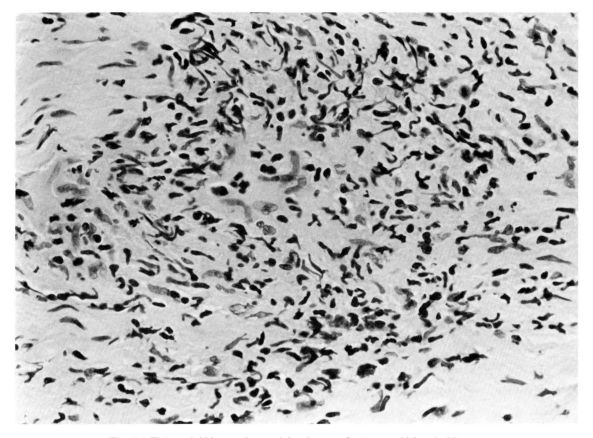

Fig. 5.4 Tuberculoid leprosy in a peripheral nerve of a 50 year-old female. M × 480

Notwithstanding the existence of some indeterminate or unclassifiable cases, the last mentioned authors correlated their subdivisions with histological patterns ranging from the fully lepromatous type (LL), composed of the classical lepra cells, to the tuberculoid variety (TT) showing foci of epithelioid cells with or without Langhans type giant cells. In considering the histological diagnosis, the need to distinguish from such conditions as tuberculosis or sarcoidosis will have limited application owing to the rarity of the tuberculoid form of leprosy in this location. On the other hand, masses of lepra cells should not be confused with the Mikulicz cells of rhinoscleroma.

Aetiology and pathogenesis
Although the causal organism was first demonstrated over a hundred years ago (Hansen, 1874), it still resists all attempts at culture on artificial media. It is known that the bacilli tend to congregate in certain anatomical sites such as the skin of the extremities, the lobes of the ears and the testes. It has been suggested on this basis that slightly lower temperatures are more conducive to

survival and multiplication of the organisms. It would now appear that, in the active stage of lepromatous leprosy, the organisms may be present in higher concentrations in the nasal mucosa (Barton, Davey, McDougall, Rees and Weddell, (1973). In 1960, Shepard demonstrated the proliferation of *Myco. leprae* when injected into the footpads of mice. This finding was subsequently confirmed and extended by Rees and his colleagues. These workers have not only produced a human-like disease by the experimental infection of mice (Rees, Waters, Weddell and Palmer, 1967) but have shown that, after a considerable time lapse, proliferation of *Myco. leprae* developed in locations in the animals remote from the site of injection, notably the nasal mucosa (Rees, McDougall and Weddell, 1974). They concluded that, in so far as the nose clearly represents a favourable environment for the multiplication of this organism, it is not only important as a site of exit (with its epidemiological implications) but could be, by the same token, and important portal of entry. Barton et al. (1973) pointed out that nasal changes are much more frequent than would be suspected from the general clinical picture.

The nasal discharge is not merely mucoid material but is, in fact, an inflammatory exudate containing large numbers of macrophages, often loaded with acid-fast bacilli. Dharmendra and Sen (1949) found that *Myco. leprae* was present in the nasal discharge of over 90 per cent of lepromatous cases whilst Pedley (1973) reported similar findings. Davey and Rees (1974) who emphasized the superabundance of *Myco. leprae* in the nasal discharge from early or recrudescent cases, examined the survival of the organism in voided material. They found 100 per cent survival up to 24 hours, falling to 10 per cent after nearly two days. This would imply that susceptible subjects could be infected by inhalation, affecting the anterior part of the inferior turbinate at an early stage, as indicated by Davey (1974).

The potential role of several common genera of flies in the transmission of leprosy has been demonstrated by Geater (1975) and it has been pointed out by Rees (1975) that such insects should be considered seriously as vehicles of infection.

Myco. leprae is often present in the Schwann cells, macrophages, and perineural cells of peripheral nerves (Weddell, Palmer, Rees and Jamieson, 1963; Lumsden, 1964; Dastur, Ramamohan and Shah, 1973; Job and Verghese, 1974). The organism has also been found, though less frequently, within the axons (Yoshizumi and Asbury, 1974; Boddingius, 1974; Job and Verghese, 1974). The last mentioned authors considered that intra-axonal bacilli probably do not play a very significant role in the destruction of the nerve but their location may well protect them from body defence mechanisms and drugs, thus leading ultimately to relapse.

Behaviour

Progressive destruction of nasal structures is not uncommon and attempts at healing with fibrosis may occur as in the fourth stage described by Job et al. (1966). Although chemotherapy has modified the course of the disease, it has not yet resolved the problem of treatment. McDougall, Weddell and Rees (1975) described the histopathological findings following treatment with Dapsone for one year. Although the overlying epithelium had been restored, bacilli were still present in the tissues. Rendall and McDougall (1976) reported a persistent lesion around the apex of an upper incisor in a patient who had been under chemotherapy for four years. Obviously, there are problems in reaching the infecting organisms, nevertheless, the changes induced in the nasal mucosa by drug therapy certainly render the patient less infective.

BIBLIOGRAPHY

Barton R P E 1976 Clinical manifestations of leprous rhinitis. Annals of Otology, Rhinology and Laryngology 85: 74–82

Barton R P E, Davey T F, McDougall A C, Rees R J W, Weddell A G M 1973 Clinical and histological studies of the nose in early lepromatous leprosy. International Journal of Leprosy 41: 512

Boddingius J 1974 The occurrence of Mycobacterium leprae within axons of peripheral nerves. Acta Neuropathologica 27: 257–270

British Medical Journal Editorial 1969 Leprosy in England 3: 730–731

Dastur D K, Ramamohan Y, Shah J S 1973 Ultrastructure of lepromatous nerves. Neural pathogenesis in leprosy. International Journal of Leprosy 41: 47–80

Davey T F 1974 The nose in leprosy. Leprosy Review 45: 97–103

Davey T F, Rees R J W 1974 The nasal discharge in leprosy: clinical and bacteriological aspects. Leprosy Review 45: 121–134

Dharmendra S N, Sen N 1949 Frequency of the presence of the leprosy bacillus in nasal smears of leprosy patients. Leprosy in India 21: 23–24

Fite G L, Cambre P J, Turner M H, Corville B S 1947 Procedure for demonstrating lepra bacilli in paraffin sections. Archives of Pathology 43: 624–625

Geater J G 1975 The fly as potential vector in the transmission of leprosy. Leprosy Review 46: 279–286

Hansen G A 1874 Indberetning til det Norsk medicinske selskab i Christiamia om en med Understøttelse af selskabet for tagen Reise for at anstill under søgelser angaende spedalskledens årokga tildels udfort sammen med forftander Hartwig. Norsk Magazin for Laevidenskaben 4 (Supplement): 1–88

Job C K, Karat A B A, Karat S 1966 The histopathological appearance of leprous rhinitis and pathogenesis of septal perforation in leprosy. Journal of Laryngology and Otology 80: 718–732

Job C K, Verghese H 1974 Electron microscopic demonstration of *Myco. leprae* in axons. Leprosy Review 45: 235–239

Jopling W H 1974 Leprosy. British Journal of Hospital Medicine 11: 43–50

Lumsden C E 1964 Leprosy and the Schwann cell *in vivo* and *in vitro*. In: Cochrane R G and Davey T F (eds) Leprosy in practice, 2nd edn. John Wright and Sons Ltd, Bristol, pp 221–250

McDougall A C, Rees R J W, Weddell A G M, Wajdi Kanan M 1975 The histopathology of lepromatous leprosy of the nose. Journal of Pathology 115: 215–226

McDougall A C, Weddell A G M, Rees R J W 1975 Lepromatous leprosy in the nose after one year of Dapsone treatment: histopathological findings. Leprosy Review 46: 267–277

Pedley J C 1973 The nasal mucus in leprosy. Leprosy Review 44: 33–35

Rees R J W 1975 Do flies transmit leprosy? Leprosy Review 46: 255–256

Rees R J W, McDougall A C, Weddell A G M 1974 The nose in mice with experimental human leprosy. Leprosy Review 45: 112–120

Rees R J W, Waters M F R, Weddell A G M, Palmer E 1967 Experimental lepromatous leprosy. Nature 215: 599–602

Rendall J R, McDougall A C 1976 Reddening of the upper central incisors associated with periapical granuloma in lepromatous leprosy. British Journal of Oral Surgery 13: 271–277

Ridley D S, Jopling W H 1966 Classification of leprosy according to immunity. International Journal of Leprosy 34: 255–273

Shepard C C 1960 The experimental disease that follows the injection of human leprosy bacilli into the footpads of mice. Journal of Experimental Medicine 112: 445–454

Stanton M B 1964 Leprosy presenting with nasal obstruction. Journal of Laryngology and Otology 78: 702–706

Weddell A G M, Palmer E, Rees R J W, Jamieson D G 1963 Experimental observations related to the histopathology in leprosy. In: Wolstenholm G E W, O' Connor M (eds) The pathogenesis of leprosy. Churchill, London, pp 3–15

Wheeler E A, Hamilton E G, Harman D J 1965 An improved technique for the histopathological diagnosis and classification of leprosy. Leprosy Review 36: 37–39

Yoshizumi M O, Asbury A K 1974 Intra-axonal bacilli in lepromatous leprosy. A light and electron microscopic study. Acta Neuropathologica 27: 1–10

6

Nasal syphilis and framboesia

NASAL SYPHILIS

Introduction

The control and treatment of venereal disease, particularly since the advent of the antibiotic era, has resulted in a significant diminution of syphilitic lesions. Towpik and Nowakowska (1970) drew attention to the fall in frequency of the more serious lesions of late syphilis. One of the inevitable consequences of this changing pattern has been less frequent consideration of syphilis in relation to differential diagnosis, not only clinically but also histopathologically. In 1975, the *British Medical Journal* pointed out that there are many who are unfamiliar with the protean manifestations of this disease. Although the nose is commonly involved in congenital syphilis, it may be affected at any stage in the course of the acquired disease. Nevertheless, during the past 50 years, there have been surprisingly few reports on syphilitic lesions of this region. Amongst the I.L.O. material, there has been only one case over a period of 27 years.

Clinical features

A primary lesion of the nose is very rare and is usually the result of accidental inoculation, resulting from scratching or picking the nose with an infected finger after attending to an infected patient. Nasal chancres are located anteriorly and are associated with enlargement of the pre-auricular or submandibular lymphnodes.

Secondary lesions are essentially of the same type as those that occur on the mucous membranes of other orifices, particularly the mouth. They appear as the white so-called mucous patches and almost certainly would be associated with oral and cutaneous lesions. Secondary lesions also occur in congenital syphilis and are encountered at or shortly after birth when attenion is drawn to them by the persistent catarrhal signs known as 'snuffles'. There may be nasal discharge which is occasionally bloodstained.

Tertiary lesions have been more commonly observed and may represent either acquired or congenital disease. These lesions may appear at any time following the secondary stage and their onset may even be recognizable before the symptoms or signs of the latter have fully subsided. In most cases, however, they appear about five years following the primary infection but their manifestation may be delayed for twenty years or more. Destructive extension of the lesion often leads to ultimate collapse of the bridge of the nose producing the characteristic saddle-back deformity. The phenomenon is a particular feature of the tertiary type of congenital lesion which tends to appear during the early years of life or at the time of the second dentition when the characteristic Hutchinsonian incisors may be observed. Nasal obstruction and bloodstained discharge are common forms of presentation. Involvement of the anterior nares may take the form of indolent, brawny, ulcerating granulations, the appearance of which may suggest, clinically, a variety of alternatives such as lupus vulgaris, rodent ulcer, squamous carcinoma or the midfacial granuloma syndrome. Destruction of the columella with subsequent retraction of the tip of the nose produces a peculiarly ugly deformity.

Anatomical site of origin

Primary lesions involve the vestibule and the anterior part of the septum whilst secondary manifestations may appear anywhere on the nasal mucosa. The sites commonly affected in tertiary syphilis are the septum, inferior turbinates, the floor of the nose and the alae nasi. Schwartz (1923) drew attention to a consistent early finding of bilateral thickening of the septum. The collapse of the bridge of the nose is not the outcome of destruction of the septum but is due to involvement of the nasal bones forming the arch which gradually founders because of the traction by the shrinking scar tissue. Syphilitic caries of the lateral nasal wall may lead to involvement of the maxillary sinus or destruction of the lachrymal duct and even invasion of the cranial cavity.

Histopathology

In the rare primary lesion, polymorphonuclear leucocytosis is rapidly replaced by lymphocytic and plasma-

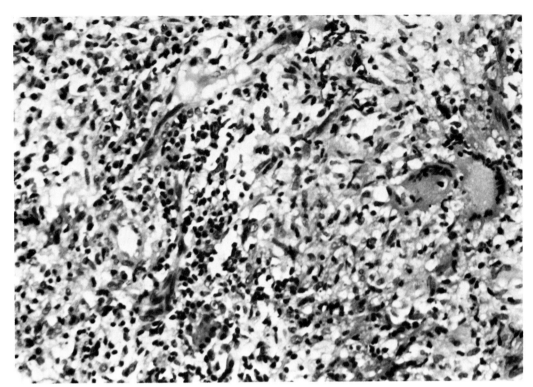

Fig. 6.1 Syphilis of the nasal cavity in a 52 year-old female, showing multinucleated giant cells with epithelioid cells mimicking tuberculosis. M × 350

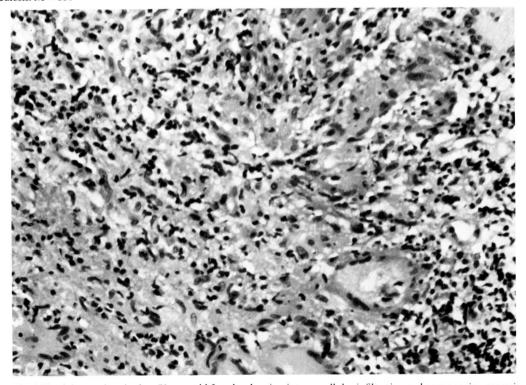

Fig. 6.2 Syphilis of the nasal cavity in a 52 year-old female, showing intense cellular infiltration and commencing necrosis. M × 350

cytic infiltration which tends to aggregate around vessels. The latter structures may show narrowing of their lumina due to endothelial proliferation. Epithelial hyperplasia occurs at the periphery of the ulcerated area. The mucous patches of the secondary lesions show epithelial proliferation with subsequent ulceration.

Tertiary lesions are of particular interest since they may present problems of differential diagnosis. The gummatous infiltration may or may not be associated with ulceration. Areas of necrosis alternate with granulation tissue which ranges from non-specific appearance to epithelioid manifestations including multinucleated giant cells which may be of the Langhans type, thereby mimicking a tuberculoid granuloma (Figs. 6.1 & 6.2). Lesions of this type quite clearly call for the standard serological tests for syphilis and culture to exclude mycobacterial infection.

Behaviour
Untreated lesions tend to extend with progressive destruction of the nasal framework. Perforation of the posterior part of the septum commonly occurs and such a finding is generally regarded as a manifestation of syphilis whereas an anterior deficiency is more likely to be the result of trauma or tuberculosis. The syphilitic perforation is usually near to the floor of the nasal cavity and a similar type of deficiency may appear in the hard palate. External fistulae in the lateral wall of the nose may also occur. Anti-syphilitic treatment arrests the progress of the lesion though residual deformities persist.

YAWS (FRAMBOESIA)

This spirochaetal infection (Treponema pertenue) produces a very similar clinical and histological pattern to that of acquired syphilis. By contrast, transmission is believed to be through the medium of insect vectors and there is no congenital manifestation. The disease is widespread in the world but confined to tropical zones. Nicolas (1924) reviewed tertiary lesions of Yaws in the nose and throat. He pointed out that the lesions were hardly distinguishable from those of syphilis and, furthermore, many cases showed positive Wasserman reactions. The suggestion by this author that reliance must be placed on the case history is still valid. Fischman and Mundt (1971) examined the sera of over 500 Pacific Islanders immigrants in New Zealand and found that about one third showed positive serological tests for syphilis which they attributed to residual Yaws antibodies.

BIBLIOGRAPHY

British Medical Journal, Annotation 1975 Never forget syphilis. 2: 460–461
Fischman A, Mundt H 1971 Test patterns of Yaws antibodies in New Zealand. British Journal of Venereal Diseases 47: 91–94
Gil Tutor E 1971 Tertiary syphilis of the nasal fossa and pharynx. Acta Otorinolaryngologica Iberio-Americana 22: 366–384

Nicolas F 1924 Notes on the nose and throat manifestations of tertiary Yaws. Journal of the Philippine Islands Medical Association 4: 140–142
Schwartz E M 1923 Gumma of the nasal septum. New York Medical Journal 118: 289–290
Towpik J & Nowakowska E 1970 Changing pattern of late syphilis. British Journal of Venereal Diseases 46: 132–134

7

Rhinoscleroma

RHINOSCLEROMA

Introduction

This disease was first described as a nasal affliction by Hebra in 1870. Mikulicz (1877) presented a detailed account of the histological picture and, in particular, the large vacuolated cells which bear his name as a characteristic feature of the lesion. In 1882, von Frisch observed organisms within the Mikulicz cells, a finding which provoked much speculation and argument which has only been resolved in recent years.

Terminology

Although the condition was first reported in the nasal cavity, it has long been recognized that the condition has a tendency to involve other parts of the upper respiratory tract, particularly the larynx and trachea. For this reason it has been commonly argued that the prefix 'rhino' should be omitted and the disease be henceforth known as 'scleroma' (International Congress in Oto-rhino-laryngology, Madrid, 1932).

Incidence

Scleroma is a chronic disease with a world-wide distribution through many degress of latitude (Fig. 7.1). Numerous endemic centres are now recognized, the largest being in Europe, involving Poland, Czechoslovakia, Hungary, Rumania, White Russia and the Ukraine. In fact, over 80 per cent of published cases have been reported from these countries and, in over 100 cases reported from North America, a similar proportion involved European immigrants (Cunning and Guerry, 1942) although an increasing number of native born

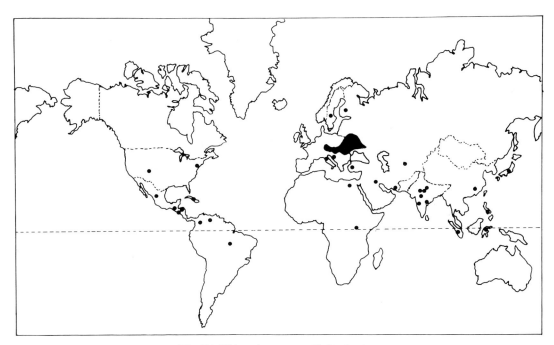

Fig. 7.1 Rhinoscleroma: world distribution.

cases are now being recognized (Shaw and Martin, 1961; Steffen and Lierle, 1961).

In Central America there is a concentration of the disease in south eastern Guatemala (Quevedo, 1949) and adjoining El Salvador (Reyes, 1946). In South America, the disease is endemic in Columbia (Lucchesi, 1955).

In the African continent, the disease is endemic in Egypt (Handousa and Elwi, 1958; Badrawy, 1966) whilst Roland (1961) reported 16 cases from Uganda and Edwards, Roberts, Storrs (1977) three cases from Nigeria. Wahi and Misra (1964) reviewed the distribution of scleroma in the northern half of India, recording nearly 300 cases encountered over a period of five years. The condition is also endemic in Indonesia (Oomen, 1952; Barten, 1956).

In Europe, Zwiefach (1955) reviewed pre-war cases in Poland whilst Woyke, Domagala and Olszewski (1969) noted that the disease still remained more common in the eastern part of Poland. In Czechoslovakia the disease is also more common in the eastern regions. A few cases have been reported from Scandinavia including one case in Finland (Grahne, Siirala, Meurman and Kunnes, 1972). Alavi, Kohout and Dutz (1971) reported two cases in Iran. Lucas and Negus (1942) reported what they believed to be a primary case in the United Kingdom but, although the clinical presentation was highly suggestive of scleroma, the diagnosis was not confirmed either histologically or bacteriologically. Endemic foci and sporadic cases have been reported in at least 68 countries (Kerdel-Vegas, Convit, Gordon and Goihman, 1963; Muzyka and Gubina, 1971).

Cases encountered in England are invariably amongst immigrants, thus representing 'imported ills'. This has been reflected in the I.L.O. experience where a small number of cases have been concentrated in recent years.

Clinical features
Age distribution shows a peak during the third decade which tallies with the observation made by Cunning and Guerry (1942) that the greatest number of cases occur during the most reproductive period of life. There has been some difference of opinion regarding the sex incidence but, in all probability, both are equally affected. Three clinical stages of the disease are recognized: (i) the catarrhal rhinitis stage, (ii) the inflammatory and proliferative granulomatous stage and (iii) the cicatricial, deformative stage. The second and third clinical phases have been well illustrated by Lucchesi (1955) and Furnas (1968). Common presenting symptoms are discharge, epistaxis and nasal obstruction. Initially, crusting of drying mucosa may resemble atrophic rhinitis but later infiltration leads to mucosal thickening which may be of cartilage-like consistency. As the disease enters the granulomatous stage, discrete nodular lesions of a reddish-violet colour may involve the interior of the nose and the skin around the external nares. Coalescence of these slowly growing masses results in the development of an unpleasant proliferative and destructive clinical picture. There may or may not be evidence of extension to other parts of the upper respiratory tract.

Anatomical site of origin
Although the nasal cavity is the common site of election, other parts of the respiratory tract may be involved either primarily or secondarily, e.g. nasopharynx, palate, larynx, trachea and bronchi. According to Kouwenaar (1956), laryngeal infection develops independently of nasal lesions. Semczuk, Hencner and Klinowski (1968) noted tracheal scleroma in 12 per cent of cases whilst bronchial infection occurred in only 7 per cent. In the nose, the mucosa and skin may both be involved and in the second phase the cavity may be completely blocked by coalescent granulomatous masses arising from the septum and turbinates.

Histopathology
Microscopically, the disease exhibits three phases corresponding to the three clinical stages. The first phase presents an essentially non-specific pattern of chronic inflammatory infiltration with lymphocytes predominating. In the second phase, diffuse subepithelial chronic inflammatory infiltration is always present and the infiltrate becomes markedly plasmacytic with lymphocytes and focal accumulations of polymorphonuclear leucocytes. Phagocytosis of the causal organism by macrophages is a common event and these cells become enlarged, vacuolated and foamy to form the characteristic Mikulicz cells. Such cells, which are of the order of 30 microns in diameter, become numerous and are interspersed amongst the predominantly plasmacytic element (Figs. 7.2 & 7.3). The Mikulicz cells contain varying numbers of bacilli which may be demonstrated by Gram staining or, more effectively, by Paragon staining of Araldite-embedded material prepared for electron microscopy. The presence of these intracellular organisms, first demonstrated by von Frisch (1882), have been repeatedly confirmed both by light and electron microscopy (Cornil and Alvarez, 1885; Welsh, Correa and Herran, 1963; Hoffmann, Loose and Harkin, 1973).

Plasmacytes often show a notable degree of activity in which the accumulation and coalescence of globules of secretory product present a characteristic appearance commonly known as Cornil or Mott cells (Fig. 7.4). Such cells are encountered in a variety of inflammatory lesions (Mott, 1905; Thiery, 1960) and are in no way specific for scleroma. As in other chronic inflammations, the cell may degenerate and be cast off leaving a naked,

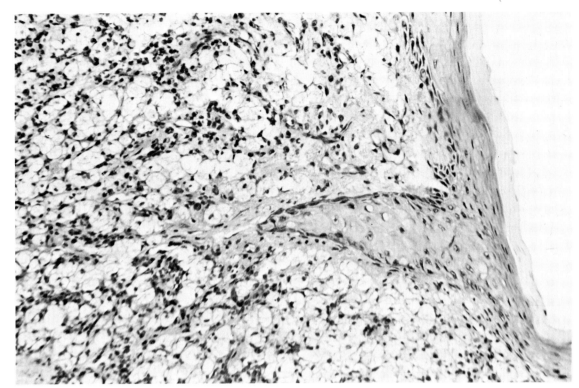

Fig. 7.2 Scleroma of the nose in a Polish patient, showing large numbers of clear Mikulicz cells underlying squamous metaplastic epithelium. M × 250

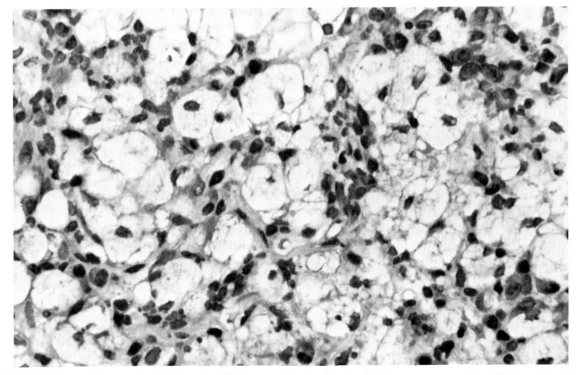

Fig. 7.3 Scleroma of the nose in a Polish patient. Higher magnification showing the foamy appearance of the Mikulicz cells and numbers of plasmacytes. M × 800

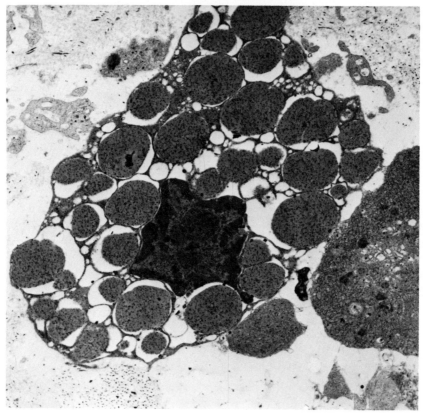

Fig. 7.4 Scleroma of the nose in an adult male Egyptian. Plasmacyte (Cornil or Mott cell) showing multiple globules of secretory product. M × 8000

eosinophilic hyaline mass known as a Russell body (Fig. 7.5).

The overlying epithelium may be either thin and atrophic or markedly proliferated, producing a pseudo-epitheliomatous hyperplasia, depending on the stage of the disease. During the second phase, Mikulicz cells may be seen infiltrating the epithelium and appearing on the surface where rupture may lead to dissemination of the organisms.

In the third phase there is much fibrosis (Fig. 7.6) with consequent distortion whilst the cellular component, particularly the Mikulicz cells, become less evident leading to difficulties in histological diagnosis.

Ultrastructural studies of scleroma have been carried out by many workers (Friedmann, 1963; Welsh et al., 1963; Fisher and Dimling, 1964; Gonzalez-Angulo, Marques-Monter, Greenberg and Cerbon, 1965; Woyke et al., 1969; Shokeir and Osman, 1972; Hoffmann et al., 1973). Under the electron microscope the Mikulicz cell is seen to contain numerous distended vesicular structures in which, apart from micro-organisms (Fig. 7.7), there

appears a variable quantity of granular material. Hoffmann and his co-workers noted the resemblance of this material to that seen surrounding the intracellular organisms and also *K. rhinoscleromatis* in culture. By fluorescent microscopy, they were able to demonstrate a similar antigenic composition. It would appear that the Mikulicz cell contains indisposable mucopolysaccharide. Osmosis causes inhibition of water with coalescence of vesicles or phagosomes leading ultimately to rupture of the cell, thus accounting for the unstained structureless material often observed under the light microscope.

Steffen and Lierle (1961) pointed out that large macrophages resembling the Mikulicz cell and containing bacteria are to be found in a variety of granulomatous lesions including lepromatous leprosy, glanders, granuloma inguinale and plague. Thus the individual cellular components of scleroma are not in themselves specific features but, in combination, they produce a characteristic morphological pattern that may be described as specific. Bacteriological confirmation must also be sought in order to support the histological diagnosis.

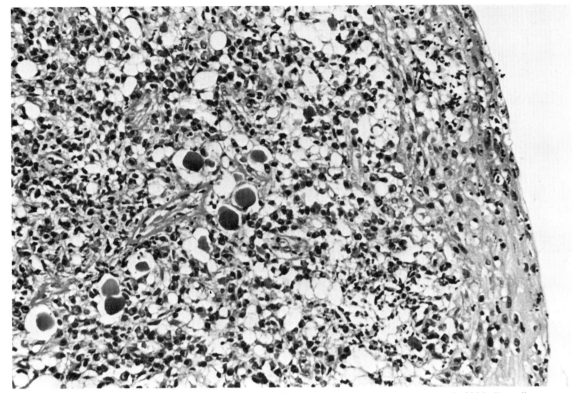

Fig. 7.5 Scleroma of the nose in a Polish patient. Note Russell bodies in granulation tissue composed of Mikulicz cells, plasmacytes and lymphocytes. M ×250

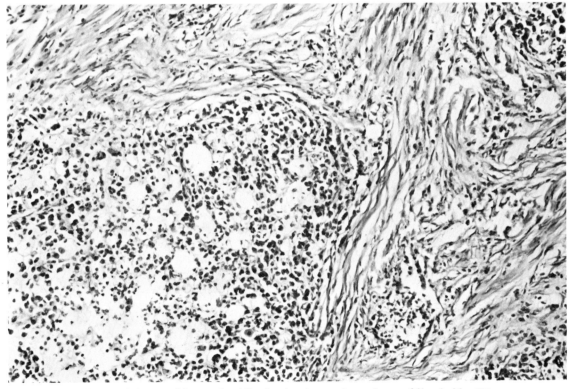

Fig. 7.6 Scleroma of the nose in a Nigerian showing an advanced stage of fibrosis. M ×180

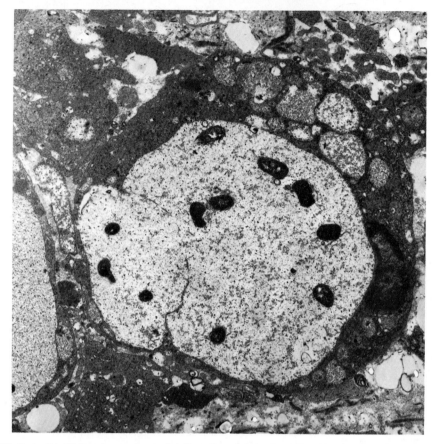

Fig. 7.7 Mikulicz cell in Rhinoscleroma in an adult Egyptian, showing bacteria within the foamy cytoplasm. M × 8000

Aetiology and pathogenesis

In 1882, Frisch isolated from the lesion a bacillus which he observed within the vacuolated cells. The organism was subsequently classified as belonging to the Klebsiella group but, although his findings have been confirmed by many other workers, the aetiological role of von Frisch's bacillus remained controversial for many decades, notwithstanding the demonstration of agglutinating and complement-fixing antibodies to the organism (Goldzieher and Neuber, 1909; Kouwenaar, Maasland and Wolff, 1934; Levine and Hoyt, 1947; Oomen, 1952), the causal nature of the bacillus remained in dispute. One of the major problems was bacteriological identification. The various members of the Klebsiella group have been distinguished on the basis of biochemical and serological tests (Levine, Hoyt and Peterson, 1947; Kauffmann, 1949). Levine et al, (1947) established a biochemical pattern for *K. rhinoscleromatis* which they claimed to be consistent in all the organisms isolated from cases of scleroma. Furthermore, although they isolated Klebsiella organisms from non scleroma cases, they did not show the same biological behaviour. In 1951, Levine reported an extension of this investigation, failing to find Klebsiella organisms in nose and throat cultures of over 500 non-scleroma subjects. On the other hand, Berger, Pollock and Richmond (1977) found *K. ozaenae* or *rhinoscleromatis* from various anatomical locations in non-scleroma cases, including sputum, blood and wound infections. Hencner (1967) examined the sera of 54 patients with clinical scleroma. Using *K. rhinoscleromatis* as the antigenic source, this author found that complement fixation tests were positive in 47 cases, high titres of agglutination in 41 and positive Coombs' anti-globulin test in 51, indicating the presence of incomplete antibodies to the organism. More recently, it has been found that the organisms isolated from clinically and histologically proven cases of scleroma are not exclusively *K. rhinoscleromatis* but includ *K. ozaenae* and *K. pneumoniae* (Rees and Gregory, 1977).

Although the possibility was indicated at a very early

stage in the history of this disease, the acceptance of the Gram negative, encapsulated bacillus of von Frisch as the aetiological agent has been a slow reluctant process. Many observers have remained sceptical, partly because of the difficulties in distinction between various members of the Klebsiella group but particularly because it was argued that Koch's postulates had not been fulfilled. The earliest attempt at experimental infection was by Galli-Valerio (1911) who produced a chronic inflammatory lesion but without the characteristic Mikulicz cells. Reyes (1946) failed to reproduce the disease either in experimental animals or human subjects and began to think along the lines of a possible virus infection. Steffen and Smith (1961) inoculated mice with *K. rhinoscleromatis* by various routes including intranasal administration. They failed to produce local lesions in the nose but the animals developed pneumonia and the pulmonary lesions showed chronic inflammation with large bacteria-containing macrophages resembling Mikulicz cells. The organism was recovered from the lungs. Talaat, Soliman and Belal (1978) produced similar results in rabbits but there is a certain lack of validity in these results in so far as lower respiratory infection in scleroma is uncommon and involvement of the pulmonary parenchyma is virtually unknown.

In more recent times, however, the disease has been reproduced in the skin of experimental animals (Hoffmann, 1967; Hoffmann and Duque, 1971). These authors, working in Colombia, succeeded in producing a lesion which was histologically identical with that found in the human disease. Their technique involved repeated inoculation of *K. rhinoscleromatis* mixed with hog gastric mucin. After many weeks, mice produced typical lesions including the classical Mikulicz cells and the organism was subsequently recovered from the lesion, thus fulfilling Koch's postulates. It would appear that the artificially cultured organism produces less capsular substance (Hoffmann, Loose and Harkin 1973) and this may account for the failure of injection of the organisms alone to produce typical Mikulicz cells. There seems to be little doubt now that the causal agent belongs to the Klebsiella group although there may be variants as indicated by Rees and Gregory (1977). Nevertheless, the majority of Klebsiellae isolated from cases of scleroma appear to be antigenically and biochemically homogeneous. There has been much speculation regarding the nature and origin of the Mikulicz cell. Streit (1935) suggested that they might be derived from any type of cell which was 'invaded' by the organism. Some workers have even suggested origin from plasmacytes (Fisher and Dimling, 1964) but the generally accepted view is that they are derived from macrophages, a view which is supported particularly by ultrastructural studies (Friedmann, 1963; Welsh et al., 1963; Hoffmann et al., 1973). Hoffmann has pointed out that the foamy

mononuclear cell has all the basic morphological structures characteristic of macrophages. Although plasma cells may occasionally appear to be vacuolated, their distinctive fine structure distinguishes them readily from macrophages and they never contain bacteria. Mikulicz cells often contain bacteria and mucopolysaccharide derived from the causal organism. This material which often lies within phagosomes has been shown to have antigenic identity with the capsular substance. The apparently indisposable substance may well protect the organism against antibodies or antibiotics. Cain and Kraus (1972) studied a 49 year-old Ukranian patient in whom scleroma persisted for over 25 years in spite of prolonged treatment and ultrastructural findings revealed the persistence of Mikulicz cells containing the organisms.

It would seem that socio-economic conditions are more important than climate in the distribution of this disease. Over 90 per cent of cases occur amongst the less well endowed (Belinoff, 1938). A familial incidence has been observed by a number of workers (Hara, Pratt, Levine and Hoyt, 1947; Oomen, 1952; Barten, 1956; Krasnilnikov, Igraitel, and Krylov, 1971), a fact which offers a clue to the mode of transmission. Krasnilnikov et al. (1971) carried out epidemiological studies in 19 villages in Byelorussia. The pattern of familial incidence was related to common residence and indicated clearly the mode of interhuman transmission. An interesting observation was made by Alvarez in 1898 who discovered a bacillus, resembling von Frisch's bacillus, on the leaves of the indigo plant and, according to Quevedo (1949) dye workers in El Salvador were particularly prone to scleroma.

Behaviour

Kouwenaar (1956) pointed out that the clinical picture varies according to the geographical location. The enormous swelling and distortion known as the 'Hebra nose' is common in Indonesia but rare in other locations, whilst laryngeal lesions are said to be more common in Europe and America. Spread to the pharynx, larynx, lachrymal duct, upper lip and paranasal sinuses may occur. Semczuk et al. (1958) found pharyngeal involvement in 43 per cent whilst the larynx was affected in 80 per cent of nasal cases in Eastern Europe. Yassin and Safwat (1966) reported three out of 25 cases in which spread to the maxillary sinus had occurred. In the granulomatous phase, masses of inflammatory tissue may cause pressure erosion on bone (Badrawy, 1966; Yassin and Safwat, 1966; Alavi et al., 1971). Extension into the orbit and the cranial cavity may be encountered (Bahri, Bessi and Rohatgi, 1972).

There are variable reports on the response to streptomycin therapy. Some cases have responded well to antibiotic treatment (Zakrzewski and Durska-

Zakrzewska, 1964) whilst in other cases the infection has persisted (Grahne et al., 1972; Cain and Kraus, 1972). Although the organism is normally sensitive to streptomycin, the essential problem is access of the antibiotic to the organism which may be impeded by the presence of the capsular mucopolysaccharide.

BIBLIOGRAPHY

Alavi K, Kohout E, Dutz W 1971 Two cases of scleroma in Iran. Journal of Clinical Pathology 24:360–362

Badrawy R 1966 Affection of bone in rhinoscleroma. Journal of Laryngology and Otology 80:160–167

Bahri H C, Bessi N K, Rohatgi M S 1972 Scleroma with intracranial extension. Annals of Otology, Rhinology and Laryngology 81: 856–859

Barten J J C 1956 Scleroma respiratorium in Indonesia. Documenta de Medicina Geographica et Tropica 8: 101–116

Belinoff S 1938 Epidemiology of scleroma (2nd. International Congress of Otorhinolaryngology, Madrid, 1932) Archives of Otolaryngology, 18: 398

Berger S A, Pollock A A, Richmond A S 1977 Isolation of Klebsiella rhinoscleromatis in a general hospital. American Journal of Clinical Pathology 67: 499–502

Cain H, Kraus B 1972 Feinstrukturelle Befunde und Probleme bei langjähriger Skleromerkrankung. Zur Morphogenese der Mikulicz-Zelle. Virchows Archiv für pathologische Anatomie 357: 345–348

Cornil V, Alvarez E 1885 Mémoire pour servir à l'histoire du rhinosclerome. Archives de Physiologie normale et pathologique, Série 3, 6: 11–40

Cunning D S, Guerry D P 1942 Scleroma. Archives of Otolaryngology 36: 662–678

Edwards M B, Roberts G D D, Storrs T O 1977 Scleroma rhinoscleroma in a Nigerian maxillo-facial practice. Review and case reports. Int J Oral Surg 6: 270–279

Fisher E R, Dimling C 1964 Rhinoscleroma. Archives of Pathology 78: 501–512

Friedmann I 1963 Electron microscopy of rare diseases of the nose. Transactions of the American Academy of Ophthalmology and Otolaryngology 67: 261–279

Frisch A 1882 Zur Aetiologie des Rhinoskleroms. Wiener medizinische Wochenschrift 32: 969–972

Furnas D W 1968 Recognition of scleroma (rhinoscleroma). Laryngoscope 78: 1948–1952

Galli-Valerio B 1911 L'Etat actuel de nos connaisances sur l'étiologie du rhinosclerome. Zentralblatt für Bakteriologie, Parasitenkunde und Infektionskrankheiten, 57: 481–490

Goldzieher M, Neuber E 1909 Untersuchungen über das Rhinosklerom. Zentralblatt für Bakteriologie, Parasitenkunde und Infektions-krankheiten 51: 121–136

Gonzalez-Angulo A, Marques-Monter H, Greenberg D S, Cerbon J 1965 Ultrastructure of nasal scleroma (emphasizing the fine structure of Klebsiella rhinoscleromatis within the lesion). Annals of Otology, Rhinology and Laryngology 74: 1022–1033

Grahne B, Siirala U, Meurman L, Kunnes K 1972 Rhinoscleroma in Finland. Acta Otolaryngologica 74: 430–435

Handousa A, Elwi A M 1958 Some clinicopathological observations on scleroma. Journal of Laryngology and Otology 72: 32–47

Hara H J, Pratt O B, Levine M G, Hoyt R E 1947 Scleroma: a clinicopathological study of seven cases in one family. Annals of Otology, Rhinology and Laryngology 56: 769–783

Hebra F 1870 Über ein eigenthümliches Neugebilde an der Nase – Rhinosklerom. Wiener medizinische Wochenschrift 20: 1–5

Hencner Z 1967 Studies on incomplete antibodies in infection with Klebsiella rhinoscleromatis. Bulletin de l'Academie Polonaise des Sciences 15: 73–77

Hoffmann E O 1967 The etiology of rhinoscleroma. International Pathology 8: 74–77

Hoffmann E O, Duque E 1971 Rhinoescleroma experimental. Revista Latinoamericana de Patologia 10: 57–70

Hoffmann E O, Loose L D, Harkin J L 1973 The Mikulicz cell in rhinoscleroma. American Journal of Pathology 73: 47–58

Kauffmann E 1949 On the serology of the Klebsiella group. Acta Pathologica et Microbiologica Scandinavica 26: 381–406

Kerdel-Vegas F, Convit J, Gordon B, Goihman M 1963 Rhinoscleroma. C C Thomas, Springfield, Illinois

Kouwenaar W 1956 Rhinoscleroma: a review of the present situation. Documenta de Medicina Geographica et Tropica 8: 13–22

Kouwenaar W, Maasland J H, Wolff J W 1934 Onderzoekingen over het rhinosclerom op Sumatra. V de waards eer complement-bindingsreactie bij het rhinoscleroomonderzoek. Geneeskundig Tijdschrift voor Nederlandsch-Indie 74: 1447–1454

Krasnilnikov A P, Igraitel N A, Krylov I A 1971 Focal incidence of scleroma. Journal of Hygiene, Epidemiology, Microbiology and Immunology 15: 243–257

Levine M G 1951 Scleroma (rhinoscleroma). American Journal of Clinical Pathology 21: 546–549

Levine M G, Hoyt R E 1947 Scleroma: complement fixation test. Proceedings of the Society of Experimental Biology and Medicine 65: 70–72

Levine M G, Hoyt R E, Peterson J E 1947 Scleroma: an etiological study. Journal of Clinical Investigation 65: 281–286

Lucas H A, Negus V E 1942 Scleroma of nose, larynx, trachea and bronchi. Journal of Laryngology and Otology 57: 447–449

Lucchesi G 1955 Statistica dello scleroma in Colombia (Sud America). Minerva Medica, 46 (Part 1): 345–348

Mikulicz J 1877 Über das Rhinosklerom (Hebra). Archiv für klinische Chirurgie 20: 485–534

Mott F W 1905 Observations of the brains of man and animals infected with various forms of trypanosomes. Proceedings of the Royal Society, Series B 76: 235–242

Muzyka M M, Gubina K M 1971 Problems of the epidemiology of scleroma. Journal of Hygiene, Epidemiology, Microbiology and Immunology 15: 233–242

Oomen H A P C 1952 Clinical course of rhinoscleroma. Documenta de medicina geographica et Tropica 4: 124–133

Quevedo J 1949 Scleroma in Guatemala. Annals of Otology, Rhinology and Laryngology 58: 613–645

Rees T A, Gregory M M 1977 Causative organisms in rhinoscleroma. Lancet 1: 650

Reyes E 1946 Rhinoscleroma. Archives of Dermatology and Syphilology 54: 531–537

Roland P E 1961 Scleroma in Uganda. Journal of Laryngology and Otology 75: 1040–1047

Semczuk B, Hencner Z, Klonowski S, Parnas J 1968 Epidemiologische, klinische und mikrobiologische Forschungen über Sklerom. Archiv für Hygiene und Bakteriologie 152: 54–61

Shaw H J, Martin H 1961 Rhinoscleroma – a clinical perspective. Journal of Laryngology and Otology 75: 1011–1039

Shokeir A A, Osman M 1972 Rhinoscleroma: an electron microscopic study. Journal of Hygiene, Epidemiology, Microbiology and Immunology 16: 1–7

Steffen T N, Lierle D M 1961 Scleroma in a non-endemic area. Laryngoscope 71: 1386–1401

Steffen T N, Smith I M 1961 Scleroma: Klebsiella rhinoscleromatis and its effect on mice. Annals of Otology, Rhinology and Laryngology 70: 935–952

Streit H 1935 Die für Sklerom charakteristischen Degenerationseirscheinungen innerhalb das Epithels. Schweizerische medizinische Wochenschrift 16: 240–242

Talaat M, Soliman H G, Belal A 1978 Experimental scleroma. Journal of Laryngology and Otology 92: 489–498

Thiéry J P 1960 Microcinematographic contributions to the study of plasma cells. In: Wolstenholm, G E W and O'Connor, M (eds) Cellular aspects of immunity. J A Churchill Ltd. London, pp 59–91

Wahi A L, Misra R N 1964 A note on the geographical distribution of scleroma. Journal of Laryngology and Otology 78: 573–577

Welsh R A, Correa P, Herran R 1963 Light and electron microscopic observations of scleroma. Experimental and Molecular Pathology 2: 93–101

Woyke S, Domagala W, Olszewski W 1969 Electron microscopic studies of scleroma granulation tissue. Acta Medica Polona 10: 231–242

Yassin A, Safwat F 1966 Unusual features of scleroma. Journal of Laryngology and Otology 80: 524–532

Zakrzewski A, Durska-Zakrzewska A 1964 On scleroma. Acta Otolaryngologica 57: 281–286

Zwiefach E 1955 Rhinoscleroma. Journal of Laryngology and Otology 69: 321–330

8

Rhinosporidiosis

RHINOSPORIDIOSIS

Introduction

This disease and its causal organism were first reported from South America by Seeber (1900). O'Kinealy (1903) described a nasal affliction in an Indian, to which he gave the name 'psorospermosis' but the condition was clearly identical with that presented by Seeber. Although the existence of the disease was first established in the New World, subsequent accounts have emanated largely from Asia.

Incidence

Vanbreuseghem (1976), in a review of over one thousand published cases, found that over 90 per cent were from Asia whilst South America accounted for less than five per cent. Asian origin is largely comprised of India (Satyanarayana, 1960; David, 1974; Grover, 1975; Gupta, Darbari, Dwivedi, Billore and Arora, 1976), Ceylon (Karunaratne, 1964) and Pakistan (Khan, Khaleque and Huda, (1969). In India, the cases are largely concentrated in the central and southern regions. In the South American continent, Seeber subsequently found a number of other cases in Argentina while Rolon (1974) published a series of cases from Paraguay. Sporadic cases have been reported from many parts of the world within the warmer latitudes (Fig. 8.1). The first case in North America was reported by Wright in 1907 whilst Marks and Johnstone (1948) reported two cases from Texas and Missouri respectively. There are many case reports scattered throughout the African continent including Ghana (Christian and Covi, 1966), Kenya (McClatchie, 1965; Cameron, Gatei and Bremner, 1973), Uganda (Mowat and Hennessy, 1941; Tamale and Hutt, 1964; Engzell and Jones, 1973), Sudan (Wahab and Talaat, 1976) and Natal (Smith, 1977).

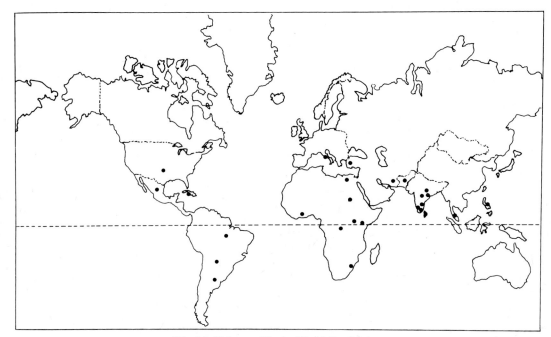

Fig. 8.1 Rhinosporidiosis: World distribution

Clinical features

The disease may be encountered at almost any age but most often in the early decades of life. Satyanarayana (1960) found a peak distribution in the third decade whilst Norman (1960) reported the disease in a three-year-old Texan boy. Most series show a predominance of males though Gupta et al. (1976) found no significant sex difference in their 21 cases collected from a population survey.

Nasal involvement presents with obstruction, discharge and epistaxis. Polypoid masses within the nasal cavity may present at the anterior nares. Conjunctival or cutaneous lesions may also occur.

Anatomical site of origin

The nose is the main location, being involved in approximately 70 per cent (Karunaratne, 1964). Satyanarayana (1960) found the maxillary sinus to be affected in two cases, whilst afflication of the nasopharynx occurred in nearly six per cent of his series. The conjunctiva is not infrequently involved (Ingram, 1910; Karunaratne, 1964; Tamale and Hutt, 1964; McClatchie, 1965; Christian and Covi, 1966). The skin may also be affected (Satyanarayana, 1960, Kameswaran, Jaiswal and Mahure, 1970; Chatterjee, Khatua, Chatterjee and Dastidar, 1977). Involvement of other parts of the respiratory tract have also been reported, including the larynx (Satyanarayana, 1960; Pillai, 1974), the trachea (Grewal and Rangam, 1959; Satyanarayana, 1960; Subramanyam and Ramano Rao, 1960) and the bronchus (Thomas, Gopinath and Betts, 1957; Subramanyam and Ramano Rao, 1960). Other less common sites have also been observed: the ear (Beattie, 1907), the penis (Ingram, 1910), the tonsil and palate (Satyanarayana, 1960). Chatterjee et al. (1977) reported involvement of bone.

Within the nasal cavity, the common sites are the septum, inferior turbinate, floor and lateral wall.

Gross appearances

To the naked eye, the polypoid granular masses are often described as having a strawberry appearance. This is due to the highly vascular composition and the presence of sporangia close to or actually on the surface of the epithelium where they present as pale, sharply defined dots. The appearance is well illustrated in the case reported by Ashworth and Logan-Turner (1923).

Histopathology

Vascular inflammatory granulation tissue is covered by partly ulcerated, metaplastic squamous epithelium (Fig. 8.2) which frequently exhibits infolding to form crypts.

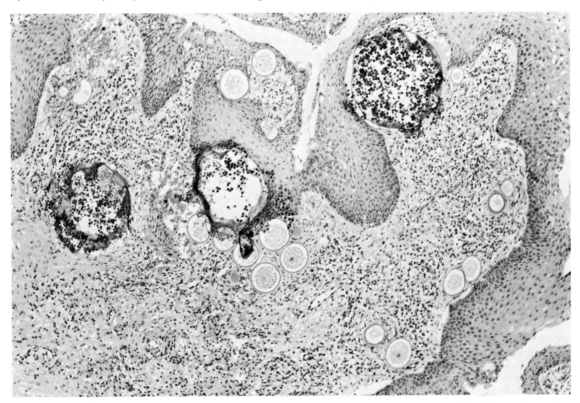

Fig. 8.2 Rhinosporidiosis in a young Ugandan female, showing subepithelial granulation tissue containing the causal organism. M × 90

The various stages in the life cycle of the organism may be found in the tissues but most readily recognizable are the sporangia in varying stages of maturity and size, ranging from about 120 to 300 microns in diameter (Fig. 8.3). They are characterized by an outer chitinous shell with an inner cellulose wall (Fig. 8.4) enclosing thousands of spores. Pressure on the epithelium leads to thinning and ultimately ulceration when the sporangia may be extruded intact onto the surface. Rupture of the sporangia occurs either on the surface or within the mucosa and the mature spores, liberated into the tissues develop into trophic forms which may be found in close association with the epithelium or occasionally engulfed by phagocytes. An intense chronic inflammatory infiltration is always present, sometimes with the formation of small abscesses whilst foreign body giant cell reaction is a common feature with engulfment of the remains of ruptured sporangia (Fig. 8.5). Engzell and Jones (1973) distinguished two histological patterns representing earlier and later stages. In the early stages, trophocytes, sporangia and spores are present in the tissues with chronic inflammatory infiltration, polymorphonuclear foci and eosinophils, particularly in relation to ruptured sporangia. In the later stages, few viable forms of the organism may be seen but numerous collapsed chitinous

shells provoke a foreign body giant cell reaction.

Electron microscopy is now providing details of the life cycle of the organism (Kannan-Kutty and Teh, 1974; Kannan-Kutty and Teh, 1975; Teh and Kannan-Kutty, 1975; Vanbreuseghem, 1976).

Aetiology and pathogenesis

The consistent presence of the parasite in its various forms is irrefutable evidence in favour of the cause of the lesion but animal inoculation has completely failed to reproduce the disease nor has the organism been grown on artificial media. Seeber (1900) believed the organism to be of fungal origin noting its resemblance to the coccidia. Other writers, however, considered that the parasite was protozoal in character (Minchin and Fantham, 1905; Beattie, 1906). Ashworth (1923) carried out an extensive study of the parasite in material removed on several occasions from an Indian medical student. Seeber did not name the organism and some early reports referred to it as Rhinosporidium kinealyi but precedence was eventually established and Ashworth named it Rhinosporidium seeberi which he believed belonged to the order Phycomycetes, sub-order Chytri-disease which do not produce hyphae. He also noted that its life cycle resembled that of the family Olpidiaceae.

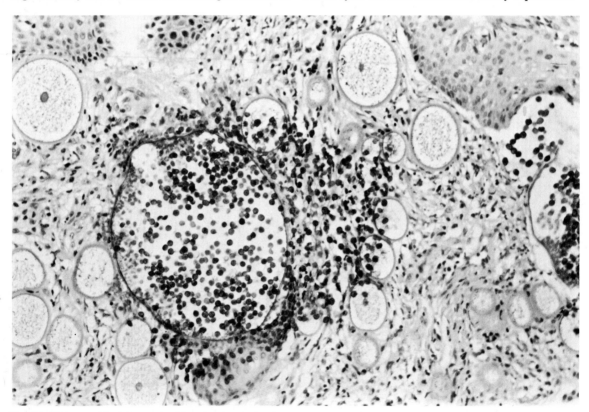

Fig. 8.3 Rhinosporidiosis in a young Ugandan female (see Fig. 8.2) showing detail of a large ruptured sporangium containing vast numbers of darkly staining spores. The smaller 'cysts' are trophic forms. M × 225

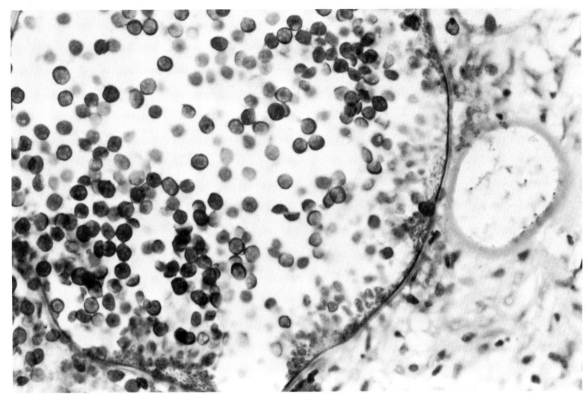

Fig. 8.4 Rhinosporidiosis in a young Ugandan female. Higher magnification of Fig. 8.3. Note double layer in the wall of the sporangium. M ×595

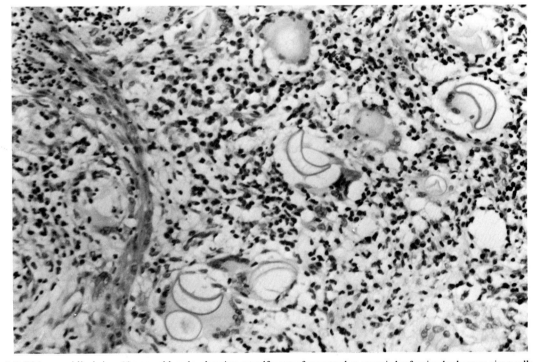

Fig. 8.5 Rhinosporidiosis in a 39 year-old male, showing engulfment of ruptured sporangia by foreign body type giant cells. M ×260

The morphology and life cycle have been studied by a number of workers (Minchin and Fantham, 1905; Beattie, 1906; Ashworth, 1923; Shrewsbury, 1933; Karunaratne, 1964; Kannan-Kutty and Teh, 1974, 1975; Bader and Bader, 1975; Vanbreuseghem, 1976). Although there was a fair measure of agreement, there were also differences in observations and interpretation but the majority of Ashworth's observations have been generally accepted.

The young form of the parasite (trophocyte) is about the size of a red blood cell, possessing a vesicular nucleus and a clearly marked border which is believed to be composed of chitin. With increase in size, the wall thickens while the cytoplasm develops vesicles, granules and spherular bodies. At a diameter of about 45 microns, the nucleus divides with subsequent repetitions and after 14 divisions, during which the cytoplasm becomes condensed around the nuclei, a total of about 16,000 young spores are produced within a sporangium of the order of 140 microns in diameter. The wall of the sporangium becomes markedly thickened due to the laying down within the chitinous shell of a thick layer of material indistinguishable from cellulose, except at one point identified as the pore. As the spores mature, the sporangium increases in size and the wall becomes stretched. Maturation predominates in the centre and each spore becomes surrounded by mucoid material which appears fibrillary under the electron microscope (Kannan-Kutty and Teh, 1974). A chitinoid shell develops between the mucoid layer and the cytoplasm. The sporangium eventually ruptures at the pore, releasing the spores. Within the tissues the spores undergo further development with the formation of vacuoles which ultimately contain electron-dense spherular bodies. Ashworth noted that these bodies were proteinaceous and believed that they had a nutritive function but it was later demonstrated that they contained DNA. This fact correlates with the observation of Teh and Kannan-Kutty (1975) that the spores undergo multiple budding, each bud separating with a spherular body and finally developing into a trophocyte.

The mode of transmission has not been finally settled. Although there has been complete failure to produce experimental disease, the condition occurs naturally in a variety of animals including horses, mules, cattle, goats, dogs, wild ducks and geese and the bird Psitaccus ondulatus (Ramachandra, Jain and Hanumantha Rao, 1975). It is of interest to note that the distribution of animal infections presented by the last mentioned authors in India corresponds closely with the distribution of the human disease in the same country. A very high proportion of reported human cases have been agricultural or farm workers (Allen and Dave, 1936; Karunaratne, 1964, Engzell and Jones, 1973; David, 1974; Grover, 1975). Allen and Dave (1936) suggested that the mechanism of transmission was via dust or water. Karunaratne noted a high incidence amongst paddy field workers. Certainly, the lack of familial incidence would appear to rule out interhuman transmission.

Behaviour

There being no effective medicinal treatment, excision of diseased areas is the only expedient. In the more radical procedures, elimination of the disease may sometimes be achieved but recurrence is common. Multiple lesions may sometimes be encountered (Desmond, 1953; Kameswaran et al., 1970; Chatterjee et al., 1977). Fatal cases with widespread dissemination have been reported (Rajam, Viswanathan, Rao, Rangiah and Anguli, 1955; Subramanyam and Ramano Rao, 1960).

BIBLIOGRAPHY

Allen F R W F, Dave M L 1936 The treatment of rhinosporidiosis in man, based on the study of sixty cases. Indian Medical Gazette 71: 376–394

Ashworth J H 1923 On rhinosporidium seeberi (Werniche 1903) with special reference to its sporulation and affinities. Transactions of the Royal Society of Edinburgh 53: 301–342

Ashworth J H, Logan-Turner A 1923 A case of rhinosporidiosis. Journal of Laryngology and Otology 38: 285–299

Bader G, Bader N G 1975 Morphologie der Gewebsformen von Erregern viszeraler Mykosen. Untersuchungen zur Polysaccharid und Proteinhistochemie. Mykosen 18: 61–80

Beattie J M 1906 Rhinosporidium kinealyi: a sporozoon of the nasal mucous membrane. Journal of Pathology and Bacteriology 11: 270–275

Beattie J M 1907 A sporozoon in aural polypi. British Medical Journal 2: 1402–1403

Cameron H M, Gatei D, Bremner A D 1973 The deep mycoses in Kenya. East African Medical Journal 50: 413–416

Chatterjee P K, Khatua C R, Chatterjee S N, Dastidar N 1977 Recurrent multiple rhinosporidiosis with osteolytic lesions in hand and foot. Journal of Laryngology and Otology 91: 729–734

Christian E C, Covi J 1966 Three cases of rhinosporidiosis in Ghana. Ghana Medical Journal 5: 63–64

David S S 1974 Nasal rhinosporidiosis. Journal of the Indian Medical Association 62: 301–306

Desmond A F 1953 A case of multiple rhinosporidiosis. Journal of Laryngology and Otology 67: 51–55

Engzell U C G, Jones A W 1973 Rhinosporidiosis in Uganda. Journal of Laryngology and Otology 87: 1217–1223

Grewal G S, Rangam C M 1959 Rhinosporidiosis of the trachea. An unusual case. Journal of Laryngology and Otology 73: 849–852

Grover S (1975) Rhinosporidiosis. Journal of the Indian Medical Association 64: 93–95

Gupta R L, Darbari B S, Dwivedi M P, Billore O P, Arora M M 1976 An epidemiological study of rhinosporidiosis in and around Raipur. Indian Journal of Medical Research 64: 1293–1299

Ingram A C (1910) Rhinosporidium kinealyi in unusual situations. Lancet 2: 726

Kameswaran S, Jaiswal S L, Mahure M N 1970 Bizarre presentation in rhinosporidiosis. Journal of Laryngology and Otology 84: 1083–1092

Kannan-Kutty A, Teh E C 1974 Rhinosporidium seeberi: cell wall formation in sporoblasts. Pathology 6: 183–185

Kannan-Kutty M, Teh E C 1974 Rhinosporidium seeberi: an electron microscopic study of its life cycle. Pathology 6: 63–70

Kannan-Kutty M, Teh E C 1975 Rhinosporidium seeberi. Archives of Pathology 99: 51–54

Karunaratne N O E 1964 Rhinosporidiosis in man. Athlone Press, London

Khan A A, Khaleque, K A, Huda M N 1969 Rhinosporidiosis of the nose. Journal of Laryngology and Otology 83: 461–473

McClatchie S E (1965) Rhinosporidiosis in Kenya. East African Medical Journal 42: 722–723

Marks R F, Johnstone H G 1948 Nasal rhinosporidiosis. Laryngoscope 58: 1108–1117

Minchin E A, Fantham H B 1905 Rhinosporisium kinealyi: a new sporozoon from the mucous membrane of the septum nasi of man. Quarterly Journal of Microscopical Science 49: 521–532

Mowat A H, Hennessy R S F 1941 Rhinosporidiosis in a native of Uganda. East African Medical Journal 18: 118–120

Norman W B 1960 Rhinosporidiosis in Texas. Archives of Otolaryngology 72: 361–362

O'Kinealy F 1903 Microscopic section of localized psorospermosis of the mucous membrane of the septum nasi. Proceedings of the Laryngological Society of London 10: 109–112

Pillai O S R 1974 Rhinosporidiosis of the larynx. Journal of Laryngology and Otology 88: 277–280

Rajam R V, Viswanathan G S, Rao A R, Rangiah P N, Anguli V C 1955 Rhinosporidiosis: a study with report of a fatal case of systemic dissemination. Indian Journal of Surgery 17: 269–298

Ramachandra P V, Jain S N, Hanumantha Rao T V 1975 Animal rhinosporidiosis in India with case reports. Annales de la Société belge de médecine Tropicale 50: 119–124

Rolon P A 1974 Rinosporidiosis. Epidemiologia en la Republica del Paraguay. Mycopatologia et Mycologia Applicata 52: 155–171

Satyanarayana C 1960 Rhinosporidiosis. Acta Otolaryngologica 51: 348–366

Seeber G R 1900 Un nuevo esporazario parásito de hombre. Dos casos encontrados en polipos nasales. Tesis, Universidad Nacionale de Buenos Aires

Shrewsbury J F D 1933 Rhinosporidiosis. Journal of Pathology and Bacteriology 36: 431–434

Smith P L 1977 Rhinosporidiosis. South African Medical Journal 51: 281

Subramanyam C S V, Ramano Rao A V 1960 A fatal case of tracheobronchial rhinosporidiosis. British Journal of Surgery 47: 411–413

Tamale J A K, Hutt M S R 1964 Five cases of rhinosporidiosis in Ugandan Africans. East African Medical Journal 41: 459–464

Teh E C, Kannan-Kutty A 1975 Rhinosporidium seeberi: spherules and their significance. Pathology 7: 133–137

Thomas T, Gopinath N, Betts R H 1957 Rhinosporidiosis of the bronchus. British Journal of Surgery 44: 316–319

Vanbreuseghem R 1976 Rhinosporidiose: klinische Aspekte, Epidemiologie und ultrastrukturelle Studien von Rhinosporidium seeberi. Dermatologische Monatsschrift 162: 512–526

Wahab S M A, Talaat T A 1976 Rhinosporidiosis in Sudan. Tropical and Geographical Medicine 28: 60–62

Wright J 1907 A nasal sporozoon (Rhinosporidium kinealyi). New York Medical Journal 86: 1149–1152

Additional references

Kutnick S L, Kerth J D 1976 Rhinosporidiosis. Laryngoscope 86: 1579–1583

Lasser A, Smith H W 1976 Rhinosporidiosis. Archives of Otolaryngology 102: 108–110

Myers D D 1964 Rhinosporidiosis in a horse. Journal of the American Veterinary Medical Association 145: 315–317

Rao M A N 1938 Rhinosporidiosis in bovines in the Madras Presidency with a discussion on the probable modes of infection. Indian Journal of Veterinary Science and Animal Husbandry 8: 187–198

Ruchman J 1939 Rhinosporidiosis: first occurrence in a female in North America. Archives of Otolaryngology 30: 239–246

Sharp H S, Biggs R 1944 A case of rhinosporidiosis. Journal of Laryngology and Otology 59: 457–458

Zschokle E 1913 Ein Rhinosporidium beim Pferd. Schweizer Archiv für Tierheilkund 55: 641–650

9

Other mycotic and parasitic infections

MYCOTIC DISEASES

General introduction

Mycotic disease of the upper respiratory tract has been increasing both as 'imported ills' due to the greatly enhanced international traffic and as 'opportunistic infections' in consequence of the use of powerful cytotoxic drugs (as applied to the treatment of neoplasms) and also steroid and antibiotic therapy. Rose and Varkey (1975) reviewed 123 cases of deep mycotic infection collected over a decade and noted that the frequency had almost doubled during the latter five years. Symmers (1965) defined 'opportunistic infection' as a serious disease, usually progressive and caused by organisms which under normal conditions would have little or no pathogenetic capacity. He illustrated the point with a fatal case in which multiple infections occurred.

Many common saprophytic organisms may become pathogenic, producing diseases in debilitated or compromised patients, e.g. uncontrolled diabetics. Such diseases may be diagnosed only at autopsy but biopsy, culture and occasionally serological tests (Smith, 1976) may assist in establishing a clinical diagnosis. Mycetal infections may be due to Eumycetes (true fungi) or Pseudomycetes which include bacteria, Actinomyces and Nocardia. Many true fungi have been incriminated in infective granulomas of the nose and sinuses (Table 9.1).

The general incidence of the deep mycoses has not been completely assessed but it undoubtedly shows geographical variation. Keye and Magee (1956) found 0.55 per cent amongst nearly 16,000 autopsies whilst Rose and Varkey (1975) recorded 0.14 per cent of hospital admissions over a period of ten years. Martin and Berson (1973) noted a high incidence in South Africa which they attributed particularly to malnutrition. The largest series of cases involving the nasal and paranasal region have emanated from Sudan (Milošev, Mahgoub, Abdel Aal and Hassan, 1969; Rudwan and Sheikh, 1976). Reports of nasal or paranasal involvement in the United Kingdom are not very common.

Table 9.1 Simplified classification of the relevant pathogenic mycetal organisms

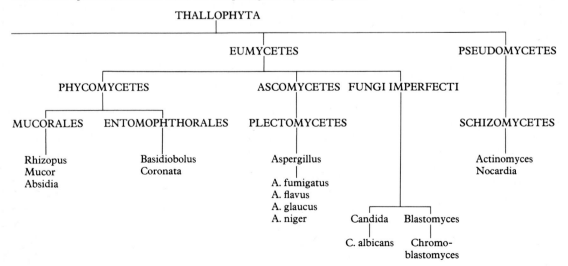

PHYCOMYCOSIS

Introduction

By definition, this disease is caused by fungi belonging to the Class Phycomycetes. Excluding Rhinosporidium seeberi, there are two important Orders in this Class; namely Mucorales which causes Mucormycosis and Entomophthorales giving rise to Entomophthorosis. It is important to distinguish between these two conditions because there are significant clinical and histopathological differences. Lichtheim (1884) established the pathogenicity of the Order Mucorales in rabbits whilst Paltauf (1885) described a disseminated Mucormycosis in a human subject. So far, it would appear that Mucormycosis is more common than Entomophthorosis but the two conditions will be considered together which will facilitate the distinction between them.

Clinical features

Mucormycosis is usually superimposed on some other disease such as uncontrolled diabetes mellitus or prolonged treatment with cytotoxic drugs, steroids or antibiotics. On the other hand, Entomophthorosis is more likely to occur in otherwise healthy subjects.

In rhinomucormycosis, the age distribution is very broadly based ranging from infancy to old age and there is no significant sex difference. In entomophthorosis involving the nasal region there would appear to be a more limited age distribution in early adult life (Martinson, 1963).

In rhinomucormycosis the disease develops rapidly, the duration of symptoms being numbered in days. It may present with nasal discharge, loss of sensation in the cheek, proptosis and even blindness. X-ray may reveal opacity of the paranasal sinuses with evidence of bone destruction. Cerebral involvement may manifest itself with headache, pyrexia and lethargy. Entomophthorosis develops more slowly and the clinical presentation is less dramatic than in mucormycosis. The general condition of the patient is usually good and the common form of presentation is nasal obstruction together with swelling of the nose and cheek, often of many months' duration which contrasts sharply with the fulminant progress of mucormycosis.

Anatomical site of origin

Mucormycosis commonly involves the ethmoid sinuses (Gregory, Golden and Haymaker, 1943; Stratemeier, 1950; Bauer, Ajello, Adams and Hernandez, 1955; Baker, 1957; Yanagisawa, Friedman, Kundargi and Smith, 1977). Although there is clinical and radiological evidence of involvement of the maxillary sinus, it has rarely been confirmed in reported cases. The nasal cavity is frequently involved (Gregory et al., 1943; Stratemeier, 1950; Kurrein, 1954; La Touche, Sutherland and Telling, 1963). Involvement of the sphenoid sinus has been reported on several occasions (Baker, 1957; La Touche et al. 1963; Yanagisawa et al., 1977) whilst the frontal sinus was affected in one of the cases reported by Bauer et al. (1955).

In rhino-entomophthorosis, the nasal cavity is invariably involved (Martinson, 1963; Bras, Gordon, Emmons, Prendegast and Sugar, 1965; Martinson and Clark, 1967; Andrade, Araújo Paula, Sherlock and Cheever, 1967; Grueber, 1969; Symmers, 1972). The maxillary sinus is not infrequently affected (Bras et al., 1965; Martinson and Clark, 1967). The last mentioned authors also reported involvement of the ethmoid sinuses in three cases and the sphenoid sinus in one case.

Histopathology

The lesion in mucormycosis consists of inflammatory granulation tissue with haemorrhage and necrosis. There is infiltration by polymorphonuclear leucocytes, histiocytes, foam cells and multinucleated giant cells, sometimes of Langhans type thereby simulating tuberculoid tissue reactions (Symmers, 1968). Aseptate fungal hyphae with or without sporangia are found lying in the inflammatory tissue (Fig 9.1) and portions of hyphae may be engulfed by giant cells. A particular characteristic of mucormycosis is involvement of blood vessels. The mycelium of Mucorales shows a predilection for penetration of arterial walls and when the hyphae reach the lumen they induce intravascular thrombosis with inevitable infarction which largely accounts for the areas of necrosis.

Entomophthorosis presents a somewhat different microscopical picture. The cellular infiltration consists predominantly of eosinophils with histiocytes, lymphocytes and plasma cells. Giant cells of foreign body type are also present. The fungus is represented by aseptate hyphae which are characteristically surrounded by an eosinophilic granular zone with or without a peripheral palisade of histiocytes (Fig. 9.2). This eosinophilic sleeve has been studied by both light and electron microscopy (Williams, 1969; Williams, Lichtenberg, Smith and Martinson, 1969). The material contains lipid substances and is autofluorescent, whilst ultrastructural examination has revealed nuclear and cytoplasmic debris derived from the cellular infiltrate. Williams and his colleagues also allege that some of the amorphous material is probably antigen-antibody complex similar to that in the Arthus type hypersensitivity reaction. Microabscesses and pseudotubercles may be present but the fungus never penetrates blood vessels.

Aetiology and pathogenesis

The genera of Mucorales involved in mucormycosis are Rhizopus, Absidia and Mucor. Rhizopus (oryzae, arrhizius and corymbifer) appears to be the commonest

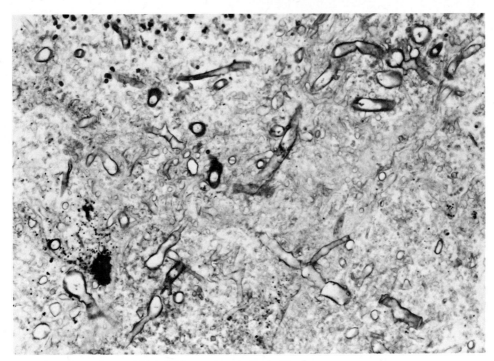

Fig. 9.1 From Systemic Pathology (ed W St C Symmers) 2nd ed vol 1 Fig. 4.10.
Field in renal infarct in a case of nasoorbitocerebral phycomycosis by a species of MUCOR. The variable width of the hyphae is characteristic. M × 215.

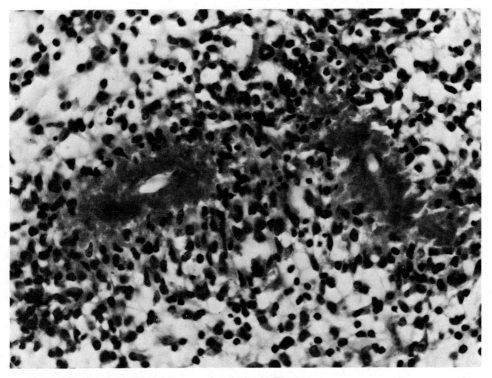

Fig. 9.2 From Systemic Pathology (ed W St C Symmers) 2nd ed vol 1 Fig. 4.9.
Entomophthorosis showing the clear, sharply outlined hyphae surrounded by a broad eosinophilic deposit (from a pulmonary granuloma in a case of nasal infection by *Entomophthora coronata*). M × 340.

cause of the disease (Baker, 1957). The hyphae which are characteristically aseptate range from 4 to 20 microns in width and up to 200 microns in length. Branching may be found both in culture and in the tissues. Although culture has not been carried out in many reported cases, these fungi are easily grown on artificial media. In culture, arial hyphae bear sporangia at their extremities, representing asexual reproduction but in tissue lesions sporangia may or may not be found. When seen, they appear as rounded, expanded ends of hyphae which in the mature state contain numerous spores of the order of 6 microns in diameter. The finding of these fungi in secretions does not necessarily have any significance since they are normally saprophytes. They are normally found in the soil and on decaying food material. However, in the presence of lowered body resistance, they may become pathogenic. Reports relating to predisposing causes are variable due to selection. Hutter (1959) reviewed mucormycosis as a complication of treatment of cancer patients and emphasized the prolonged use of antibiotics, steroids, chemotherapeutic agents and altered metabolic states such as diabetes mellitus. He claimed that the latter disease was present in 19 per cent of cases of mucormycosis. Bauer, Flanagan and Sheldon (1955) demonstrated that Alloxan-induced diabetes in rabbits predisposed to invasive mucormycosis, the fungus being introduced via the intranasal route. The fungus invaded the nasal mucosa and the infection extended to the orbit and brain. Similar conclusions were drawn from further animal experiments (Elder and Baker, 1956). Nevertheless, mucormycosis has been reported as occurring naturally in animals (Gleiser, 1953; Davis, Anderson and McCrory, 1955). Genera of the Mucorales readily break down carbohydrate (sugar fungi) and Bauer et al. (1955) suggested that these normally saprophytic fungi may become pathogenic in carbohydrate enriched tissues of uncontrolled diabetes. Long and Weiss (1959) believed that acidosis, with or without diabetes, might be an important factor. With more efficient control of diabetes mellitus, one would expect this disease to be a less frequent predisposing factor but Pillsbury and Fischer (1977) reported 13 cases rhinocerebral mucormycosis who in all but two were diabetics. It is interesting to note that the two non-diabetic patients were severely acidotic and dehydrated. On the other hand, Keye and Magee (1956), in a review of secondary fungal infections, found that diabetes mellitus was present in less than 10 per cent.

Baker, Schofield, Elder and Spilo (1956) showed that pre-treatment of experimental animals with cortisone resulted in an increased susceptibility to infection by Rhizopus oryzae. Torack (1957) reported three fatal cases of mucormycosis who had received steroid therapy. Hutter (1959) pointed out that patients with cancer,

particularly involving the lymphoreticular system are at risk during treatment. Keye and Magee (1956) found six cases of mucormycosis complicating Hodgkin's Disease and leukaemias and all had pulmonary involvement. A common factor is probably the use of cytotoxic drugs. Baker (1956) reported two cases of fatal pulmonary mucormycosis complicating leukaemia. Both cases had received steroids, cytotoxic drugs and antibiotics. It is generally believed that the prolonged use of antibiotics may disturb the biological balance of saprophytic flora in the body, thereby encouraging a more aggressive behaviour of certain organisms.

Entomophthorosis has two manifestations, subcutaneous lesions and infection of the upper respiratory tract. The organism responsible for the former condition has been identified as Basidiobolus ranarum (Joe, Eng, Pohan, van der Meulen and Emmons, 1956) whilst the nasal and paranasal infection is caused by Entomophthora coronata (Martinson and Clark, 1967). The infection appears to be a primary disease, there being no obvious predisposing cause. Rhino-entomophthorosis is essentially a tropical infection (Nigeria, Jamaica, Brazil and India).

In the present anatomical context, the portal of entry for both types of Phycomycetal infection is obviously the nasal cavity.

Behaviour

Baker (1952) expressed the view that mucormycosis is the most acutely fatal mycosis. Once the fungus becomes aggressively invasive, the infection spreads from the nasal cavity into the ethmoid sinuses and thence to the orbit where the eye is attacked and blindness ensues (Baker, 1957). Subsequent spread from the orbit may cause thrombosis of the cavernous sinus (Gregory et al., 1943; Wolf and Cowan, 1949; McCall and Strobos, 1957; La Touche et al., 1963). Extension to the cranial cavity may occur either through the orbit and cavernous sinus or direct from the nasal cavity via the cribriform plate (Kurrein, 1954). Meningo-encephalitis develops in which the fungus can be found and the condition is generally referred to as rhinocerebral mucormycosis (La Touche et al., 1963; Pillsberg and Fischer, 1977; Yanagisawa et al., 1977). Many cases of cerebral involvement have had a fatal outcome but 11 out of the 13 cases reported by Pillsberg and Fischer survived, which they attributed to aggressive surgery and use of Amphotericin B. The infection is liable to become systematized with involvement of internal organs (Fig. 9.3), especially the lungs. The lowered body resistance that permits establishment of the infection clearly plays a part in the fatal progression.

By contrast, Entomophthorosis affecting the nose and sinuses develops more slowly against higher resistance and tends to be limited in its extent. Spread from the

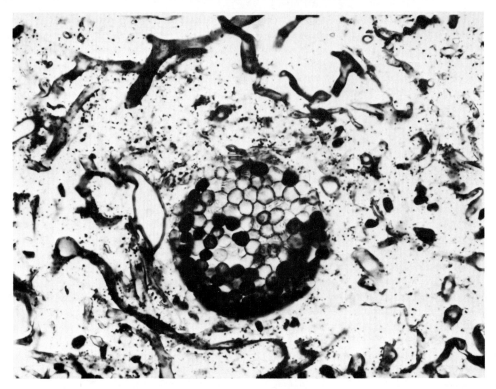

Fig. 9.3 From Systemic Pathology (ed W St C Symmers) 2nd ed vol 1 Fig. 4.11.
Hyphae and sporangium of RHIZOPUS species in nasal biopsy of leukaemic patient with extensive phycomycotic infection.
M × 630.

nose to the paranasal sinuses often occurs but the infection is usually confined to these regions. Symmers (1972) reported a case of nasal infection which developed secondary involvement of both lower lobes of the lungs. One could reasonably assume that the pulmonary infection was inhalatory rather than systematized. It is clear that rhino-entomophthorosis has a better prognosis than mucormycosis.

ASPERGILLOSIS

Introduction

The first record of paranasal infection by this fungus was by Zarniko (1891) who reported involvement of the maxillary sinus in a 15 year-old female. Two years later, Mackenzie (1893) published another case of antral infection. Following the turn of the century, Harmer (1913) reported yet another case of aspergillosis of the maxillary sinus and Tilley (1915) collected a further five cases of paranasal infection.

Incidence

The majority of reports of paranasal involvement in the English language literature have been solitary cases and,

in 1978, Stevens estimated that the total number of examples was under fifty. The largest series of cases so far published have been from Sudan (Milošev, Mahgoub, Abdel Aal and Hassan, 1969; Rudwan and Sheikh, 1976).

Clinical features

The infection is essentially in adults and most of the individual cases have occurred in middle-aged adults with a predominance of females. On the other hand, the 17 cases reported by Milošev et al. (1969) ranged in age from the second to the seventh decade with a majority of males.

Patients with this type of infection may present with sneezing, nasal obstruction, discharge and intermittent epistaxis. Pain is a variable symptom and may be related to invasive tendency. The majority of patients developing this type of local infection are otherwise in reasonably good health. X-rays reveal sinus opacities and occasionally evidence of bone destruction.

Anatomical site of origin

Although lesions are found in the nose, no cases have been reported as confined to the nasal cavity. The majority of cases involve the maxillary sinus but infection of the ethmoid sinuses has also been reported (Tilley, 1915; Milosev et al., 1969; Warder, Chikes and Hudson, 1975; Rudwan and Sheikh, 1976). Infection of the frontal sinus is less common (Warder et al., 1975; Rudwan and Sheikh, 1976; Stevens, 1978) whilst the sphenoid sinus is very occasionally involved (Wright, 1927; Rudwan and Sheikh, 1976).

Gross appearances

Nasal and paranasal mucosa may be thickened and granular and localized masses may be present in the respective cavities. The finding of greenish gelatinous material in a paranasal sinus should lead one to suspect the possibility of Aspergillosis. There are two types of infection by this fungus: (i) the fungal ball, often referred to as 'aspergilloma', may be found in the maxillary or frontal sinuses, associated with secondary infection causing ulceration of the mucosa but usually no fungal invasion and (ii) the invasive or granulomatous lesion which is more typical of infection occurring in the tropical regions. Warden et al. (1975) described two cases of 'aspergilloma' of the maxillary sinus and one case of invasive infection.

Histopathology

The fungal ball consists essentially of a mass of mycelium composed of branching septate hyphae together with varying amounts of necrotic material and inflammatory infiltration. The granulomatous lesion consists of a non-specific granulation tissue containing micro-abscesses and multinucleated giant cells. There may also be areas of necrosis. The fungus is represented by septate hyphae, with or without branching, giving a positive Periodic acid Schiff reaction but it is shown up particularly well with the methenamine silver stain. The hyphae may be found lying in micro-abscesses or within the giant cells (Figs. 9.4, 9.5, 9.6 & 9.7) and may sometimes be observed penetrating arterial walls with induction of thrombosis though this tendency is not as marked as in mucormycosis. As the lesion progresses, fibrosis develops and areas may become almost completely sclerosed.

Aetiology and pathogenesis

Aspergillosis is the most common fungal infection in the antrum (Levine, 1977). Aspergillus (also known as Eurotium) is an ubiquitous saprophyte which is found in the soil and on decaying food material. It is also said to be a cause of a common infection in birds (Savetsky and Waltner, 1961). The common species involved in human paranasal infections are *A. fumigatus* and *A. flavus*. Five paranasal cases investigated at the Mycological Reference Laboratory in London were found to be caused by *A. fumigatus* and *A. flavus* in two cases each and *A. glaucus* in one, whilst a subsequent antral infection

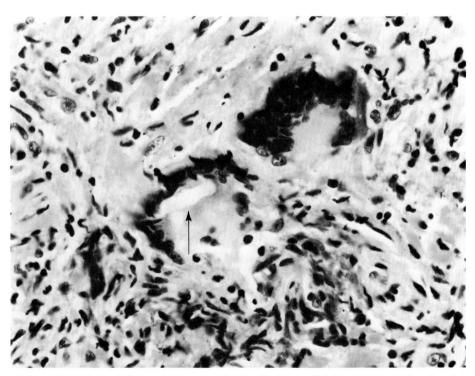

Fig. 9.4 Orbital aspergillosis due to A. flavus, showing unstained hypha (arrowed) lying within a multinucleated giant cell. M × 500. By courtesy of W St C Symmers.

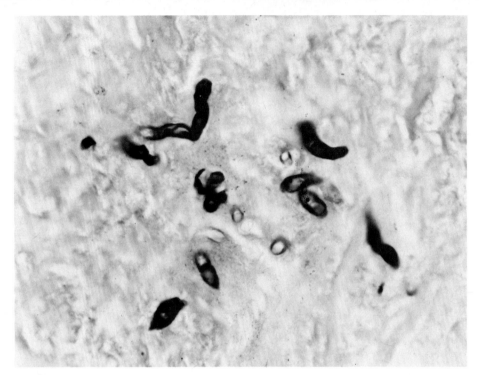

Fig. 9.5 Orbital aspergillosis (see Fig. 9.4), showing fragments of hyphae stained with methenamine silver. M ×500. By courtesy of W St C Symmers.

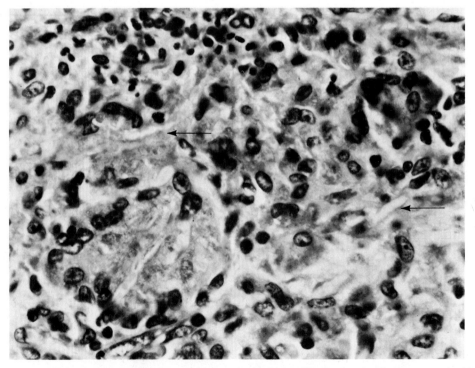

Fig. 9.6 Orbital aspergillosis from a rare case of naso-orbito-cerebral infection. Hyphae (arrowed) appear unstained by H and E technique and are seen lying within multinucleated giant cells. M ×630. By courtesy of W St C Symmers.

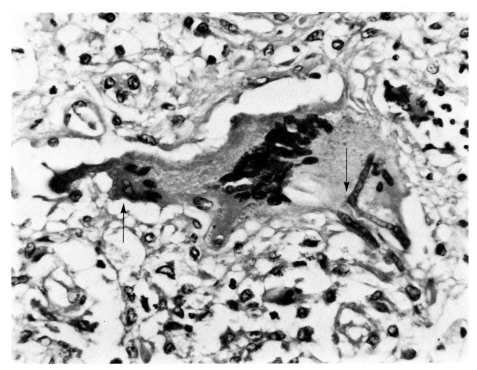

Fig. 9.7 Orbital aspergillosis (see Fig. 9.6) showing hyphae (arrowed) exhibiting positive periodic-acid Schiff reaction and lying within a multinucleated giant cell. M × 400. By courtesy of W St C Symmers.

was found to be due to *A. niger* (British Medical Journal, 1977). The Sudanese cases (Milošev et al., 1969; Rudwan and Sheikh, 1976) were all caused by *A. flavus*.

Aspergillus is an opportunistic fungus which can give rise to a variety of forms of human infection: Pulmonary, cutaneous, cerebral and systemic dissemination in addition to paranasal lesions. Many infections with Aspergillus are often superimposed on some other debilitating disease and the predisposition may be aggravated by therapy, as in mucormycosis (McGill, Simpson and Healy, 1980). Spens and Tattersall (1965) reported a fatal case of meningo-encephalitis due to Aspergillus following treatment of pulmonary tuberculosis with anti-tuberculous drugs and also a steroid compound. Immuno-suppressants may allow formerly saprophytic aspergillus to reach blood vessels which they penetrate, resulting in a septicaemia. Turner, Papadimitriou, Hackshaw and Wetherall (1975) injected *A. fumigatus* intravenously into rats which developed a cerebral infection whilst Epstein, (1968) produced experimental intracranial aspergillosis by an intranasal route coupled with intensive cortisone administration. By contrast, many paranasal infections by this fungus appear to be primary rather than superimposed upon other diseases. The series reported by Milošev et al. (1969) certainly fit into this category.

The organism, which may well be present in the inspired air, clearly gains entry through the nose and Milošev et al. suggested that the saprophyte becomes pathogenic under anaerobic conditions. These authors found precipitating antibodies in four out of six cases tested but frequently there are no antibodies detectable which is probably a reflection of a localized lesion. Andersen and Stenderup (1956) obtained a strongly positive skin reaction to an extract of the fungus in an antral infection but this has not been followed up by other workers.

Behaviour

The disease shows a marked tendency to develop slowly, the duration of symptoms often being numbered in years. Paranasal aspergillosis shows a greater tendency to remain localized which is a reflection of the greater body resistance in many cases. Nevertheless, it spreads from the nose to the sinuses and may involve the orbit. Wright (1927) reported two cases of orbital involvement secondary to nasal infection. The majority of cases reported by Milošev et al. (1969) exhibited proptosis, implying orbital spread, whilst one of the cases reported by Warder et al. (1975) had fronto-ethmoidal and orbital involvement. This appears to be the limit of extension in the majority of paranasal infections. None of Milošev's cases developed pulmonary infection but one died with involvement of the base of the skull. Rhinocerebral or widely disseminated disease is more likely to result from immuno-suppression as in the case reported by Spens and Tattersall (1965) in which there was meningo-encephalitis comparable with the more common event in mucormycosis.

Although the prognosis in paranasal aspergillosis is appreciably better than in mucormycosis, anti-fungal drugs are not very effective in the absence of surgical excision of diseased tissue.

CANDIDIASIS

In the general context, this is the commonest fungal infection. Keye and Magee (1956) found that Candidiasis was the most frequent fungal infection in a general hospital, accounting for 28 per cent of all fungal diseases identified in autopsy material. Candida albicans is the most common opportunist and may cause widespread lesions, involving the skin, mucous membrane of the alimentary tract, internal organs and may also become systematized. Infection of the lower respiratory tract is well recognized but reports of involvement of the nose and sinuses are extremely rare. One of the present

authors (Osborn, 1963) reported a case of infection of the frontal sinus in a Sikh. The patient had been diagnosed previously, in India, as having tuberculosis of the frontal sinus for which anti-tuberculous drugs were given. The disease persisted and a further exploration of the frontal sinus was performed in London. The tissue removed showed extensive caseation with Langhans type giant cells, many of which contained fungal elements.

Candida albicans, which is included in the Class Fungi Imperfecti, exists in two forms: (i) yeast-like bodies and (ii) pseudo-hyphae that give the impression of being septate. Material from the frontal sinus lesion was not available for culture but, on a morphological basis, it was concluded that the lesion was due to infection by Candida species in the pseudo-hyphal form (Fig. 9.8). It is a matter for conjecture whether the fungal disease was primary or whether the initial infection was tuberculous with secondary fungal infection influenced by prolonged antibiotic treatment.

BLASTOMYCOSIS

This disease is largely of New World origin though there are examples in Europe and Asia. Blastomyces belongs

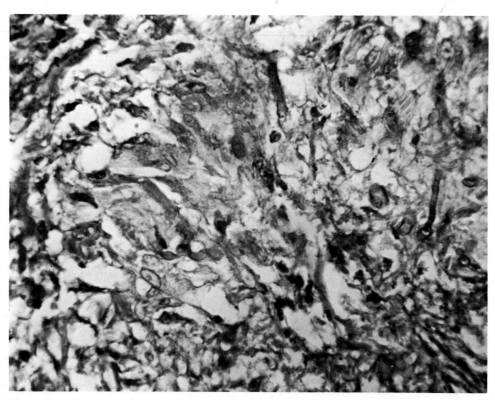

Fig. 9.8 Candidiasis of the frontal sinus in a 31 year-old male, showing pseudohyphae lying in granulation tissue. M × 550.

to the Fungi Imperfecti and consists of two main types – the North and South American varieties. The North American fungus (Blastomyces dermatitidis) produces skin lesions but may also cause pulmonary infection which tends to become generalized. So far, there are no accounts of involvement of the nose and sinuses.

The South American variety has a tendency to involve mucous membranes. Chromoblastomycosis is due to a naturally pigmented fungus which mainly affects the skin and the cerebral tissues. Symmers (1960) reported a nasal lesion in a male student from Ceylon. The clinical diagnosis was rhinosporidiosis but biopsy revealed dark golden brown bodies about 10 microns in diameter whose appearance was identical with the fungus causing cutaneous chromoblastomycosis (Phialophora pedrosoi).

ACTINOMYCOSIS

Over 50 per cent of cases of this pseudomycetal infection occur in the head and neck region but reports of involvement of the nose and sinuses are not very common.

The condition may develop over a period of weeks or months and swelling of the cheek with facial pain are common presenting symptoms. The usual site of infection is the maxillary sinus (Kernan, 1936; Voss, 1939; Hersh, 1945; Stanton, 1966). Antral irrigation may reveal foul pus containing the causal organism.

The cause of the disease is an anaerobic species of Actinomyces, sometimes identified as *A. bovis* which has long been established as the cause of the granulomatous lesion of the tongue and jaw in cattle. Some of the anaerobic Actinomyces (especially *A. israelii*) are common saprophytes in the human oral cavity. Lewy and Manning (1949) reported an actinomycotic infection of the maxillary and ethmoid sinuses in a steel worker following dental extraction. Culture revealed *A. bovis* and it would appear that this organism must have been present as a saprophyte prior to the dental operation. On the other hand, Stanton (1966) published a case of antral infection in a housewife living in an agricultural area.

Again, culture revealed *A. bovis* and the possibility of direct inhalation of the organism seems likely.

The mycelium of Actinomyces is often jointed and may break up to form numerous short rods, 3 to 4 microns in length. Many of these organisms (especially the anaerobic variety) form compact mycelial colonies in liquid media or in tissues. The peripheral threads often have expanded ends around which may be deposited products of inflammatory exudate, producing a radial arrangement of clubs – hence the name 'ray fungus'. These compact colonies may appear in the purulent exudate within the sinus cavity. The anaerobic group are non-acid-fast.

Erosion of bone may occur even at an early stage (Lewy and Manning, 1949) and longstanding infection may develop the classical brawny swelling of the cheek with the appearance of fistulae (Kernan, 1936). Cases with early diagnosis appear to respond to repeated lavage (Hersh, 1945; Stanton, 1966).

NOCARDIASIS

It has been suggested that the aerobic varieties of Actinomyces should be called Nocardia. Some members of this group, like the anaerobic organisms, are non-acid-fast but others, such as 'asteroides' are acid-fast and rod forms may simulate Mycobacterium tuberculosis.

Nocardia infection of the nose and sinuses is even more rare than Actinomycosis and the present authors have only knowledge of one case: An eighty year-old woman first presented with epistaxis of two months' duration. Subsequently, granular lesions were found on the left middle and inferior turbinates and she developed a fluctuant abscess in the neck. Biopsies were taken from the nose and the neck and cultures for Mycobacterium tuberculosis were negative. Histopathology of the nose revealed granulation tissue containing many multinucleated giant cells, often of Langhans type and sometimes forming tuberculoid lesions. A Fite modification of the Ziehl-Neelsen stain revealed acid-fast rods and culture produced an aerobic actinomyces (Nocardia). After a year of chemotherapy, the nose appeared normal.

BIBLIOGRAPHY

Andersen H C, Stenderup A 1956 Aspergillosis of the maxillary sinus. Acta Otolaryngologica 46: 771–773

Andrade Z A, Araújo Paula L, Sherlock I A, Cheever A W 1967 Nasal granuloma caused by entomophthora coronata. American Journal of Tropical Medicine and Hygiene 16: 31–33

Baker R D 1952 Resectable mycotic lesions and acutely fatal mycoses. Journal of the American Medical Association 150: 1579–1581

Baker R D 1956 Pulmonary mucormycosis. American Journal of Pathology 32: 287–307

Baker R D 1957 Mucormycosis – a new disease? Journal of the American Medical Association 163: 805–808

Baker R D, Schofield R A, Elder D T, Spoto A P 1956 Alloxan diabetes and cortisone as modifying factors in experimental mucormycosis (Rhizopus infection). Federation Proceedings of American Societies for experimental biology 15: 506–507

Bauer H, Ajello L, Adams E, Hernandez D U 1955 Cerebral mucormycosis: pathogenesis of the disease. American Journal of Medicine 18: 822–831

Bauer H, Flanagan J F, Sheldon W H 1955 Experimental cerebral mucormycosis in diabetic rabbits. American Journal of Pathology 31: 600

Bras G, Gordon C C, Emmons C W, Prendegast K M, Sugar M 1965 A case of phycomycosis observed in Jamaica: infection with entomophthora coronata. American Journal of Tropical Medicine and Hygiene 14: 141–145

British Medical Journal 1977 Paranasal fungal infections 1: 1291

Davis C L, Anderson, W A, McCrory B R 1955 Mucormycosis in food producing animals. Journal of the American Veterinary Medical Association 126: 261–267

Elder D T, Baker R D 1956 Pulmonary mucormycosis in rabbits with alloxan diabetes. Archives of Pathology 61: 159–168

Epstein S M, Miale T D, Moossy J, Verney E, Sidransky H 1968 Experimental intracranial aspergillosis. Journal of Neuropathology and Experimental Neurology 27: 473–482

Gleiser C A 1953 Mucormycosis in animals. Journal of the American Veterinary Medical Association 123: 441–445

Gregory J E, Golden A, Haymaker W 1943 Mucormycosis of the central nervous system. Bulletin of the Johns Hopkins Hospital 73: 405–419

Grueber H L E 1969 Rhino-entomophthoromycosis. Journal of the Christian Medical Association of India 44: 20–24

Harmer D 1913 Suppuration of the antrum due to aspergillus fumigatus. Journal of Laryngology and Otology 28: 494–495

Hersh J H 1945 Primary infection of the maxillary sinus by actinomyces necrophorus. Archives of Otolaryngology 41: 204–207

Hutter R V P 1959 Phycomycetous infection (mucormycosis) in cancer patients: a complication of therapy. Cancer 12: 330–350

Joe L K, Eng N I T, Pohan A, van der Meulen H, Emmons C W 1956 Basidiobolus ranarum as a cause of subcutaneous mycosis in Indonesia. Archives of Dermatology and Syphilis 74: 378–383

Kernan J D 1936 Case of actinomycosis of the left antrum treated by diathermy. Laryngoscope 46: 483–484

Keye J D, Magee W D 1956 Fungal diseases in a general hospital. American Journal of Clinical Pathology 26: 1235–1253

Kurrein F 1954 Cerebral mucormycosis. Journal of Clinical Pathology 7: 141–144

La Touche C J, Sutherland T W, Telling M 1963 Rhinocerebral mucormycosis. Lancet 2: 811–813

Levine P A 1977 Aspergillosis of the maxillary sinus. Archives of Otolaryngology 103: 560–562

Lewy R B, Manning E L 1949 Actinomycosis involving ethmoid and maxillary sinuses. Archives of Otolaryngology 49: 423–430

Lichtheim L 1884 Über pathogene Mucorinen und die durch sie erzeugten Mykosen des Kaninchens. Zeitschrift klinische Medizin 7: 140–177

Long E L, Weiss D C 1959 Cerebral mucormycosis. American Journal of Medicine 26: 625–635

McCall W, Strobos R R J 1957 Survival of a patient with central nervous system mucormycosis. Neurology 7: 290–292

Mackenzie D 1893 Preliminary report on aspergillus mycosis of the antrum maxillare. Johns Hopkins hospital Bulletin 4: 9–10

Martin P M D, Berson S D 1973 Fungus disease in southern Africa. Mycopathologia et Mycologia applicata 50: 1–84

Martinson F D 1963 Rhinophycomycosis. Journal of Laryngology and Otology 77: 691–705

Martinson F D, Clark B M 1967 Rhinophycomycosis entomophthorae in Nigeria. American Journal of Tropical Medicine and Hygiene 16: 40–47

Milošev B, El Mahgoub S, Abdel Aal O, El Hassan A M 1969 British Journal of Surgery 56: 132–137

Osborn D A 1963 Mycotic infection of the frontal sinus. Journal of Laryngology and Otology 77: 29–33

Paltauf A 1885 Mycosis mucorina. Virchows Archiv für patholohische Anatomie 102: 543–564

Pillsbury H C, Fischer N D 1977 Rhinocerebral mucormycosis. Archives of Otolaryngology 103: 600–604

Rose H D, Varkey B 1975 Deep mycotic infection in the hospitalized adult: a study of 123 patients. Medicine (Baltimore) 54: 501–507

Rudwan M A, Sheikh H A 1976 Aspergilloma of the paranasal sinuses – a common cause of unilateral proptosis in Sudan. Clinical Radiology 27: 497–502

Savetsky L, Waltner J 1961 Aspergillosis of the maxillary antrum. Archives of Otolaryngology 74: 695–698

Smith H 1976 Opportunistic fungal infections. Hospital Update 2: 573–579

Spens N, Tattersall W H 1965 Fungal infection of the central nervous system supervening during routine chemotherapy for pulmonary tuberculosis. British Medical Journal 2: 862

Stanton M B 1966 Actinomycosis of the maxillary sinus. Journal of Laryngology and Otology 80: 168–174

Stevens M H 1978 Aspergillosis of the frontal sinus. Archives of Otolaryngology 104: 153–156

Stratemeier W P 1950 Mucormycosis of the central nervous system. Archives of Neurology and Psychiatry 63: 179–180

Symmers W St C 1960 Chromoblastomycosis simulating rhinosporidiosis in a patient from Ceylon. Journal of Clinical Pathology 13: 287–290

Symmers W St C 1965 Opportunistic infections. Proceedings of the Royal Society of Medicine 58: 341–346

Symmers W St C 1968 Aspects of the contributions of histopathology to the study of deep-seated fungal infections. Ciba Foundation Symposium on Systemic Mycoses 26–37

Symmers W St C 1972 Histopathology of phycomycoses. Annales de la Société Belge de Médecin Tropicale 52: 365–389

Tilley H 1915 Aspergillosis of the maxillary antrum. Proceedings of the Royal Society of Medicine 8: 14–22

Torack R M 1957 Fungus infections associated with antibiotics and steroid therapy. American Journal of Medicine 22: 872–882

Turner K J, Papadimitriou J, Hackshaw R, Wetherall J D 1975 Experimental aspergillosis in normal rats infected intravenously. Journal of the Reticuloendothelial Society 17: 300–312

Voss H G W 1939 Actinomycosis. Journal of the American Dental Association 26: 260–263

Warder F R, Chikes P G, Hudson W R 1975 Aspergillosis of the paranasal sinuses. Archives of Otolaryngology 101: 683–685

Williams A O 1969 Pathology of phycomycosis due to entomophthora and basidiobolus species. Archives of Pathology 87: 13–20

Williams A O, Lichtenberg F, Smith J H, Martinson F D 1969 Ultrastructure of phycomycosis due to entomophthora, basidiobolus and associated 'splendore-hoeppli' phenomenon. Archives of Pathology 87: 459–468

Wolf A, Cowen D 1949 Mucormycosis of the central nervous system. Journal of Neuropathology and Experimental Neurology 8: 107

Wright R E 1927 Two cases of granuloma invading the orbit due to an aspergillus. British Journal of Ophthalmology 11: 545

Yanagisawa E, Friedman S, Kundargi R S, Smith H W 1977 Rhinocerebral phycomycosis. Laryngoscope 87: 1319–1335

Zarniko C 1891 Aspergillusmykose der Kieferhöhle. Deutsche medizinische Wochenschrift 17: 1222

NASAL LEISHMANIASIS

Introduction

Leishmaniasis is an endemic infectious disease caused by a protozoon of the family Trypanosomatidae, genus Leishmania. This parasite infests the blood of various vertebrates including Man and is transmitted by an insect vector. There are three main forms of Leishmaniasis, caused by three designated species of Leishmania which are, in fact, morphologically indistinguishable: (i) visceral involvement, known as Kala Azar (Leishmania donovani), (ii) cutaneous infection, commonly known as Oriental Sore (Leishmania tropica) and (iii) mucosal lesions affecting particularly the nasal and oral cavities, referred to as Espundia (Leishmania braziliensis).

Incidence

In the general context, Leishmaniasis is endemic in widely distributed tropical and subtropical countries of Asia, Southern Europe, Africa, Central and South America. The nasal lesions are found largely in Mexico, the Guianas, Brazil, Peru, Paraguay, Argentina and the West Indies. Klotz and Lindenberg (1923) reported 15 nasal cases from South America whilst Jaffé (1944) published 25 cases of 'American Leishmaniasis' including a number of nasal lesions. It has been stated that mucosal involvement is found only in the New World (Jaffé, 1954) but, according to Manson-Bahr (1944), the Oriental Sore in Sudan may involve the nose producing a picture indistinguishable from Espundia. In Europe, reports of nasal affliction are confined to either immigrants or patients who have spent some time particularly in South America (Partenheimer, 1947; Reipen, 1951; Emslie, 1962).

Clinical features

The age distribution covers a wide range from childhood to old age and there is no significant sex difference. The

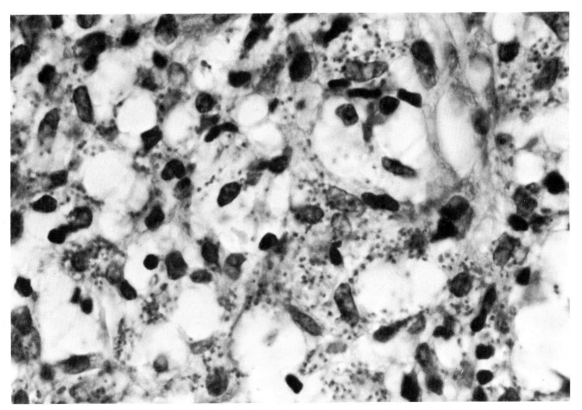

Fig. 9.9 Leishmaniasis of the nose, showing largely intracellular parasites. M × 1250. By courtesy of S Haim.

nasal lesions of Espundia or bubas braziliana may present four clinical varieties: (i) atrophic (ii) ulcerative and destructive with mutilation, (iii) infiltrative and (iv) polypoid (Pupo, 1946). Ulcerative or nodular lesions involve the anterior nares spreading backwards into the nasal fossa and downwards into the upper lip. Fine nodularity may involve the nasal mucosa extending to the nasopharynx and the soft palate (Emslie, 1962). The anterior nose may become grossly deformed (tapir nose) or destroyed (Pupo, 1946) and the lesion may be painful. Plaques of infiltration and ulceration may occur, as described by Haim (1976). There may be a primary cutaneous lesion, particularly on the lower limb.

Anatomical site of origin

The anterior nares and upper lip are always involved. Within the nasal cavity, the disease affects the septum, lateral wall and the floor.

Histopathology

Klotz and Lindenberg (1923) carried out a microscopical study of the lesions in their 15 cases. They noted certain important points: perivascular lymphocytic infiltration, progressive increase in the number of plasmacytes, development of 'endothelial', necrosing and fibrous nodules, marked endarteritis and the presence of the parasite within endothelial cells at all stages of the disease. Leishmania are also found in histiocytes (Figs. 9.9 & 9.10), polymorphonuclear leucocytes and fibroblasts. At a later stage, a strikingly tuberculoid picture, with Langhans type giant cells, replaces the phase of the infected macrophages (Jaffé, 1944). There are fewer parasites though some may be seen inside the giant cells and this may be an expression of a change in the patient's state of immunity (Friedmann and Osborn, 1976).

Klotz and Lindenberg noted that the parasites were less easily found in formalin-fixed tissue and they recommended fixation in Zenker's solution. The protozoon stains well with the Leishman modification of the Romanowsky stain with which it was first identified at the beginning of the present century. Giemsa stain is also effective and the parasite gives a positive Periodic acid Schiff reaction.

Jaffé (1944) noted proliferation of the epithelium covering the lesion and pseudo-epitheliomatous hyperplasia coupled with fairly fast growth of the lesion may

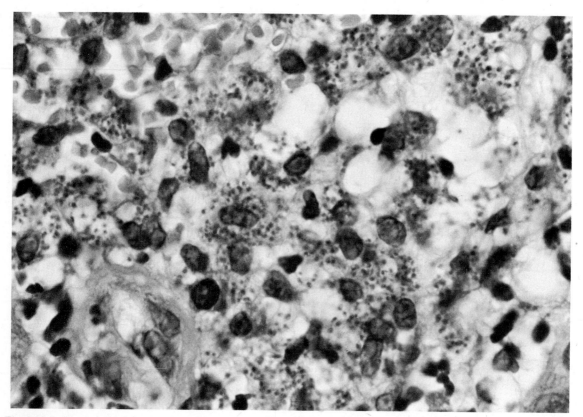

Fig. 9.10 Leishmaniasis of the nose showing intracellular parasites with involvement of endothelial cells (upper left). M × 1250. By courtesy of S Haim.

arouse some suspicion of malignancy. A knowledge of geographical pathology is helpful and any tuberculoid lesion in the nose of patients coming from endemic areas should be examined for Leishmania.

Aetiology and pathogenesis

The protozoon causing nasal Leishmaniasis is known as Leishmania braziliensis though it is indistinguishable from the other species. The infection is transmitted by the bite of a sandfly (Phlebotomus intermedius). When seen in the tissues, the protozoon appears as an ovoid body between two and four microns in diameter. With the modified Romanowsky stain, the parasite is blue with a red nucleus and a kinetoplast. There may also be a small vacuole. In culture on Nicolle's medium and also in the gut of the insect vector the protozoon assumes a flagellate form.

The incubation period is said to be between two to four weeks (Emslie, 1962) and there is an initial

cutaneous lesion which may heal in a matter of months. Some of the earlier observers believed that the nasal mucosal lesions constituted a metastatic infection but a more recent alternative is that the nasal disease is the result of auto-inoculation by a contaminated finger (Jaffé, 1954). Montenegro (1926) showed that an extract of the parasite produced a strongly positive reaction when injected intradermally.

Behaviour

Although the primary cutaneous lesion may heal spontaneously, the mucosal infection becomes a chronic condition and does not heal unless treatment is applied. In the early stages, the lesions do respond to antimony compounds but at a later stage the disease is liable to produce serious disfigurement. Not only may the nose become deformed but may undergo massive destruction which has been well illustrated by Pupo (1946). In severe cases, death may occur as a result of secondary infection such as bronchopneumonia.

BIBLIOGRAPHY – NASAL LEISHMANIASIS

Emslie E S 1962 South American Leishmaniasis in London. British Medical Journal 1 : 299–300
Friedmann I, Osborn D A 1976 In : Symmers W St C (ed) The nose and sinuses in systemic pathology, 2nd edition. Churchill-Livingstone, Edinburgh. Vol 1, ch 4, pp 211–212
Haim S 1976 Involvement of mucous membranes in cases of Leishmania tropica. The Family Physician Israel 6 : 13 ff
Jaffe L 1954 Nasal Leishmaniasis americana in Panama. Archives of Otolaryngology 60 : 601–611
Jaffe R 1944 Histopathological picture of American Leishmaniasis. Practica Oto-rhino-laryngologica 6 : 45–56
Klotz O, Lindenberg H 1923 The pathology of Leishmaniasis of the nose. American Journal of Tropical Medicine 3 : 117–141
Manson-Bahr P, 1944 Synopsis of Tropical Medicine. Cassell and Co Ltd, p 22
Montenegro J 1926 Cutaneous reaction in Leishmaniasis. Archives of Dermatology and Syphilis 13 : 187–194
Partenheimer K 1947 Ein Beitrag zur Kenntnis der südamerikanischen Schleimhautleishmaniose (Espundia). Archiv für Ohren-, Nasen und Kehlkopfheilkunde, 155 : 116–124

Pupo J A 1946 Estudo clinico da leishmanióse tegumentar americana (Leishmania brasiliensis – Vianna 1911). Revista do Hospital das Clinicas 1 : 113–164
Reipen W 1951 Leishmania – Erkrankung der Nase. Zeitschrift für Laryngologie, Rhinologie und Otologie 30 : 177–180

Additional references

Bader G 1972 Morphologie der Gewebsformen von Erregern viszeraler Mykosen und der Variabilität der Gewebsreaktionen. Beiträge zur Pathologie 147 : 111–118
McGill T J, Simpson G, Healy G B 1980 Fulminant aspergillosis of the nose and paranasal sinuses : a new clinical entity. The Laryngoscope 90
Pototschnig B 1964 Leishmaniosi della laringe. Otorinolarungologia Italiana 33 : 235–249
Ribuffo A, e Raschella D 1964 Leishmaniosi del cavo orale. Valsalva 40 : 125–133
Stipic A, Wey W 1976 Ein Beitrag zur Klinik der Leishmaniose. ORL, Supplementum 1 : 143–147

10

Midfacial granuloma syndrome

THE MIDFACIAL GRANULOMA SYNDROME

The nose and paranasal sinuses are the site of election of some dramatic ulcerative granulomatous processes of obscure aetiology and consequently known by a variety of labels which include three possible clinico-pathological entities to be described.

McBride (1897) described a patient with a rapid destruction of the nose and face, proceding to a fatal termination. Under the heading of 'malignant granuloma', Woods (1921) reported two cases presenting with nasal lesions, one of which died while the other responded to irradiation. Kraus (1929) desribed three patients with granulomas and extensive destruction of the nose, oral cavity and pharynx and suggested the diagnostic term 'Granuloma gangraenescens'. Stewart (1933) gave a detailed account of destructive granulomas in the nose whilst another form of nasal granuloma was defined by Wegener (1936 and 1939) who described it as a rhinogenic form of polyarteritis. Wegener's granulomatosis, in contrast with the 'Stewart type' of granuloma, was frequently found to exhibit widespread involvement, particularly of the lungs and kidneys but, subsequently, a localized or limited form was reported (Carrington and Liebow, 1966).

Many attempts have been made to clarify the conflicting concepts, both biological and histological, of this quasi-neoplastic disease. The three supposed entities, i.e. Stewart's type, the systemic and limited forms of Wegener's granulomatosis could conceivably be variants of a single disorder, probably vascular in its basis and possibly due to a disturbance that is immunologically determined (Friedmann and Osborn, 1976). This concept has received support from DeRemee, McDonald, Harrison and Coles (1976) who believe that there are compelling considerations in favour of a unification incorporating all three conditions into a continuum as previously suggested by Nieberding, Schiff and Harmeling (1963). The generic term 'Respiratory' vasculitis' has also been suggested by DeRemee, Weiland and McDonald (1980) for Wegener's and Stewart's granuloma. Nevertheless, it is convenient to

begin by describing the Stewart type and the Wegener forms separately.

IDIOPATHIC, MIDFACIAL, PLEOMORPHIC GRANULOMA (STEWART TYPE)

It seems likely that the case described by McBride in 1897 was the forerunner in the literature of this disease. With the passage of time it has become clear that the common causes of tissue destruction are not identifiable in this condition.

Terminology
The ever growing number of publications make it difficult to compile a complete list. A plethora of terms has been introduced including 'malignant granuloma' (Woods, 1921), 'granuloma gangraenescens' (Kraus, 1929), 'progressive lethal granulomatous ulceration' (Stewart, 1933), 'lethal midline granuloma' (Williams, 1949), 'non-healing midline granuloma' (Walton, 1959), 'polymorphic reticulosis' (Eichel, Harrison, Devine, Scanlon and Brown, 1966), 'midline malignant reticulosis' (Kassel, Echevarria and Guzzo, 1969), 'idiopathic midline granuloma' (Fauci, Johnson and Wolff, 1976). Frequently, the expression 'Stewart's type' is used because of the extensive account given by that author. Woods' term 'malignant granuloma' has been losing favour and, although Williams' expression 'lethal midline granuloma' has the merit of directing attention to the topographical region of the presenting lesion, it has been criticized for implying a hopeless prognosis which is now inappropriate, as is the term 'non-healing'. Furthermore, the expression 'midfacial' is considered more acceptable than 'midline'. The substitution of 'reticulosis' for 'granuloma' has received support from other authors (Fechner and Lamppin, 1972; Schäfer and Schuster, 1975). Moncades, Hagege and Marchand (1977) suggested the comprehensive expression 'rhino-sinusites nécrosantes lethales plurilesionelles' and recently Tsokos, Fauci and Costa (1980) have described twelve patients displaying the features of

Stewart's type midline granuloma as 'Idiopathic Midline Destructive Disease'.

Incidence

The lesion is an uncommon one and in much of the literature the nature of the condition has taken precedence over its frequency. In the I.L.O. material, seven cases have been positively identified as belonging to this group. These cases were collected over a period of 27 years during which time 425,989 new patients were seen in the associated hospital. The condition is undoubtedly less common than the Wegener type.

Clinical features

The age distribution is broadly based, ranging from 15 to 80 years with an average of about 45 years. In the series studied by DeRemee, Weiland and McDonald (1978), there was a male predominance of more than 3:1 but in the I.L.O. material there was an excess of females. The initial clinical manifestation of this lesion is the development of an indurated swelling of the tissues of some part of the nose, such as the vestibule, septum or, more rarely, the turbinates. Ulcerations spread inexorably, destroying the soft tissues, cartilage and bone. The ulcerated mucosa is covered by sticky black or brownish yellow crusts, removal of which reveals what looks like simple granulation tissue. Exposure of bone

may lead to the formation of sequestra whilst ulceration of the turbinates and septum spreads rapidly through the nose, often involving the hard palate which may become perforated. Bacterial infection of the ulcerated tissue leads to inflammatory oedema of the lips, cheeks and eyelids and subcutaneous abscesses may follow. Extensive destruction of the nose, face and hard palate may result in exposure of the roof of the maxillary sinus, involvement of orbit and loss of teeth. (Figs. 10.1 & 10.2). Similar destruction may involve the oro, naso- and hypopharynx (Ellis, 1957). Cachexia, haemorrhage or intercurrent infection may ultimately lead to death of the patient (McKinnon, 1970). There is often a sharply contrasting discrepancy between the dramatic clinical picture and the apparently trivial histopathological findings.

Histopathology

The microscopical picture of 'polymorphic reticulosis' as described by DeRemee et al. (1978) does not differ from the account of 'midline granuloma' given by Friedmann (1955). Various histological patterns can be recognized:

1. Non-specific pleomorphocellular granulation tissue containing 'waves' of fibrous tissue.
2. Non-specific granulation tissue with histiocytes predominating.

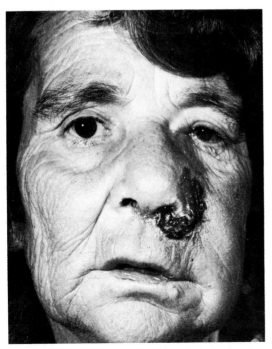

Fig. 10.1 Midfacial pleomorphic granuloma (Stewart type) in a 63 year-old female, showing extensive destruction of the wall of the nose.

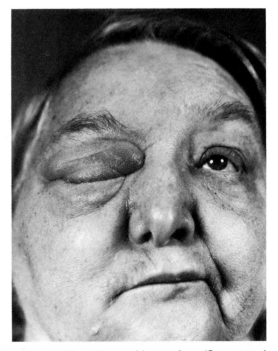

Fig. 10.2 Midfacial pleomorphic granuloma (Stewart type) in a 65 year-old female showing nasal and orbital involvement.

3. Non-specific granulation tissue with necrotic changes predominating.

These variants may represent stages of the same underlying process and have been implied by subsequent authors in the term polymorphic. The essential change is a dense accumulation of the pleomorphic cells in the affected tissues. The cells are predominantly lymphocytes but there is a considerable admixture of plasma cells whilst elongated or spindle shaped histiocytes with round or ovoid nuclei are present and may constitute a major component (Figs. 10.3, 10.4, 10.5, 10.6, 10.7). DeRemee et al. (1978) described mature and stimulated lymphocytes, plasma cells and immunoblasts. Some of the cells certainly show a moderate degree of immaturity and the infiltrate has a pronounced tendency towards vascular orientation (Friedmann, 1955). Necrosis is not limited to the ulcerated surface but may affect a very considerable part of the tissue. Small haemorrhages are numerous and dense fibrous granulation tissue is laid down in the deeper layers during periods of organization or following treatment. Vascular thrombosis and infec-

tion of soft tissue and bones may occur (Moschella, 1973).

The heterogeneity of the proliferating cells accompanying the histiocytic elements and the lack of well defined neoplastic characteristics make it unlikely the disease represents a true tumour. The presence of atypical cells in this lesion is not an indication of its neoplastic nature. Too much emphasis should not be placed on the presence of atypical cells, as has been advocated by some authors (Michaels and Gregory, 1977). In the context of skin lesions, Clark, Mihm, Reed and Ainsworth (1974) emphasized that histologically atypical and even disturbing lymphoreticular infiltrates do not necessarily imply or predict malignant change, hence the diagnosis of malignant lymphoma should not be made on the basis of skin biopsies alone. In so far as there is an element of non-specificity in the cellular infiltrate, diagnostic difficulties may well arise through lack of representative tissue. Furthermore, the clinical picture may be of great importance in assessing the histological findings. This is evident also from the description of the clinicopathological features of 'idi-

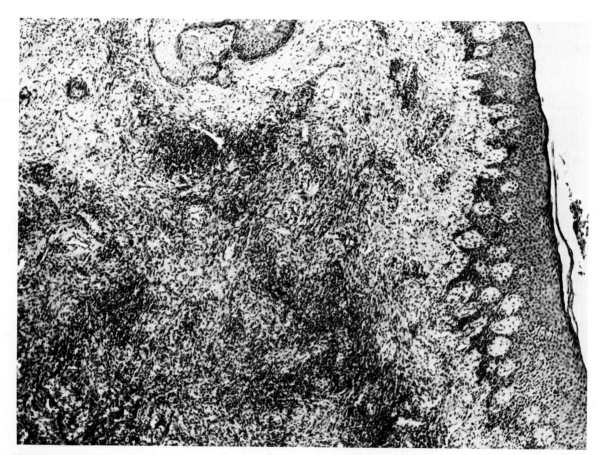

Fig. 10.3 Midfacial pleomorphic granuloma (Stewart type) in a 65 year-old female (see Fig. 10.2), showing intense cellular infiltration. M ×90

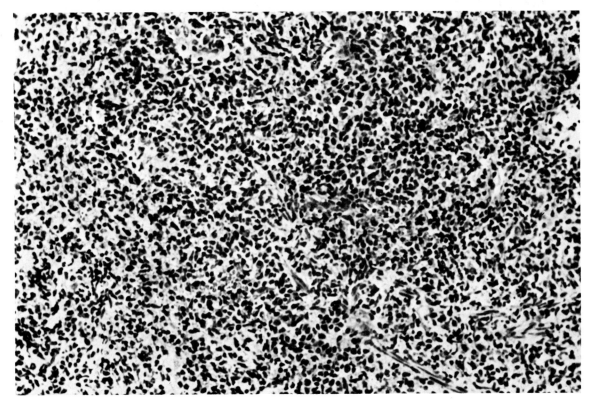

Fig. 10.4 Midfacial pleomorphic granuloma (Stewart type) in a 50 year-old female, showing pleomorphocellular infiltrate. M ×285

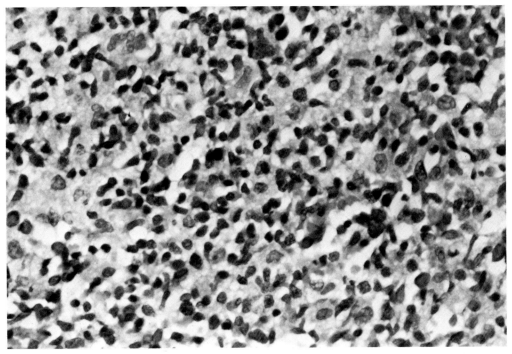

Fig. 10.5 Midfacial pleomorphic granuloma (Stewart type) in a 63 year-old female (see Fig. 10.1) showing pleomorphic exudate. M ×520

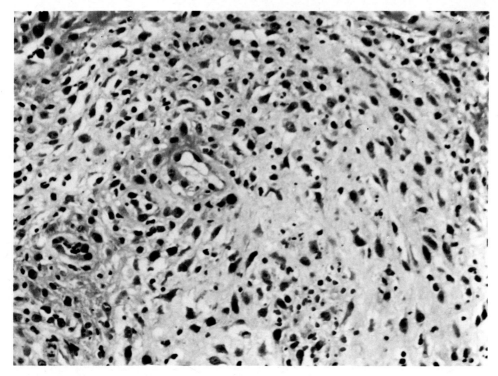

Fig. 10.6 Midfacial pleomorphic granuloma (Stewart type) in a 51 year-old female, showing pleomorphic pattern. M × 305

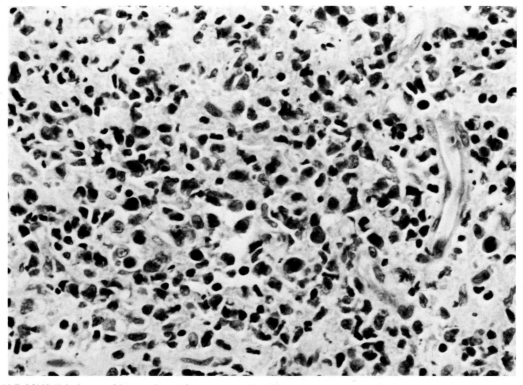

Fig. 10.7 Midfacial pleomorphic granuloma (Stewart type) in a 48 year-old female (see Fig. 10.17), showing pleomorpho-cellular infiltrate. M × 520

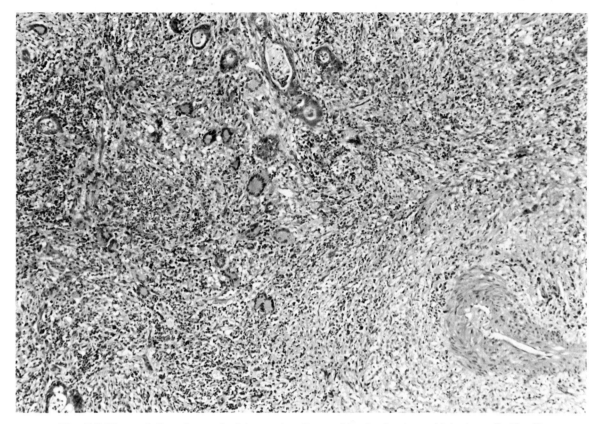

Fig. 10.8 Wegener's Granulomatosis of the nose in a 43 year-old male, showing multiple giant cells. M × 90

opathic midline destructive disease' (mentioned earlier) by Tsokos et al. as follows: A locally destructive lesion always restricted to the upper respiratory tract and no systemic disease developing during a follow-up period of 1 to 8 years (mean 4.5 years). Repeated biopsy findings show non-specific acute and chronic inflammation with some necrosis, occasionally with granuloma formation. Malignant or atypical cells are absent and there is, as a rule, no vasculitis; although in 50 per cent of cases inflammatory cells seen in the wall and occasionally around small vessels. Repeated cultures and special stains for infectious causes are negative.

Aetiology and pathogenesis
A variety of views have been expressed on the causal factors of this disease. Bergquist and Koch (1949) believed that the condition was neoplastic whilst Mills (1958) suggested an infective origin on the grounds of the high frequency of isolation of staphylococci. Noma neonatorum, a usually fatal gangrenous process affecting the midfacial tissues, seems to develop in and around blood vessels. Ghosal, Sen Gupta, Mukherjee, Choudhury, Dutta and Sarkar (1978) reported 35 cases

apparently caused by *Pseudomonas aeruginosa*. In the present context, however, it is clear that whatever organisms are isolated merely represent secondary infection since the disease does not respond to appropriate antibiotics. Hypersensitivity reaction has been suggested by a number of authors (Blatt, Seltzer, Rubin, Furstenberg, Maxwell and Schull, 1959; Friedmann, 1964; Fauci et al., 1976). Although it is generally recognized that the disease is not a lymphoma, its relationship to other lymphoreticular diseases has to be considered and will be discussed in connection with the unifying concept of pathogenesis.

Behaviour
In the absence of effective treatment the disease shows a marked tendency to progress with massive destruction of the nose and face leading ultimately to the death of the patient, frequently as a result of intercurrent infection. The earlier concept was that of a strictly localized lesion but it soon became clear that remote involvement could occur. Dickson (1960) described a fatal case in which, in addition to involvement of the nose and sinuses, there were similar infiltrative lesions

in the skin, muscle, cervical lymphnodes and suprarenal glands. Involvement of the larynx (McKinnon, 1970) is not uncommon.

The introduction of low dosage irradiation (Glass, 1955; Howells, 1955; Ellis, 1955; Dickson, 1960; Ardouin, 1964) transformed the survival pattern. In the I.L.O. material, about two thirds survived for over five years and about half the cases survived more than ten years. Of the two longest survivors, one died after 20 years from an unrelated cause whilst the other has survived 15 years with one recurrence. Eight additional cases were collected by the present authors through the medium of the Ear, Nose and Throat Tumour Panel and of these two are known to be alive and well 7 and 22 years after presentation. It is noteworthy that those cases which did not receive irradiation have fared badly. Irradiation can produce quite dramatic results, especially in the earlier stages of the disease but, in the context of low dosage, histological misinterpretation could lead to a malignant lymphoma being inadequately treated.

It has been suggested that some of these pleomorphic midfacial granulomas may ultimately become malignant lymphomas but follow-up of cases studied by the present authors has not, so far, revealed convincing evidence of such an event. Initial histological misinterpretation might account for some instances of apparent neoplastic change but, in view of the possible relationship to lymphomatoid granulomatosis (to be discussed later), the issue must be regarded as unresolved.

WEGENER'S GRANULOMATOSIS

This condition was defined by Wegener (1936, 1939) and has retained its eponymous title, although an earlier report by Klinger appeared in 1931.

Incidence

As in the case of the Stewart type granuloma, frequency of the condition has often been passed over in the literature. In the I.L.O. material, 17 cases were identified over a period of 27 years. On this basis, Wegener's Granulomatosis would appear to be more common than the midfacial pleomorphic granuloma.

Clinical features

Age distribution is broadly based with equal involvement of the sexes. The disease is encountered most commonly in the fourth and fifth decades but is not infrequently found in younger subjects. The I.L.O. cases ranged from 15 to 64 years. Patients usually present with constitutional symptoms out of all proportion to the clinical findings. Almost invariably, they are febrile, lose weight, become anaemic and exhibit leucocytosis and elevated sedimentation rate. It is important to emphasize the

rhinogenous origin of this form of granuloma although the presenting signs may be located elsewhere, in the larynx, orbit or skin. Systemic manifestations such as purpura may overshadow the apparently trivial nasal discharge and sinusitis which is often of long duration and may be indicative of a prodromal stage of the disease. Bloodstained discharge, symptoms of sinusitis, hoarseness or signs of middle ear infection may develop. The disease progresses in spite of antibiotic treatment whilst oedema of the face and eyes, proptosis, antro-alveolar fistula or even saddle-back deformity of the nose may develop. On the other hand there may be no external manifestation of the disease in spite of considerable intranasal involvement. Examination may reveal a crusted bleeding granularity of the septal or turbinal mucosa whilst later frank granulomatous lesions may be found, especially on the septum with extensive destruction of intranasal structures. Spreading ulcers may develop in the mouth, tongue, pharynx and larynx (Friedmann, 1964; McKinnon, 1970). The genital organs may also be affected (Friedmann, 1971; Matsudo, Mitsukawa, Ishii and Shirai, 1976). The ear may also be involved (Friedmann and Bauer, 1973).

Atypical cases may occur. Pritchard and Gow (1976) described two cases of Wegener's Granulomatosis presenting as rheumatoid arthritis with subsequent development of nasal lesions. Neurological involvement, which occurs in more than a quarter of cases, has been described by Anderson, Jamieson and Jefferson (1975) who noted granulomatous lesions of the central nervous system and vasculitis of both central and peripheral systems. Neurological lesions are less common in the Stewart type of granuloma. Pambakian and Tighe (1971) described two cases in which the early and predominating lesions were formed in the breast prior to the development in the upper respiratory tract of the characteristic clinical features.

There is a growing recognition of the fact that classical features of this disease are not always present. Many cases ultimately exhibit evidence of renal involvement but a concept of limited Wegener's Granulomatosis, in which the kidneys appear to be unaffected, has been put forward by Carrington and Liebow (1966) with subsequent support from Cassan, Coles and Harrison (1970). The main site of election in this group is in the lungs with limited remote lesions occasionally including the nose. Fienberg (1953) suggested the existence of intermediate cases between the classical disseminated disease and the more localized form. On the other hand, Cassan et al. (1970) regarded the issue of a separate entity or a modified form of the classical disease as being unresolved. Carrington and Liebow (1966) believed that localized vasculitis with granulomatosis may be much more frequent than the original disease described by Wegener. It is important to recognize the disease in its early limited form in the upper respiratory tract (Friedmann, 1976).

Histopathology

The presence of multinucleated giant cells, although not pathognomonic, is helpful in the correct interpretation of the presenting lesion. The giant cells of Wegener's disease resemble those of tuberculosis (Langhans type) but their nuclei are often peculiarly compact, appearing dense, ovoid and intensely haematoxyphilic (Figs. 10.8, 10.9, 10.10 & 10.11) and may often be clustered in two semicircular groups at opposite poles of the cell. The cytoplasm is more compact, homogeneous and eosinophilic than in the giant cells of other tuberculoid granulomas. In all cases giant cells can be found in the biopsy material although their number varies considerably. They may be widely scattered throughout the tissue and numerous enough to be readily found or they may be scanty with a tendency to be grouped adjacent to blood vessels, presenting a picture similar to that of giant cell arteritis but in the latter lesion the giant cells represent a reaction to the elastic tissue breakdown whereas in Wegener's disease this situation does not obtain.

Necrotizing arteritis is an essential component of the microscopical picture. Vessel walls are infiltrated by acute inflammatory cells and show a partial fibrinoid necrosis (Figs. 10.12, 10.13 & 10.14), which contrasts with the usual appearance in polyarteritis nodosa where destruction of the artery is complete. Focal haemorrhage and necrosis are the inevitable consequences of the vascular lesions. Patchy necrosis is a common feature, the necrotic material having a characteristic granular appearance with conspicuous stippling by haematoxyphilic particulate debris of nuclear origin. Organization and fibrosis proceed simultaneously with destruction and the scar tissue may in its turn become involved in the necrotizing process. Destruction of tissue is not as extensive as in the pleomorphic granuloma, there being less tendency for involvement of cartilage but saddle deformity of the nose may develop. The kidneys show focal glomerulitis, periglomerulitis and vasculitis whilst some of the vascular lesions with granuloma formation and necrosis may be found in the lungs, spleen and other viscera.

In the limited form of Wegener's Granulomatosis, Carrington and Liebow (1966) observed similarities to and differences from the classical disease. Vasculitis

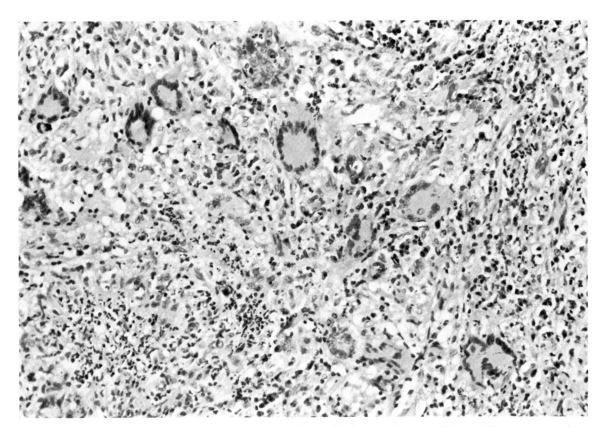

Fig 10.9 Wegener's Granulomatosis of the nose in a 43 year-old male. Higher magnification of Fig. 10.8. Note tendency towards Langhans type of giant cell. M × 225

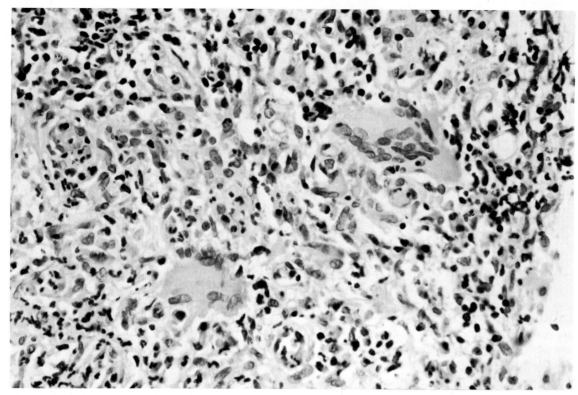

Fig 10.10 Wegener's Granulomatosis of the nose in a 41 year-old male. Note resemblance to foreign body type of giant cell. M ×480

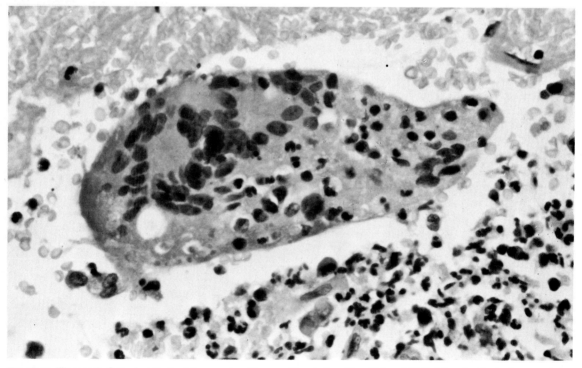

Fig 10.11 Wegener's Granulomatosis of the nose in a 43 year-old male (see Figs. 10.8 and 10.9). Note foreign body type of giant cell. M ×595

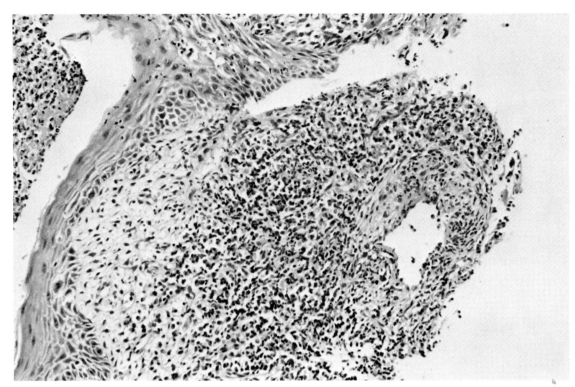

Fig. 10.12 Wegener's Granulomatosis of the nose in a 41 year-old male (see Fig. 10.10), showing subepithelial granulation tissue with arteritis. M × 180

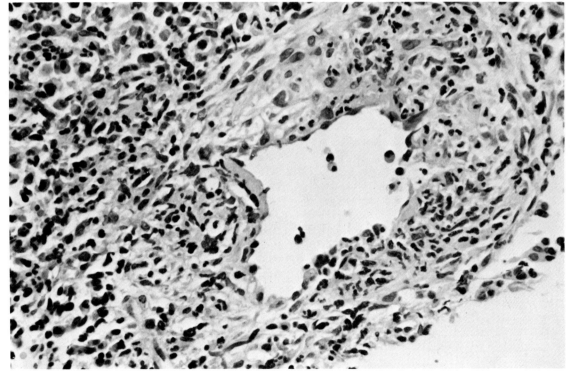

Fig. 10.13 Wegener's Granulomatosis of the nose in a 41 year-old male. Higher magnification of Fig. 10.12. Note acute inflammatory infiltration of the arterial wall. M × 480

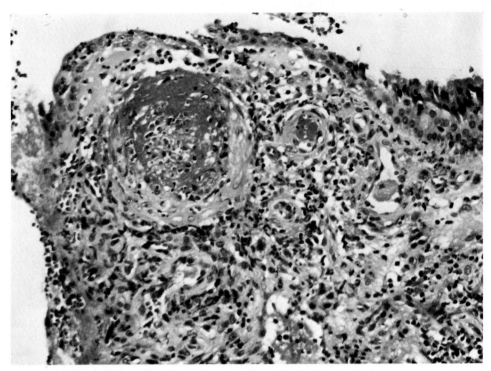

Fig. 10.14 Wegener's Granulomatosis of the nose in a 37 year-old male, showing necrotizing arteritis with partial fibrinoid necrosis. M × 200

tends to affect both arteries and veins whilst bizarre cells resembling those seen in Hodgkin's Disease may be present.

Aetiology and pathogenesis

The cause of this disease is still not known. The infective theory proposed by Mills (1958), who did not distinguish between the Wegener and Stewart types, has received no support from bacteriological studies. Walton (1958) concluded that the disease was the result of a hypersensitivity reaction, possibly to drugs or the products of tissue breakdown. Blatt, Seltzer, Rubin, Furstenberg, Maxwell and Schull (1959) regarded the disease as being due to an auto-immune reaction. On the other hand, Shillitoe, Lehner, Lessof and Harrison (1974) found a depression of certain immunological reactions and concluded that the disease was probably due to a cell mediated immune deficiency.

Many forms of vasculitis, idiopathic or iatrogenic, are believed to be triggered off by the deposition of immune complexes (antigen-antibody combinations) in the vessel wall (Schroeter, Copeman, Jordon, Sams and Winkelmann, 1971; Parish, 1972; Wolff, Fauci, Horn and Dale, 1974; Sams, Thorne, Small, Mass, McIntosh and Stanford, 1976). Circulating immune complexes

have been reported in Wegener's Granulomatosis with varying frequency. Travers (1979) claimed that they had been found in about two-thirds of cases. On the other hand, Shillitoe et al. (1974) found immune complexes in one out of seven cases but many had been receiving chemotherapy before the tests were made. Howell and Epstein (1976) found that immune complexes may be present during the active phase of Wegener's disease but tend to disappear during remission brought about by immuno-suppressive therapy. Following the deposition of these substances in the vascular wall, inflammatory damage ensues and the disintegration of the accumulated neutrophils is followed by secondary tissue destruction due to the release of lysosomal enzymes (Leucocytoclasis). The latter phenomenon is believed to be an early event in the pathogenesis of Wegener's Granulomatosis. Donald, Edwards and McEvoy (1976) carried out ultrastructural studies of tissue injury in limited Wegener's Granulomatosis of the lung. The lysis of leucocytes resulted in the liberation of cytoplasmic organelles into the circulation, leading to platelet aggregation and fibrin deposition in vessels with intact endothelium. Necrosis of the vascular endothelium and obstruction of the lumen also occurred but these vascular phenomena were suppressed by cyclophosphamide treatment.

Behaviour

Modern chemotherapy has certainly modified the natural history of this disease. The earlier cases tended to be progressive although local destruction was never as extensive as in the Stewart type granuloma. Nevertheless, nasal deformity and involvement of the orbit occurred. Systemic involvement was a common event, affecting the lungs, kidneys (Fig. 10.15), skin, spleen and other viscera. In the I.L.O. material, at least 50 per cent exhibited remote lesions and the greater proportion died within periods ranging from three months to three years. Later cases have fared better, having received intensive treatment with immuno-suppressive drugs (steroids, axothiaprine and cyclophosphamide). Seven cases have survived with controlled disease for periods ranging from 5 to 17 years. Most of the last mentioned cases presented with disease apparently limited to the nasal region. Carrington and Liebow (1966) suggested that the limited form of the disease might have a better prognosis. Pulmonary involvement occurred in nearly one-third of the cases whilst two cases were known to have affected kidneys. In an additional ten cases collected through the medium of the Ear, Nose and Throat Tumour Panel, survival was less encouraging and renal involvement had occurred in over 50 per cent. Clearly, the earlier diagnosis of Wegener's Granulomatosis in the apparent absence of systemic lesions has acquired an added urgency since the introduction of potent drugs capable of arresting the disease. Death caused by the disease is usually the result of renal failure or intercurrent infection.

The unifying concept of pathogenesis

In the early literature of the midfacial granuloma syndrome, the histological distinctions were not always made or appreciated. Friedmann (1955) separated the Stewart from the Wegener type although he thought that they might be similar in character. Eichel and Mabery (1968) did not accept the 'lethal midline granuloma' as a specific entity but, on the other hand, Wetmore and Platz (1978) considered that it was an entity distinct from Wegener's Granulomatosis and also from malignant lymphoma.

There are often blurred margins between the two main types of midfacial granuloma and their correct histological identification in the presenting lesion may

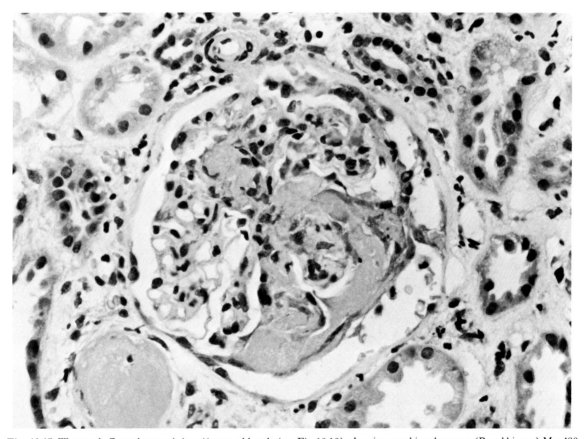

Fig. 10.15 Wegener's Granulomatosis in a 41 year-old male (see Fig. 10.10), showing renal involvement. (Renal biopsy) M × 480

well prove to be difficult. The lesion in Wegener's disease may sometimes resemble that of the Stewart type with an occasional giant cell embedded in the granulations, yet systemic lesions may develop (Appaix, Pech and Codaccioni, 1959). On the other hand, such granulomas may fail to produce the characteristic systemic lesions of Wegener's Granulomatosis and remain entirely localized.

Pulmonary involvement, especially in the systemic and limited forms of Wegener's Granulomatosis, has focussed attention on the existence of a spectrum of ill-defined and rare primary lymphoreticular proliferative lesions of that organ. Gibbs and Seal (1978) suggested that such lesions ranged from obvious benign disease to malignant lymphoma. Among the lesions to be considered are the so-called pseudolymphoma and lymphomatoid granulomatosis. Saltzstein (1963) drew attention to a much better prognosis in many 'lymphomas' of the lung and he distinguished a large group, characterized by mature lymphocytic infiltration combined with other inflammatory cells and the presence of lymphoid follicles with true germinal centres, to which he gave the name pseudolymphoma. Liebow, Carrington and Friedman (1972), under the heading of lymphomatoid granulomatosis, reported 40 cases of granulomatous lesions with

vasculitis involving primarily the lungs but, in addition, many other locations (kidneys, skin, liver, heart, central nervous system and very occasionally lymphnodes). The lesions are characterized by a pleomorphic cellular infiltrate (small and large mononuclear cells, lymphocytes, plasmacytes, polymorphonuclear leucocytes, eosinophils and often many histiocytes) combined with a vasculitis involving both arteries and veins. The surrounding infiltrate invaded the vessel walls giving an appearance of disruption although fibrinoid change was rare. Not unsimilar appearances have been observed in the Stewart type granuloma (Figs. 10.16 & 10.17). Of the 40 cases more than half died, a small proportion exhibiting features of terminal lymphoma. Gibbs (1977) believed that lymphomatoid granulomatosis had affinities with both Wegener's Granulomatosis and malignant lymphoma. Part of the basis for this view is the 'angiocentric and angiodestructive' pattern as defined by Liebow et al. (1972) and this could represent a link with the concept of a unified approach to the midfacial granuloma syndrome although the vascular lesions are not typical of those usually found in Wegener's disease. However, the relationship to malignant lymphoma remains doubtful and ill-defined since neither lymphomatoid granulomatosis nor the Stewart type granuloma

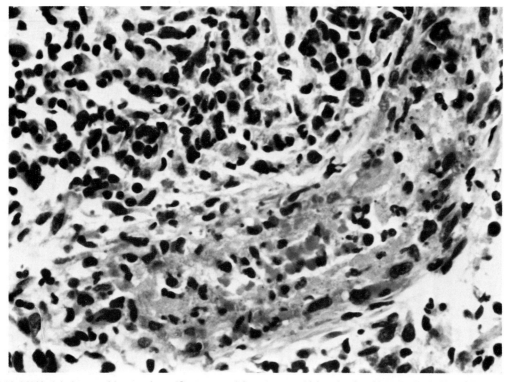

Fig. 10.16 Midfacial pleomorphic granuloma (Stewart type) in a 53 year-old female, showing vascular infiltration resembling that seen in lymphomatoid granulomatosis. M × 650

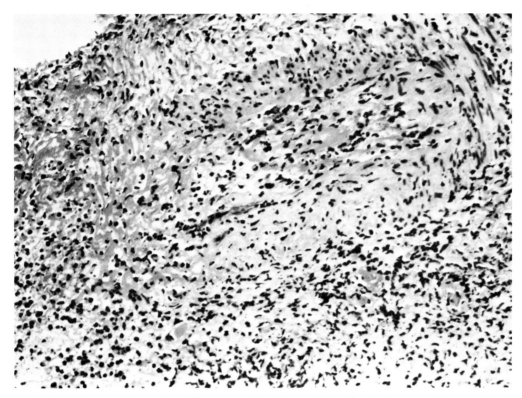

Fig. 10.17 Midfacial pleomorphic granuloma (Stewart type) in a 48 year-old female, showing necrotizing vasculitis. M × 260

commonly affects lymphnodes although 'atypical hyperplasia' has been reported by Liebow (1973) in some patients with pulmonary granulomas. Clearly there are a number of lesions with identical or vaguely similar histological features which may or may not indicate a common pathogenesis.

The dynamic behaviour of granulomatous lesions cannot be interpreted through the histological pattern and varies greatly according to the nature of the causal agent (Spector, 1969 and 1971). The cellular turnover in a granuloma, i.e. the rate of replacement of cells by either emigration for the circulation or mitosis in situ, ranges from a high to a low order. According to Spector, high turnover granulomas are dependent particularly on emigration from the circulation, whereas low turnover granulomas are more self sufficient and presumably depend for their continued existence on multiplication of macrophages within the lesion. This would seem to correlate well with the natural history of midfacial granulomas which are probably largely of low turnover type. In so far as macrophages have the ability to transform into epithelioid and giant cells, it is possible that the Stewart type granuloma could evolve, enhanced by delayed hypersensitivity, into an epithelioid or giant cell granuloma. Consideration of these basic principles may assist in a better understanding of the enigma of the midfacial granuloma syndrome.

BIBLIOGRAPHY

Anderson J M, Jamieson D G, Jefferson J M 1975 Non-healing granuloma and the nervous system. Quarterly Journal of Medicine, New Series 44: 309–323

Appaix A, Pech A, Codaccioni J M 1959 Granulome malin mediofaciale et granulomatose de Wegener. Discussion nosologique à propos d'une observation. Journal Français d'Oto-Rhino-Laryngologie et Chirurgie maxillo-faciale 8: 737–771

Ardouin A P 1964 The management of malignant granuloma. Proceedings of the Royal Society of Medicine 57: 299–303

Bergquist B, Koch H S 1949 Contribution to the question of granuloma gangrenescens. Acta Otolaryngologica 37: 405–414

Blatt I M, Seltzer H S, Rubin P, Furstenberg A C, Maxwell J H, Schull W J 1959 Fatal granulomatosis of the respiratory tract (lethal midline granuloma – Wegener's granulomatosis). Archives of Otolaryngology 70: 707–757

Carrington C B, Liebow A A 1066 Limited forms of angiitis and granulomatosis of Wegener's type. American Journal of Medicine 41: 497–527

Cassan S M, Coles D T, Harrison E G 1970 The concept of limited forms of Wegener's granulomatosis. American Journal of Medicine 49: 366–379

Clark W H, Mihm M C, Reed R J, Ainsworth A M 1974 The lymphocytic infiltrates of the skin. Human Pathology 5: 25–43

DeRemee R A, McDonald T J, Harrison E G, Coles D T 1976 Wegener's granulomatosis. Anatomic correlates. A proposed classification. Mayo Clinic Proceedings 51: 777–781

DeRemee R A, Weiland L H, McDonald T J 1978 Polymorphic reticulosis, lymphomatoid granulomatosis. Two diseases or one? Mayo Clinic Proceedings 53: 634–640

Dickson R J 1960 Radiotherapy of lethal midline granuloma. Journal of Chronic Diseases 12: 417–427

Donald K J, Edwards R L, McEvoy D S 1976 An ultrastructural study of the pathogenesis of tissue injury in limited Wegener's granulomatosis. Pathology 8: 161–169

Eichel B S, Harrison E G, Devine K D, Scanlon P M, Brown H A 1966 Primary lymphoma of the nose including relationship to lethal midline granuloma. American Journal of Surgery 112: 597–605

Eichel B S, Mabery T E 1968 The enigma of the lethal midline granuloma. Laryngoscope 78: 1367–1386

Ellis M P 1955 Malignant granuloma of the nose. British Medical Journal 1: 1251–1253

Ellis M P 1957 Malignant granuloma of the nose. Annals of Otology, Rhinology and Laryngology 66: 1002–1008

Fauci A S, Johnson R E, Wolff S M 1976 Radiation therapy of midline granuloma. Annals of Internal Medicine 84: 140–147

Fechner R E, Lamppin D M 1972 Midline malignant reticulosis. A clinicopathological entity. Archives of Otolaryngology 95: 467–476

Fienberg R 1953 Necrotizing granulomatosis and angiitis of the lungs. American Journal of Clinical Pathology 23: 413–428.

Friedmann I 1955 Pathology of malignant granuloma. Journal of Laryngology and Otology 69: 331–341

Friedmann I 1964 The pathology of midline granuloma. Proceedings of the Royal Society of Medicine 57: 289–297

Friedmann I 1971 The changing pattern of granulomas of the upper respiratory tract. Journal of Laryngology and Otology 85: 631–682

Friedmann I, Bauer F 1973 Wegener's granulomatosis causing deafness. Journal of Larnygology and Otology 87: 449–464

Friedmann I 1976 Wegener's granulomatosis presenting as rheumatoid arthritis. Proceedings of the Royal Society of Medicine 69: 785

Friedmann I, Osborn D A 1976 The non-healing granulomas of unknown cause. In: Symmers W St C (ed). 2nd Ed. Churchill-Livingston, Edinburgh, pp 212–217

Friedmann I, Sando I 1978 Idiopathic pleomorphic midfacial granuloma (Stewart's type). Journal of Laryngology and Otology 92: 601–611

Ghosal S P, Sen Gupta P L, Mukherjee A K, Choudhury M, Dutta N, Sarker A K 1978 Noma neonatorum: its pathogenesis. Lancet 2: 289–291

Gibbs A R 1977 Lymphomatoid granulomatosis – a condition with affinities to Wegener's granulomatosis and lymphoma. Thorax 32: 71–79

Gibbs A R, Seal R M E 1978 Primary lymphoproliferative conditions of the lung. Thorax 33: 140–152

Glass E J G 1955 Malignant granuloma. Journal of Laryngology and Otology 69: 315–320

Howell S B, Epstein W V 1976 Circulating immunoglobulin complexes in Wegener's granulomatosis. American Journal of Medicine 60: 259–268

Howells G H 1955 Malignant granuloma. Journal of Laryngology and Otology 69: 309–314

Kassel S H, Echevarria R A, Guzzo F P 1969 Midline malignant reticulosis: so-called lethal midline granuloma. Cancer 23: 920–935

Klinger H 1931 Grenzformen der Periarteriitis nodosa. Frankfurter Zeitschrift für Pathologie 42: 455–480

Kraus E J 1929 Über drei Fälle einer eigenartigen Neubildung der Nasen-, Rachen- und Mundhöhle. Klinische Wochenschrift 8: 932–934

Liebow A A 1975 Pulmonary angiitis and granulomatosis. American Review of Respiratory Diseases 108: 1–18

Liebow A A, Carrington C B, Friedman P J 1972 Lymphomatoid granulomatosis. Human Pathology 3: 457–558

McBride P 1897 A case of rapid destruction of the nose and face. Journal of Laryngology and Otology 12: 64–66

McKinnon D M 1970 Lethal midline granuloma of the face and larynx. Journal of Laryngology and Otology 84: 1195–1203

Matsudo S, Mitsukawa S, Ishii N, Shirai M 1976 A case of Wegener's granulomatosis with necrosis of the penis. Tohoku Journal of Experimental Medicine 118: 145–151

Michaels L, Gregory M M 1977 The pathology of non-healing midline granuloma. Journal of Clinical Pathology 30: 317–327

Mills C P 1958 Malignant granuloma of the nose and paranasal sinuses. Journal of Laryngology and Otology 72: 849–887

Moncades J, Hagege C E, Marchand J 1977 Quelques cas de necrose atypique medio-faciale. Journal d'Oto-Laryngologie et de Chirurgie Faciale 94: 339–341

Moschella S L 1973 The so-called midline granuloma. Cutis (New York) 11: 650–652

Nieberding P H, Schiff M, Harmeling J G 1963 Periarteritis nodosa. Archives of Otolaryngology 77: 512–524

Pambakian H, Tighe J R 1971 Breast involvement in Wegener's granulomatosis. Journal of Clinical Pathology 24: 343–347

Parish W E 1972 Cutaneous vasculitis: antigen-antibody complexes and prolonged fibrinolysis. Proceedings of the Royal Society of Medicine 65: 276–278

Pritchard M H, Gow P J 1976 Wegener's granulomatosis presenting as rheumatoid arthritis. Proceedings of the Royal Society of Medicine 69: 501–504

Saltzstein S L 1963 Pulmonary malignant lymphomas and pseudolymphomas: classification, therapy and prognosis. Cancer 16: 928–955

Sams M V, Thorne E G, Small P, Mass M F, McIntosh R M, Stanford R E 1976 Leucocytoclastic vasculitis. Archives of Dermatology 112: 219–226

Schäfer R J, Schuster H H 1975 Granuloma Gangraenescens als maligne Retikulose. Zentralblatt für allgemeine Pathologie 119: 111–115

Schroeter A L, Copeman P W M, Jordon R E, Sams M W, Winkelmann R K 1971 Immunofluorescence of cutaneous vasculitis associated with systemic disease. Archives of Dermatology 104: 254–259

Shillitoe E J, Lehner T, Lessof M H, Harrison D F N 1974 Immunological features of Wegener's granulomatosis. Lancet 1: 281–284

Spector W G 1969 Granulomatous inflammatory exudate. In: Richter G W, Epstein M A (eds) International Review of

Experimental Pathology. Academic Press, New York, 8: 1–53

Spector W G 1971 The cellular dynamics of granulomas. Proceedings of the Royal Society of Medicine 64: 941–942

Stewart J P 1933 Progressive lethal granulomatous ulceration of the nose. Journal of Laryngology and Otology 48: 657–701

Travers R L 1979 Polyarteritis and related disorders. British Journal of Hospital Medicine 22: 38–45

Tsokos M, Fauci A, Costa J 1980 Idiopathic midline destructive disease: A subgroup of patients with midline granuloma. Laboratory Medicine (Abstract) p 156

Walton E W 1958 Giant cell granuloma of the respiratory tract (Wegener's granulomatosis). British Medical Journal 2: 265–270

Walton E W 1959 Non-healing granulomata of the nose. Journal of Laryngology and Otology 73: 242–260

Wegener F 1936 Über generalisierte, septische Gefässerkrankungen. Verhandlungen der Deutschen pathologischen Gesellschaft 29: 202–210

Wegener F 1939 Über eine eigenartige rhinogene Granulomatose mit besonderer Beteiligung des Arteriensystems und der Nieren. Beiträge zur pathologischen Anatomie und allgemeinen Pathologie 102: 36–38

Wetmore S J, Platz C E 1978 Idiopathic midface lesions. Annals of Otology, Rhinology and Laryngology 87: 60–69

Williams H L 1949 Lethal granulomatous ulceration involving the midline facial tissues. Annals of Otology, Rhinology and Laryngology 58: 1013–1054

Wolff S M, Fauci A S, Horn R G, Dale D C 1974 Wegener's granulomatosis. Annals of Internal Medicine 81: 513–525

Woods R 1921 Malignant granuloma of the nose. British Medical Journal 2: 65–66

Additional references

Abel T, Andrews B S, Cunningham P H, Brunner C M, Davis J S, Horwitz D A 1980 Rheumatoid vasculitis: effect of cyclophosphamide on the clinical course and levels of circulating immune complexes. Annals of Internal Medicine 93: 407–413

Crissman J D 1979 Midline malignant reticulosis and lymphomatoid granulomatosis. Archives of Pathology 103: 561–564

DeRemee R A, Weiland L H, McDonald T J 1980 Respiratory vasculitis. Mayo Clin Proc 55: 492–498

Hu C-H, O'Loughlin S, Winkelmann R K 1977 Cutaneous manifestations of Wegener's granulomatosis. Arch Dermatol 113: 175–182

Katzenstein A-L, Carrington Ch B, Liebow A A 1979 Lymphomatoid granulomatosis: A clinicopathologic study of 152 cases. Cancer 43: 360–373

Kay S, Fu Y, Minars N, Brady J W 1974 Lymphomatoid granulomatosis of the skin. Light microscopic and ultrastructural studies. Cancer 34: 1675–1682

McDonald T J, DeRemee R A, Kern E B, Harrison E G 1974 Nasal manifestations of Wegener's granulomatosis. Laryngoscope 84: 2101–2112

Olsen K D, Neel H B, DeRemee R A, Weiland L H 1980 Nasal manifestations of allergic granulomatosis and angitis (Churg-Strauss syndrome). Otolaryngol Head Surg 88: 85–89

Tsokos M, Fauci A, Costa J 1980 Idiopathic midline destructive disease: A subgroup of patients with midline granuloma. Lab Investigations 40/1 p 156

11

Tumours of the nose and sinuses – material and classification

TUMOURS OF THE NOSE AND SINUSES – GENERAL COMMENTS

It has been a common practice in textbooks to deal with tumours of this region without drawing a distinction between nasal and paranasal origin. Admittedly, in the context of malignancy, it may be difficult to define the precise site of origin and the common approach has undoubtedly been influenced by therapeutic considerations. Nevertheless, from a pathological point of view, identification of origin has been achieved sufficiently frequently to establish distinctive patterns. Apart from tumours peculiar to particular locations, such as the olfactory neuroblastoma, there are often marked differences in relative frequency between the nasal and paranasal regions. This is reflected in the fact that tumours of the nasal cavity are predominantly benign whilst those in the paranasal sinuses are mostly malignant. Tumours in the two regions may not only show differences of pathological frequency but may exhibit contrasting behaviour.

In over a thousand tumours of the nose and sinuses collected in the Institute of Laryngology and Otology, about three quarters were of nasal origin. In terms of primary involvement, the ratio of benign to malignant tumours in the nasal cavity was nearly 6:1 but, excluding the paranasal extensions of the transitional type papilloma of the nose, the ratio in the sinuses was completely reversed. The following chapters are based principally on this material but experience was also drawn from many external cases in which pathological opinions were sought including accession to the Ear, Nose and Throat Tumour Registry. Table 11.1 classifies the internal cases seen and treated in the associated Royal National Throat, Nose and Ear Hospital between the beginning of 1948 and the end of 1974. This does give some measure of the relative frequency of the various types of tumours but, because of the selection factor in a specialized Institute, the figures will not necessarily relate to the experience of a pathologist working in a general hospital. All 'tumours' encountered in Ear, Nose and Throat practice are not necessarily true neoplasms but certain lesions have been

Table 11.1 Tumours of the nose and sinuses. I.L.O. material

Histological type	Totals	Nose	Sinuses
Epithelial origin:			
Squamous papilloma	283	283	–
Transitional type papilloma	200	200	–
Squamous carcinoma	116	34	82
Transitional carcinoma	52	10	42
Anaplastic carcinoma	44	6	38
Melanotic tumours	43	42	1
Ameloblastic tumours	4	–	4
Mucosal gland tumours:			
Tubulocystic adenoma	2	1	1
Microcystic papillary adenoma	17	13	4
Simple adenocarcinoma	15	4	11
Mucoepidermoid tumour	7	2	5
Pleomorphic tumour	4	4	–
Cribriform adenocarcinoma	14	1	13
Basal cell tumour (malignant)	1	–	1
Vascular origin:			
Haemangioma	149	148	1
Angiosarcoma	1	1	–
Haemangiopericytoma	2	2	–
Juvenile angiofibroma	14	14	–
Lymphoreticular origin:			
Malignant lymphoma	10	4	6
Plasmacytoma	7	6	1
Neurogenic origin:			
Neurilemmoma	5	4	1
Neurofibroma	1	1	–
Olfactory neuroblastoma	2	2	–
Meningioma	1	–	1
Nasal 'glioma'	2	2	–
Common connective tissue origin:			
Fibrosarcoma	5	–	5
Fibrous histiocytoma (malignant)	2	–	2
Chondroma	1	1	–
Chrondrosarcoma	3	–	3
Osteoma	23	–	23
Osteoid osteoma	1	–	1
Osteogenic sarcoma	6	1	5
Muscular origin:			
Rhabdomyosarcoma	4	3	1
Leiomyosarcoma	2	1	1
Total	1043	790	253

included in the Table (e.g. juvenile angiofibroma) for the sake of completeness. Table 11.2 shows the proportion of nasal and paranasal tumours and the distribution between benign and malignant varieties. Table 11.3

Table 11.2 Tumours of the nose and sinuses

Location	Total	Benign	Malignant	B/M
Nasal cavity	790	672	118	5.7:1
Paranasal sinuses	253	33	220	1:6.7
Totals	1043	705	338	

Table 11.3 Tumours of the nose and sinuses

Location	Total	Epithelial	Non-epithelial	E/non-E
Nasal cavity	790	600	190	3.15:1
Paranasal sinuses	253	202	51	3.96:1
Totals	1043	802	241	

indicates the relative frequency of epithelial and non-epithelial tumours which differ slightly between the nasal and paranasal regions due to the high incidence of vascular tumours in the nasal cavity.

Soft tissue tumours may not infrequently present as 'nasal polypi' and distinction from the simple oedematous polypoid mucosa may only be established after histological examination when various neoplasms such as transitional type papilloma, carcinoma, malignant melanoma or plasmacytoma may be revealed. It should be emphasized that all tissues removed from the nose and sinuses be submitted for histology.

Inevitably, there are boderline diseases, especially in the skeletal system, which present clinically as tumour-like lesions (reparative granuloma) or may occasionally develop into neoplasms (Paget's Disease and Fibrous Dysplasia) or may be the subject of pathogenic dispute (Giant cell lesions and ossifying fibroma). Consideration of such diseases is clearly relevant to the study of fibro-osseous lesions in the region.

Where possible, under the heading of behaviour, survival patterns of malignant tumours are given. In so far as they are not precisely related to varying forms of treatment, only crude survival rates are presented with the object of giving the pathologist a general impression of behavioural characteristics.

Classification of tumours of the region under consideration inevitably involves nomenclature which is always a divisive factor. During the past decade, a subcommittee of the World Health Organization has considered terminology of tumours in the various anatomical regions and, in 1978, the International Reference Centre published their conclusions on tumours of the upper respiratory tract. The terminology used in the present work largely coincides with that of the W.H.O. but there

are a few differences which are indicated in the classification presented in Table 11.4.

Table 11.4 Classification of tumours of the nose and sinuses

Present authors	International reference centre
Epithelial origin:	
Squamous papilloma	Squamous papilloma
Transitional type papilloma	'Transitional' papilloma (Inverted and exophytic types)
Squamous carcinoma	Squamous carcinoma
Transitional carcinoma	'Transitional' carcinoma
Anaplastic carcinoma	{ Spindle cell carcinoma { Undifferentiated carcinoma
Ameloblastoma	Ameloblastoma
Ameloblastic fibroma	
Mucosal gland tumours:	
Tubulo-cystic adenoma	Oxyphilic adenoma
Microcystic papillary adenoma	'Transitional' papilloma
Eosinophilic granular cell tumour	Oxyphilic adenoma
Simple adenocarcinoma	{ Adenocarcinoma { Mucinous adenocarcinoma
Acinic cell tumour	{ Acinar cell adenocarcinoma { Clear cell adenocarcinoma
Muco-epidermoid tumour	Muco-epidermoid carcinoma
Pleomorphic tumour	Pleomorphic adenoma
Cribriform adenocarcinoma	Adenoid cystic carcinoma
Basal cell tumour	
Malignant melanoma	Malignant melanoma
Juvenile melanoma	
Vascular origin:	
Haemangioma	{ Haemangioma { Angiogranuloma
Angiosarcoma	Angiosarcoma
Haemangiopericytoma	Haemangiopericytoma
Chemodectoma	Paraganglioma
Glomus tumour	
Lymphoreticular origin:	
Malignant lymphoma	Malignant lymphoma
Hodgkin's disease	Hodgkin's disease
Plasmacytoma	Plasmacytoma
Neurogenic origin:	
Neurilemmoma or Schwannoma	Neurilemmoma
Neurofibroma	Neurofibroma
Olfactory neuroblastoma	Olfactory neurogenic tumour
Neuroepithelioma	Esthesioneuroepithelioma
Neurocytoma	Esthesioneurocytoma
Meningioma	Meningioma
Nasal 'glioma'	Nasal glial heterotopia
Common connective tissue origin:	
Fibrosarcoma	{ Fibrosarcoma { Fibromatosis
Myxoma	Myxoma
Malignant fibrous histiocytoma	Malignant fibro-xanthoma
Lipoma	Lipoma
Liposarcoma	Liposarcoma
Chondroma	Chondroma

Table 11.4 Classification of tumours of the nose and sinuses

Present authors	International reference centre
Chondrosarcoma	Chondrosarcoma
Mesenchymal chondrosarcoma	
Chondromyxoid fibroma	
Osteoma	Osteoma
Ossifying fibroma	{ Ossifying fibroma { Cementifying fibroma
Osteoid osteoma	
Benign osteoblastoma	
Osteogenic sarcoma	Osteosarcoma
Muscular origin:	
Rhabdomyosarcoma	Rhabdomyosarcoma
Embryonal	Embryonal
Alveolar	Alveolar
Pleomorphic	Pleomorphic
Leiomyoma	Leiomyoma
Leiomyosarcoma	Leiomyosarcoma

12

Papillomas of the nose and sinuses

PAPILLOMATA OF THE NOSE AND SINUSES

Benign epithelial tumours of the nasal region have been the subject of controversy since their first recognition. Relevant factors have been lack of histological correlation, confusion between simple polyps and papillomas on the one hand and between papillomas and carcinomas on the other. An early distinction between hard and soft lesions (Hopmann, 1883) presaged the present day subdivision into tumours of the vestibule (lined by skin) and tumours arising in the nasal or paranasal mucosa. The former are dismissed by most writers as being identical with the common wart of the skin whilst the latter were designated 'true papillomas' by Kramer and Som (1935). Following the sequestration of the vestibular group, interest became centred on the mucosal lesions whose variable histological characteristics have led to widely differing opinions.

Ringertz (1938) divided the nasal papillomas into squamous and those exhibiting cylindrical or transitional epithelium. This corresponds more or less to cutaneous and mucosal origin and has been adopted in the present discussion.

SQUAMOUS PAPILLOMA OF THE VESTIBULE

Terminology

Although many of these lesions bear a considerable resemblance to the common cutaneous wart, they are more frequently referred to as papillomas or hyperkeratotic papillomas. In so far as they have not yet been proved to be a uniform group from an aetiological point of view, the use of the label wart cannot always be justified and for the present the term papilloma is preferable.

Indicence

This tumour is the commonest in the nasal region. In the I.L.O. material it represents over one-third of all neoplasms in the nasal cavity.

Clinical features

The age distribution is broadly based but with a peak in middle age. In the I.L.O. material there was a predominance of females though, to some extent, this may reflect cosmetic concern rather than aetiological significance. The tumour commonly presents as a small cauliflower-like swelling in the nostril, usually less than a centimetre in diameter. It is usually solitary but occasionally bilateral tumours are encountered.

Histopathology

The microscopical picture is that of an exophytic squamous proliferation in which all the normal layers of the skin are represented, usually with marked hyperkeratosis (Fig. 12.1). The basal layer of the epithelium may exhibit some degree of dysplasia and suspicions of malignancy may have to be allayed against the background of the general histological pattern and the age of the patient. In the stratum spinosum the nuclei often show great activity, characterized by their large size, pale staining and prominence of nucleoli. The latter may be greatly enlarged, eosinophilic, irregular and sometimes multiple giving an appearance of intranuclear inclusion bodies but basophilic inclusions are not often seen. Occasional cells may show cytoplasmic vacuoles and there is usually a well marked stratum granulosum with prominent keratohyaline granules. An abundance of keratin is to be found on the surface and parakeratosis may be present.

Electron microscopical observations reveal typical squamous cells with their multiple desmosomal attachments and tonofibrils (Fig. 12.2). Solitary, intranuclear virus-like particles are not infrequently seen though their interpretation is debatable but occasionally an organized pattern is found (Fig. 12.3).

Aetiology and pathogenesis

Although the vestibular papillomata are accepted as a separate group (Snyder and Perzin, 1972) it is not necessarily a homogeneous one of viral origin, as has been generally assumed (Henriksson, 1952). Readily identifiable virus particles have only been found in a

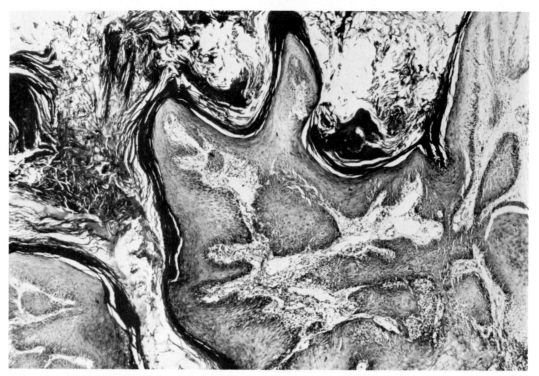

Fig. 12.1 Hyperkeratotic papilloma arising on the septum of a 39 year-old female. M ×55

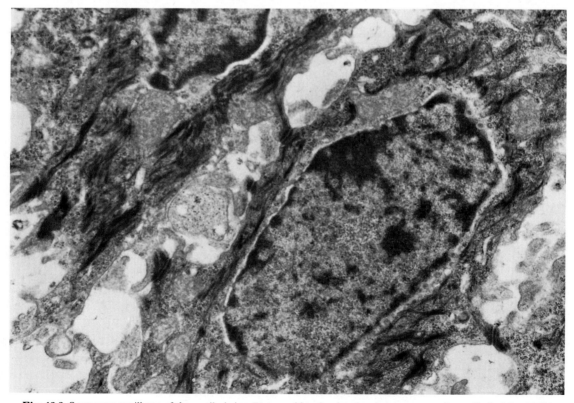

Fig. 12.2 Squamous papilloma of the vestibule in a 51 year-old male, showing desmosomes and tonofibrils. M ×17 500

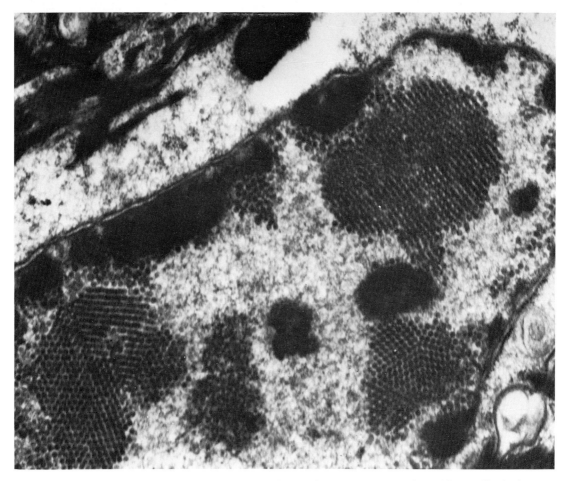

Fig. 12.3 Squamous papilloma of the vestibule in a 24 year-old male, showing intranuclear virus with crystalline lattice structure. M ×25 600

small proportion of cases. In the I.L.O. material, intranuclear viral bodies were found forming a 'crystalline lattice' in 27 per cent of cases. The interpretation of positive findings is impeded by the absence of a suitable experimental technique for reproducing the human wart. It seems likely that some vestibular papillomas are of viral origin whilst others are not. In this context, it is of interest to note that the age distribution of viral warts on the hands shows a peak in the second decade (Barr and Coles, 1970) which contrasts with the maximum in nasal lesions. The occasional multiple lesion is certainly consistent with viral origin but the possibility of other aetiological agents cannot be excluded.

Behaviour

No precise information is available regarding the natural history of these lesions. It is possible that some may undergo spontaneous regression after the manner of some cutaneous warts in other locations. Those cases

presenting at clinics almost invariably have their tumour excised and recurrence is almost unknown. Malignant change is so rare that such a diagnosis would suggest a mistaken initial assessment.

TRANSITIONAL TYPE PAPILLOMA

Introduction

The earliest description of this mucosal lesion was by Billroth (1855) in his monograph on mucous polyps and one of his drawings was a very accurate portrayal of the histological structure as we see it today. At that time, however, he labelled it as a 'villous carcinoma' and described another case as an earlier stage in its development.

Terminology

A considerable variety of names have been applied to

this lesion since Kramer and Som (1935) introduced the term 'true papilloma of the nasal cavity'. These include 'cylindrical' or 'transitional cell papilloma' (Ringertz, 1938), 'transitional cell papilloma' (Osborn, 1956), 'inverting papilloma' (Norris, 1963; Trible and Lekagul, 1971), 'inverted papilloma' (Lampertico, Russell and MacComb, 1963; Oberman, 1964; Fechner and Alford, 1968; Hyams, 1971). In his description of the development of these tumours, Ringertz (1938) used the word inverted as being synonymous with infolding. Unfortunately, the term was seized upon by other writers who interpreted it literally as the antonym of everted, as applied to the exophytic squamous papilloma and, in logical consequence, expressions such as 'downgrowth' and even 'invasion' have been used by some authors with resulting confusion. The term inverted papilloma as used by some of its protagonists may be justly regarded as a genuine attempt to emphasize the infolded character of the epithelial proliferation but misinterpretation is clearly unavoidable. In naming this lesion one may refer to either the character or the behaviour of the epithelium. The present authors have retained the former mode, using the expression 'transitional type' in order to eliminate the erroneous impression of origin from a 'transitional cell' which does not exist as an entity. If it is thought desirable to emphasize the growth pattern rather than the structure of the epithelium then the tumour would be better referred to as an 'introverted papilloma'.

Incidence

This tumour is frequently described as uncommon or even rare. Snyder and Perzin (1972) found 39 cases of 'papillomatosis' over a period of 29 years and during the same period 2204 patients were seen with simple nasal polyps. Clairmont, Wright, Rooker and Butz (1974) estimated that intransal papillomata represented 0.04 per cent of all nasal biopsies. In the context of Ear, Nose and Throat practice the transitional type papilloma is, in fact, more common than the above mentioned figures would suggest. In the I.L.O. material, this tumour accounted for 25 per cent of tumours of the nasal cavity and 19 per cent of all tumours in the nose and sinuses.

Clinical features

In table 12.1 it can be seen that the age distribution has a peak in the sixth decade. This series of 200 cases also showed a male predominance of 5:1. Other published

Table 12.1 Age distribution of transitional type papilloma in 200 I.L.O. cases

Decade	2	3	4	5	6	7	8	9
No.	4	9	21	50	60	39	16	1

data (Brown, 1964; Snyder and Perzin, 1972) show general concurrence with these findings.

The patients usually present with nasal obstruction which may be accompanied by some discharge, usually watery in character. The lesions are polypoid in appearance and may present at the anterior nares. A more solid consistency and a greater tendency to bleed following avulsion may lead the surgeon to suspect that he is dealing with something more than a simple polyp.

Anatomical site of origin

Although commonly unilateral these lesions tend to have a somewhat diffuse origin which has led to the not infrequent use of the term 'nasal papillomatosis' (Kramer and Som, 1935; Snyder and Perzin, 1972). In the I.L.O. material, the nasal cavity was always involved and the paranasal sinuses in about 25 per cent. In the nasal cavity, the lateral wall was known to be involved in more than half the cases but the nasal septum was affected in only about eight per cent. Bilateral involvement was uncommon (four per cent). The reported incidence of septal involvement varies greatly. Hyams (1971) found approximately 50 per cent but the discrepancy is probably due to differences in selection between a diagnostic reference and a treatment centre in which the latter must clearly furnish a closer approximation to the truth. As regards paranasal origin, maxillary and ethmoidal sinuses are commonly involved but the frontal and sphenoid sinuses much less frequently.

Gross appearance

Because of the frequent resemblance to simple polyps, the diagnosis may not be suspected in many cases until microscopy is performed. In some cases, however, the tissue may have a more solid appearance and consistency (Fig. 12.4) and occasionally the cut surface may reveal, even to the naked eye, the infolded structure (Fig. 12.5).

Histopathology

Epithelial proliferation leads inevitably to an increase in surface area which is accommodated most readily by infolding into the soft oedematous stroma (Fig. 12.6) and continuing invagination may reduce the connective tissue element to narrow slits between the epithelial masses (Fig. 12.7). The deep infolding may often give a false impression of downgrowth whilst the original surface cells, which may degenerate, come to lie at the centres of apparently isolated masses thereby producing the picture of pseudocentral necrosis (Fig. 12.8). The epithelial structural pattern is essentially that of proliferation and metaplasia, producing a characteristic spectrum that ranges from pseudostratified columnar

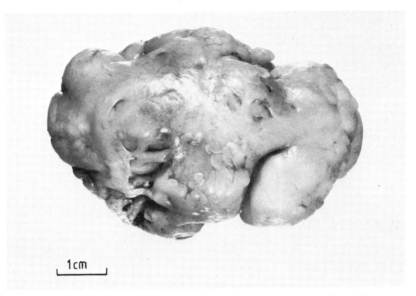

Fig. 12.4 Transitional type papilloma of the nose in a 54 year-old male, showing solid consistency.

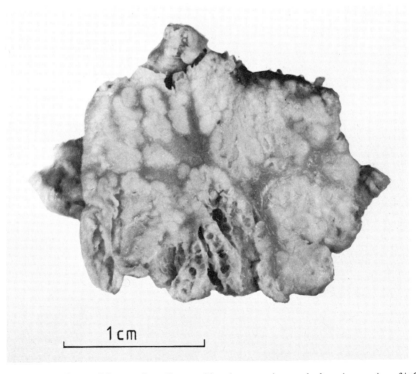

Fig. 12.5 Transitional type papilloma of the nose in a 65 year-old male presenting a naked eye impression of infolded epithelium.

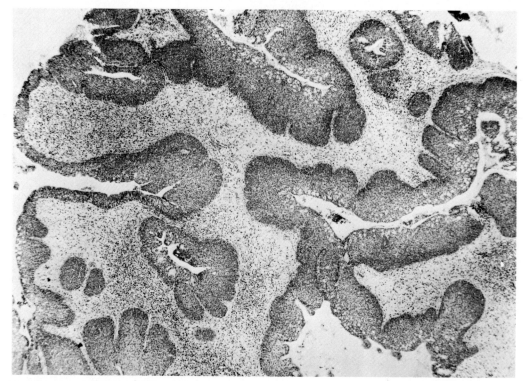

Fig. 12.6 Transitional type papilloma of the nose in a 69 year-old male, showing infolding into the stroma. M × 35

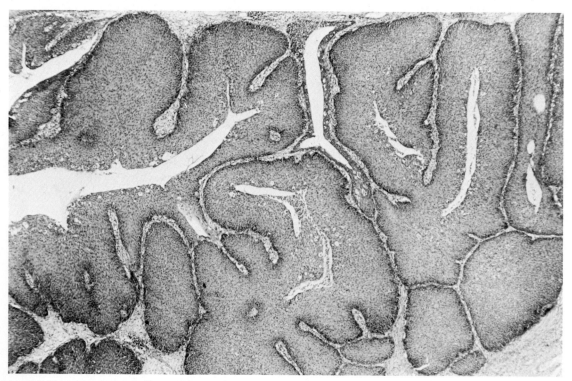

Fig. 12.7 Transitional type papilloma of the nose in a 66 year-old male, showing marked reduction of the stroma by infolding of the epithelium. M × 90

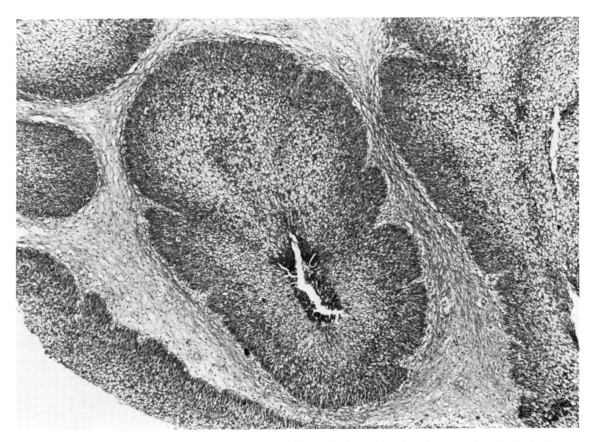

Fig. 12.8 Transitional type papilloma of the nose showing infolded epithelium which gives the impression of isolated cell mass with pseudocentral necrosis. M × 90

through true statified columnar and transitional type to completely metaplastic squamous epithelium. In consequence, a commonly seen pattern is that of transitional type epithelium (Fig. 12.9) and the expression has been adopted as an all-embracing term to indicate the epithelial character of these tumours.

The proliferated epithelium, more particularly in the asbence of complete squamous metaplasia, often contains numerous spaces presenting a 'moth-eaten' appearance (Fig. 12.10). Some of these spaces are due to incarcerated goblet cells but many are intercellular and often contain polymorphonuclear leucocytes which commonly infiltrate the epithelium. Occasionally, pseudostratification is maintained and epithelial proliferation merely contributes to the increase in surface area with consequent infolding. Such areas could be justly called cylindrical type but the pattern is quite different from that described by Hyams (1971) under this heading. Everywhere the basement membrane remains intact and, apart from the progressive changes in orientation of the cells occasioned by metaplasia, there is no significant disturbance of

polarity. The basal cells not infrequently exhibit minor degrees of anisonucleosis with hyperchromatism and varying numbers of normal mitoses. The stroma varies greatly in amount according to the degree of invagination and its substance may be largely oedematous, fibrous or chronic inflammatory whilst eosinophil infiltration is not uncommon. Occasionally, there may be small areas of exophytic growth with hyperkeratosis, resembling that seen in the vestibular papillomas though such appearances have been found to be without clinical significance.

The tumour mass may cause pressure erosion of bone and the invaginating faculty may result in the insertion of epithelium between bony trabeculae, giving a superficial impression of invasion (Fig. 12.11). It is this feature which accounts for the surgeon's impression of invasive tendency at operation.

Another structural variant which requires special mention relates particularly to the septal area. Papillomas arising on the septum do not usually exhibit the deep infolding seen in other locations and there is a notable

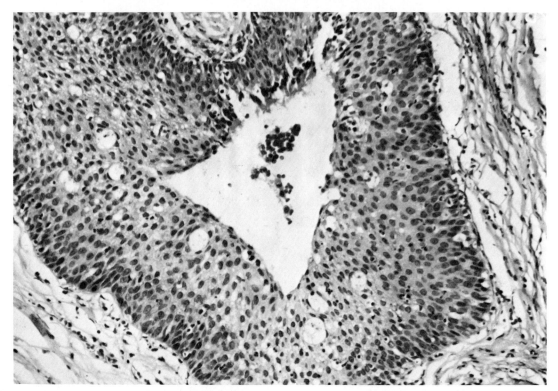

Fig. 12.9 Transitional type papilloma of the nose in a 57 year-old male. Infolded epithelium showing transitional differentiation. M × 230

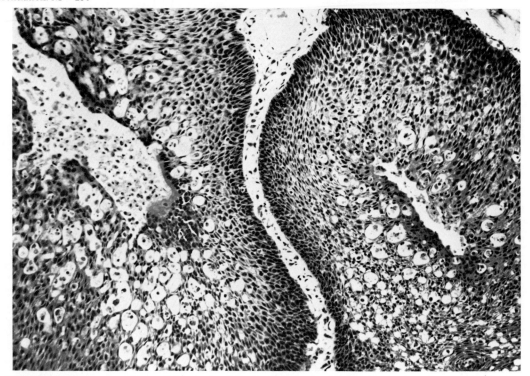

Fig. 12.10 Transitional type papilloma of the nose in a 54 year-old male, showing 'moth-eaten' appearance due to numerous intercellular spaces. M × 168

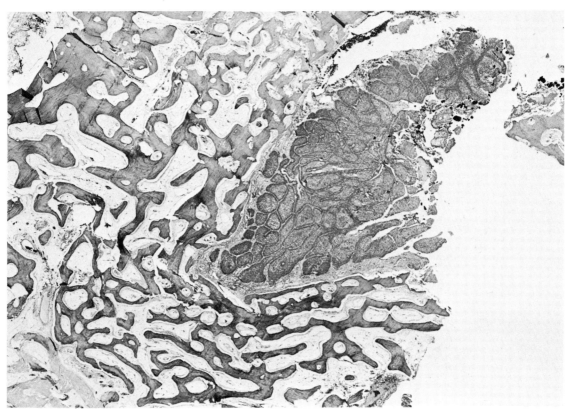

Fig. 12.11 Transitional type papilloma of the nose in a 51 year-old male. Proliferative infolding of epithelium causing pressure erosion of bone and simulating invasion. M ×17.5

tendency to outfolded or exophytic type of growth of distinctly smaller dimensions. The proliferated epithelium tends to assume transitional type structure but keratinization is uncommon (Fig. 12.12). Oberman (1964) referred to such lesions simply as septal papillomas whilst Hyams (1971) used the term 'fungiform' to denote this exophytic growth which, in his material, was almost exclusive to the septum. The significance of this pattern is debatable because (a) infolded structure is not excluded from septal growths, (b) outfolded patterns are found in other locations, including the marginal zone between the vestibule and the nasal cavity proper, (c) cases of septal involvement may have intranasal lesions in other locations and (d) there does not appear to be any significant behavioural difference between the infolded and outfolded pattern. Deep invagination will be restricted in areas where the surface epithelium is more firmly bound to underlying structures when a mixed picture of infolding and outfolding is encountered (Fig. 12.13). The rarity of simple polyps in the septal region is undoubtedly a reflection of greater structural rigidity in this site. In the view of the present authors, although septal growths may be identifiable on structural

grounds, the difference in growth pattern has no practical significance and is occasioned largely by local conditions.

The electron microscopical picture varies according to the degree of metaplasia. Many cells may be seen in a clearly transitional phase with fewer desmosomes and a relative dearth of tonofibrils whilst intercellular boundaries may be marked by interdigitating processes which separate to facilitate the infiltration by polymorphonuclear leucocytes.

Aetiology and pathogenesis
It was the variegated epithelial pattern which led Tobeck (1929) to subdivide nasal papillomas into four groups but such a classification has no practical significance and merely represents variation on the theme of metaplasia which very readily occurs in the upper respiratory tract.

Although the weight of opinion has been and still is in favour of a neoplastic process, a contrary view was held by some writers (Eggston and Wolff, 1947; Lehman, 1949) who described the lesion as a 'papillary sinusitis' in which epithelial hyperplasia resulted from a virus infection. However, no convincing evidence of viral

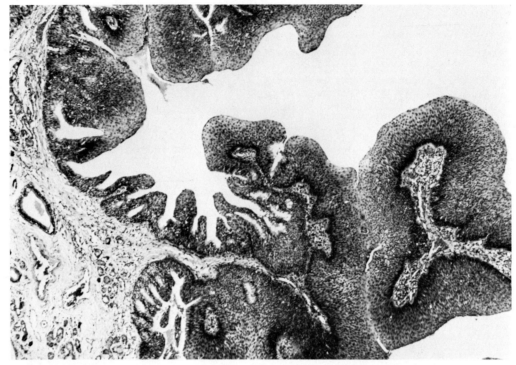

Fig. 12.12 Transitional type papilloma of the nose in a 58 year-old male, showing extroverted septal growth. M ×55

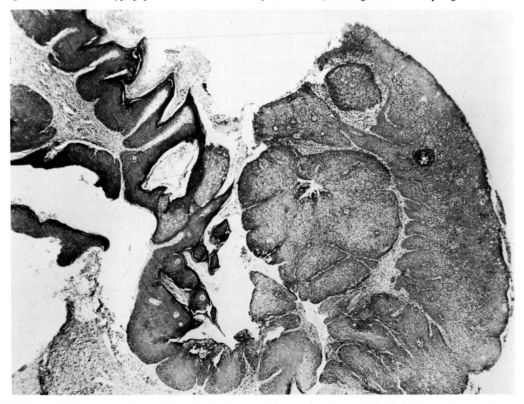

Fig. 12.13 Transitional type papilloma of the nose in a 51 year-old male, showing combined infolding and exophytic growth with keratinization. M ×35

involvement has yet been produced. Henriksson (1952) reported negative results following inoculation of rats with an ultrafiltrate from human papillomas. Gaito, Gaylord and Hilding (1965) also failed to demonstrate any evidence of viral activity either by electron microscopical studies or by inoculation of material from papillomas into tissue culture cells. The claim of Jarvi (1944) to have found inclusion bodies was unconvincing and irrelevant since the tissue demonstrated was manifestly not that of the tumour under discussion. Isolated, intranuclear, virus-like particles have been seen in the present authors' material but the crystalline pattern occasionally seen in the squamous papilloma has not, so far, been encountered and the difficulties of interpretation leave the problem unresolved.

No occupational clue to a possible environmental agent has been noted but it is not without interest that Herrold (1964) was successful in inducing papillomas in the nasal region of Syrian hamsters following the administration of diethyl nitrosamine by various routes. The papillomas bore a resemblance to the human variety in so far as they exhibited squamous metaplasia and marked infolding and her results seemed to indicate a specific sensitivity of the nasal mucosa to the oncogenic agent.

Behaviour

The transitional type or introverted papilloma presents two aspects of practical importance. Firstly, the notable tendency to recur after local removal and, secondly, occasional malignant change.

Experience based on the I.L.O. material reveals that more than one-third of the cases (including three with septal lesions) have exhibited recurrence which was not infrequently multiple and was probably underestimated because of the frequency with which removal of 'polyps' had previously been carried out without histological examination (27 per cent). The greater number of cases had one or two recurrences only but in a few the event was repeated on many occasions and, in all, covering a period of many years with a quite unpredictable pattern. Except in the event of malignant change, the histological picture shows no significant alteration. An increase in the infolding with consequent reduction of the stroma leading to greater solidity is not uncommon in recurrent tumours but, *per se*, does not have any sinister implication.

On the subject of malignant change, the issue has been confused by the application of different criteria. The simultaneous finding of a papilloma and a carcinoma at the first histological examination is a not uncommon experience (Reuys, 1932; Ringertz, 1938; Osborn, 1956 and 1970; Norris, 1963; Marcial-Rojas and DeLeon, 1963; Hyams, 1971; Snyder and Perzin, 1972). Whilst such an observation constitutes strong circumstantial evidence it is not proof. Furthermore, alleged microscopical evidence of malignant transformation should be regarded with caution against the background of apparent difficulties in distinguishing between a papilloma and a carcinoma of similar structure (Brown, 1964; Cummings and Goodman, 1970). The only unequivocal evidence of malignant change is provided by long term observation with histological control. Four previously published cases (Hellman, 1897; Saxén, 1924, Kramer and Som, 1935; Ringertz, 1938) which appeared to meet these criteria were reviewed by one of us (Osborn, 1956) and to these may be added three cases published respectively by Mabery, Devine and Harrison (1965), Worgan and Hooper (1970), Snyder and Perzin (1972). The case reported by Fechner and Alford (1968) could well be included although the period of histological control was only one year and validity rests on the claim that the whole tumour was examined at the time of the first biopsy.

In the I.L.O. material, four out of 200 cases have undergone malignant change whilst under controlled observation, intervals ranging from five to twenty years. This total of twelve cases may be related to between 700 and 800 changes of papilloma published in the literature of the Western World, giving an incidence of between 1.5 and 2.0 per cent which approximates to the present authors' experience. There is no gainsaying that malignancy can supervene in this type of papilloma but overall experience does not suggest that the lesion is necessarily premalignant. In view of the massive increase in epithelial surface, it is likely that the incidence reflects the greater amount of epithelium at risk.

Papillomas undergoing malignant change show increased nuclear irregularity and disorientation of cells (Figs. 12.14, 12.15, 12.16 & 12.17), whilst invasive elements often show metaplasia to squamous carcinoma. It is essential that all material from this type of papilloma should be examined histologically in toto and that a follow-up system be maintained.

BIBLIOGRAPHY

Barr A, Coles R B 1970 Viral warts. British Journal of Hospital Medicine 3: 831–835

Billroth T 1855 Über den Bau der Schleimpolypen. G. Reimer (Berlin)

Brown B 1964 The papillomatous tumours of the nose. Journal of Laryngology and Otology 78: 889–905

Clairmont A A, Wright R E, Rooker D T, Butz W C 1974 Papillomas of the nasal and paranasal cavities. Southern Medical Journal 68: 41–45

Cummings C W, Goodman M L 1970 Inverted papillomas of the nose and paranasal sinuses. Archives of Otolaryngology 92: 445–449

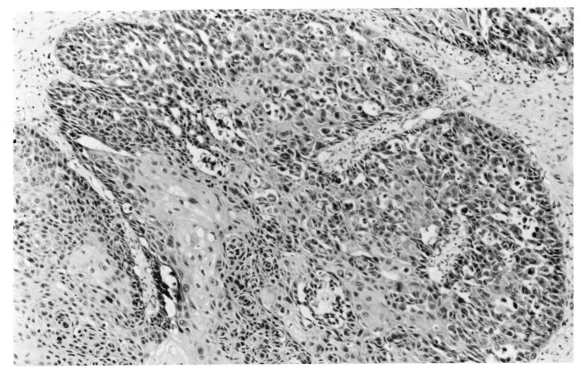

Fig. 12.14 Malignant change in a transitional type papilloma of the nose in a 66 year-old male (see Fig. 12.7), showing development of a squamoid element. M × 90

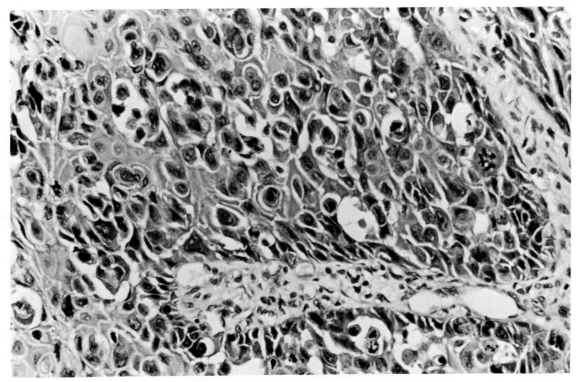

Fig. 12.15 Malignant change in a transitional type papilloma of the nose in a 66 year-old male. Higher magnification of Fig. 12.14, showing disturbed polarity. M × 225

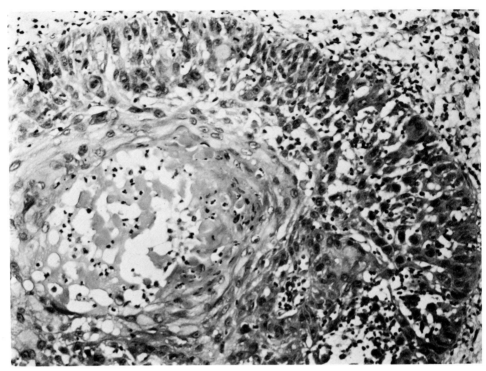

Fig. 12.16 Malignant change in a transitional type papilloma of the nose in a 78 year-old male, 19 years after the initial diagnosis of papilloma. M × 195

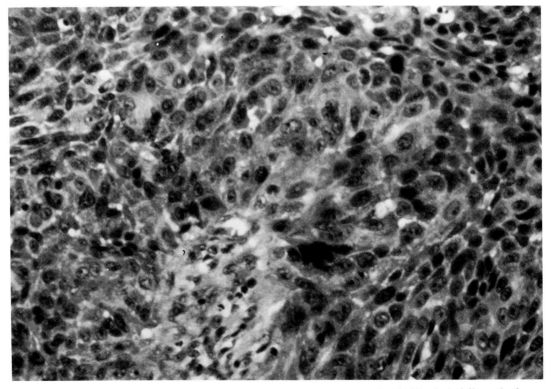

Fig. 12.17 Malignant change in a transitional type papilloma of the nose in a 75 year-old male. Histological diagnosis of transitional papilloma three years previously. M × 252

Eggston A A, Wolff D 1947 Histopathology of the ear, nose and throat. Williams and Wilkins, Baltimore, p 648 *et seq.*

Fechner R E, Alford D O 1968 Inverted papilloma and squamous carcinoma. Archives of Otolaryngology 88: 507–512

Gaito R A, Gaylord W H, Hilding D A 1965 Ultrastructure of a human papilloma. Laryngoscope 75: 144–152

Geschicter C F 1935 Tumours of the nasal and paranasal cavities. American Journal of Cancer 24: 637–660

Hellman L 1897 Papilloma durum der Nasen- und Stirnhohlenschleimhaut; Übergang in Carcinom; mit Rücksicht auf die Kasuistik des harten Papilloms. Archiv für Laryngologie und Rhinologie (Berlin) 6: 171–192

Henriksson N G 1952 Papillomas of the nose: a clinical survey and contribution to our knowledge of these tumours. Acta Otolaryngologica 42: 18–29

Herrold K M 1964 Epithelial papillomas of the nasal cavity. Archives of Pathology 78: 189–195

Hopmann L 1883 Die papillären Geschwülste der Nasenschleimhaut. Virchows Archiv für pathologische Anatomie 93: 213–258

Hyams V S 1971 Papillomas of the nasal cavity and paranasal sinuses. Annals of Otology, Rhinology and Laryngology 80: 192–206

Jarvi O 1944 Kieferhöhlenpapillom mit (virusbedingten) Cytoplasmeinschlüssen. Acta Otolaryngologia 32: 284–291

Kramer R, Som M L 1935 True papilloma of the nasal cavity. Archives of Otolaryngology 22: 22–43

Lampertico P, Russell W O, McComb W S 1963 Squamous papilloma of the upper respiratory epithelium. Archives of Pathology 75: 293–302

Lehman R H 1949 Papillary sinusitis. Annals of Otology, Rhinology and Laryngology 58: 507–511

Mabery T E, Devine K D, Harrison E G 1965 The problem of malignant transformation in a nasal papilloma. Archives of Otolaryngology 82: 296–300

Marcial-Rojas R A, DeLeon E 1963 Epithelial papilloma of the nose and accessory sinuses. Archives of Otolaryngology 77: 634–639

Norris H J 1963 Papillary leisons of the nasal cavity and paranasal sinuses; part II, inverting papilloma. Laryngoscope 73: 1–17

Oberman H A 1964 Papillomas of the nose and paranasal sinuses. American Journal of Clinical Pathology 42: 245–258

Osborn D A 1956 Transitional cell growths of the upper respiratory tract. Journal of Laryngology and Otology 70: 574–588

Osborn D A 1970 Nature and behaviour of transitional tumours in the upper respiratory tract. Cancer 25: 50–60

Reuys H 1932 Über Fibroepitheliome und ihre Beziehung zu den papillären Carcinomen. Zeitschrift für Hals-, Nasen- und Ohrenheilkunde 30: 421–432

Ringertz N 1938 Pathology of malignant tumours arising in the nasal and paranasal cavities and the maxilla. Acta Otolaryngologica, Supplement 27, chapter 4, p 31–42

Saxén A 1924 Über die pathologische Anatomie der von der Nasenkavität und der Kieferhöhle ausgehenden Karzinome und Papillome. Acta Otolaryngologica 6: 543–554

Snyder R N, Perzin K H 1972 Papillomatosis of the nasal cavity and paranasal sinuses (inverted papilloma, squamous papilloma). Cancer 30: 668–690

Tobeck A 1929 Beiträge zur Kenntnis der sogenannten harten Papillome der Nase. Beiträge zur Anatomie, Physiologie, Pathologie und Therapie des Ohres 27: 432–442

Trible W M, Lekagur S 1971 Inverting papilloma of the nose and paranasal sinuses. Laryngoscope 81: 663–668

Worgan D, Hooper R 1970 Malignancy in nasal papillomata. Journal of Laryngology and Otology 84: 309–316

KERATOACANTHOMA

This cutaneous lesion, otherwise known as *Molluscum Sebaceum*, has been recognized for nearly a hundred years, being first described by Hutchinson (1889) as a 'crateriform ulcer of the face'. Subsequently, it was noted that certain skin lesions regarded as squamous carcinoma were self-healing (Dunn and Smith, 1934).

The lesion occurs predominantly in the head and neck region (Beare, 1953; Fisher, Morgan, McCoy and Wechster, 1972). Beare (1953) found 18 out of 76 cases involving the skin of the nose of which three affected the tip. In the I.L.O. material there was one case involving the tip of the nose, ultimately developing into a massive lesion. Rapaport (1975) reported a giant keratoacanthoma of the nose.

The age incidence is essentially in adult life, the majority occurring within the fourth to the sixth decades (Rook and Whimster, 1950). The condition occurs predominantly in males.

Keratoacanthoma presents as a dome-shaped lesion with a rought surface due to the presence of keratin.

There may be histological difficulties in distinguishing the lesion from a squamous carcinoma and two essential points have to be considered:

1. The clinical history in which the keratoacanthoma develops more rapidly than a squamous carcinoma (a matter of weeks rather than months)
2. The lesion must be bisected so that the characteristic keratin-filled crater can be seen in a section with its superficial covering of a relatively normal layer of squamous epithelium.

The sides and base often contain epidermoid 'cysts' which open into the crater (Fig. 12.18). The basement membrane may be intact but the epithelium may appear to be broken up by inflammatory infiltration and irregular projections may mimic squamous carcinoma although cellular atypia are much less common in keratoacanthoma.

MacCormac and Scarff (1936) reported ten cases under the title of Moluscum Sebaceum and expressed the view that the lesion was due to inflammatory and

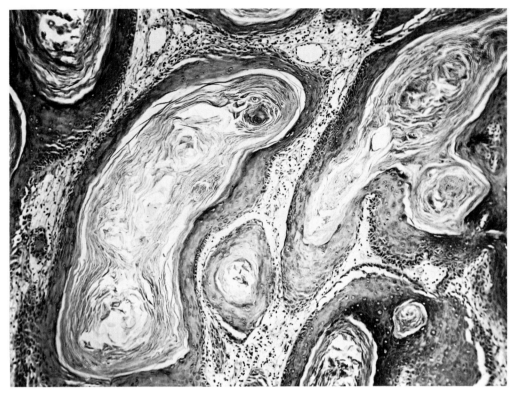

Fig. 12.18 Keratoacanthoma of the nose in a 53 year-old male. M ×65

hyperplastic changes in so-called sebaceous cysts. Nevertheless, there are persistent differences of opinion on the precise nature of the lesion. Most observers appear to have accepted the condition as benign (Fouracres and Whittick, 1953; Bowman and Pinkus, 1955; Calnan and Haber, 1959). On the other hand, Kwitten (1975) believes that the lesion is essentially malignant although he admits that the condition may exhibit self-healing.

BIBLIOGRAPHY

Beare J M 1953 Molluscum sebaceum. British Journal of Surgery 41 : 167–172

Bowman H E, Pinkus H 1955 Keratoacanthoma (molluscum sebaceum). Archives of Pathology 60 : 19–25

Calnan C D, Haber H 1959 Molluscum sebaceum. Journal of Pathology and Bacteriology 69 : 61–66

Dunn J S, Smith J F 1934 Self-healing primary squamous carcinoma of the skin. British Journal of Dermatology and Syphilis 46 : 519–523

Fisher E R, Morgan M, McCoy H, Wechster H L 1972 Analysis of histopathologic and electron microscopic determinants of keratoacanthoma and squamous carcinoma. Cancer 29 : 1387–1397

Fouracres F A, Whittick J W 1953 The relationship of molluscum sebaceum (keratoacanthoma) to spontaneously healing epithelioma of the skin. Cancer 7 : 58–64

Hutchinson J 1889 Crateriform ulceration of the face. British Medical Journal 1 : 412–413

Kwitten J 1975 A histologic chronology of the clinical course of the keratocarcinoma (so-called keratoacanthoma). Archives of Dermatology 111 : 127–135

MacCormac H, Scarff R W 1936 Molluscum sebaceum. British Journal of Dermatology and Syphilis 48 : 624–626

Rapaport J 1975 Giant keratoacanthoma of the nose. Archives of Dermatology 111 : 73–75

Rook A, Whimster I 1950 La kerato-acanthome. Archives belges de Dermatologie et Syphilologie 6 : 137–146

13

Carcinoma of the surface epithelium (including ameloblastoma)

CARCINOMA OF THE NOSE AND SINUSES

Introduction

Medical records indicate the recognition of malignant disease of the nose throughout the nineteenth century although Cornil and Ranvier (1869) asserted that there was no well authenticated case of primary carcinoma of the nasal cavity. Bosworth (1889) reviewed 30 nasal tumours collected over a period of 45 years but while undoubtedly clinically malignant, many were not confirmed microscopically and were by no means all carcinomas. One was almost certainly a malignant melanoma (an error which could still be made today) and another could well have been an olfactory neuroblastoma. The case reported by Lawrence (1856) as having no microscopic evidence of malignancy was associated with considerable destruction of tissue suggesting the possibility of a non-healing granuloma. Bosworth's own case was probably a genuine carcinoma as judged by his camera lucida drawing although it could have been of paranasal rather than nasal origin. The confusion which surrounded earlier reports of carcinoma in this region only began to be resolved at the turn of the century and even then distinction between nasal and paranasal origin was rarely made.

Terminology

The many classifications which have appeared in the literature were based on histological subdivision. Kummel (1900) recognized squamous and cylindrical cell carcinoma. Citelli and Calamida (1903) noted a blending of these two histological types and introduced the term 'papillary' which has appeared in many subsequent classifications. The failure to separate the cylindrical cell type from adenocarcinoma persisted well into the present century (Harmer and Glas, 1907; Hautant, Monod and Klotz, 1933). The term transitional cell carcinoma was first introduced by Quick and Cutler (1927) and has suffered from a confused and controversial background in which the tumour was believed to have its origin in a mythical transitional cell. The modern interpretation merely indicates the resemblance to transitional type

epithelium (Osborn, 1970). The expression 'Schneiderian carcinoma' (Ewing, 1927) has no specific meaning beyond that of carcinoma involving the lining mucosa of the region. It was never clear how it related to other types of carcinoma and the term is now obsolete.

Incidence

Carcinoma of the nose and sinuses is relatively rare and in most geographical regions it is generally accepted as being less than one per cent of all malignant tumours in all sites. In the United Kingdom, deaths from cancer of the nose and sinuses has been found to be 0.2 per cent of all malignancies (Registrar General's Statistics, 1973). In the I.L.O. material, all types of carcinoma accounted for 24 per cent of all tumours in the nose and sinuses and 72 per cent of all malignant neoplasms in the region. A higher incidence of paranasal carcinoma has been observed amongst Africans (Keen, De Moor, Shapiro and Cohen, 1955) and in Mexico (Hendrick, 1958).

Clinical features

The age distribution in both nasal and paranasal carcinoma shows a peak in the sixth decade and, with the exception of the cribriform adenocarcinoma, there is no significant difference between the various histological types. The sex ratio shows a predominance of males, ranging from 1.5:1 in paranasal to 2:1 in nasal carcinomas.

Intranasal carcinoma usually presents with nasal obstruction, with or without attendant epistaxis or discharge. When anterior in origin, there may be visible or palpable swelling in the vestibule. Paranasal carcinomas are associated with nasal obstruction, discharge, epistaxis or epiphora whilst pain may be manifest in the later stages. In advanced cases, involvement of the anterior antral wall or the orbit may give rise to swelling of the cheek or proptosis respectively.

Anatomical site of origin

The commonest site of intranasal carcinoma is the vestibule, accounting for over 40 per cent. Goepfert, Guillamondegui, Jesse and Lindberg (1974) found that most vestibular carcinomas were in the midline, involving the septum or columella. About one quarter of intranasal carcinomas involve the septum and may often arise in the region of the muco-cutaneous junction (Deutsch, 1966). Less frequently, the lateral wall, including the turbinates, may be affected. The roof and floor of the nasal cavity are less commonly involved.

Carcinoma represents about 7 per cent of nasal but 75 per cent of paranasal tumours and although precise origin may sometimes be debatable, paranasal carcinomas are primarily antral in nearly 70 per cent. The remainder are largely ethmoidal (approximately 30 per cent) with an occasional carcinoma in the frontal sinus (1–2 per cent). The latter is often absent from published series of paranasal tumours though Lewis and Castro (1972) found six cases amongst 462 paranasal carcinomas, corresponding closely with the present authors' experience. Many individual cases have been reported but lack of detail has cast doubt on the authenticity of some (Osborn and Wallace, 1967). Sphenoidal carcinoma is extremely rare. Lewis and Castro (1972) found two cases whilst the I.L.O. material contained one example.

The common site of origin within the maxillary sinus is believed to be in the antro-ethmoidal angle since this region is frequently found to be involved at presentation.

Gross appearances

The naked eye features of carcinoma of this region vary considerably. Vestibular tumours often have the appearance of wart-like or fungating masses, tending to project from the anterior nares. Tumour masses in the nasal and paranasal cavities may often present, on removal, the appearances of thickened polypoid mucosa which is not obviously neoplastic and, usually, it is only in the larger specimens resulting from radical surgery that new growth is apparent to the unaided eye (Fig. 13.1). It cannot be emphasised too strongly that material removed from these regions and submitted for pathological examination is frequently unremarkable on gross inspection and only microscopy will confirm or eliminate malignant disease.

Histopathology

The various histological types may be classified as (a) squamous, (b) transitional, (c) anaplastic and (d) carcinoma of glandular origin or gland-like structure. Although it is maintained that some simple adenocarcinomas may be of surface origin, group (d) will be discussed as a whole under the heading of mucosal gland tumours (Chapter 14).

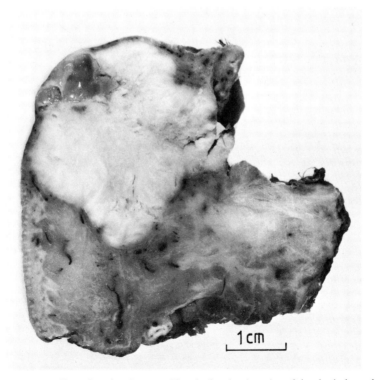

Fig. 13.1 Carcinoma of the maxillary sinus in a 71 year-old male showing invasion of the cheek through the anterior wall.

Squamous carcinoma is by far the commonest type, comprising about 63 per cent of nasal and 44 per cent of paranasal carcinomas. Vestibular tumours are exclusively squamous, as are the majority of those arising in the nasal septum. At least 50 per cent of antral carcinomas are squamous but only about 20 per cent of ethmoidal carcinomas are of this type. As in squamous carcinomas in other locations, there is a wide range of differentiation with varying degrees of keratin production and individual tumours show a mixed pattern with less well differentiated areas (Fig. 13.2) whilst necrosis is not uncommon.

Transitional carcinoma is less frequent but of greater interest and importance. It accounts for approximately 20 per cent of all carcinomas in the nose and sinuses and has been defined as exhibiting the form of transitional epithelium (Osborn, 1970). It includes the cylindrical type of Kummel (1900), Ringertz (1938) and many of those described as 'papillary', often with transition between the cylindrical and squamous type (Citelli and Calamida, 1903; Hautant et al., 1933).

Resemblance to the transitional type papilloma is readily apparent, the essential feature being the persist-ence of the basement membrane on a deeply infolded epithelium, often presenting a papillary or garland-like appearance (Fig. 13.3). As in the papilloma, a complete spectrum ranges from pure cylindrical to pure squamous structure. The distinction between the well differentiated transitional carcinoma and the transitional type papilloma may present diagnostic difficulties which can usually be resolved by careful evaluation,. The important distinguishing feature is the disorientation or disturbed polarity of the cells within the basement membrane (Figs. 13.4 & 13.5). Nuclear changes, unless of a gross nature, are liable to be misleading. The less well differentiated forms may show an extraordinary degree of de-differentiation within the basement membrane. They correspond to the transitional cell carcinoma of Quick and Cutler (1927) and possibly also to the Schneiderian carcinoma of Ewing (1927). Although much of the malignant activity appears to be intra-epithelial, invasion is always present and often assumes a squamoid structure. Nevertheless, the persistence of the basement membrane is a dominant feature which is readily discernable by both light and electron microscopy (Fig. 13.6) and would appear to have significance from

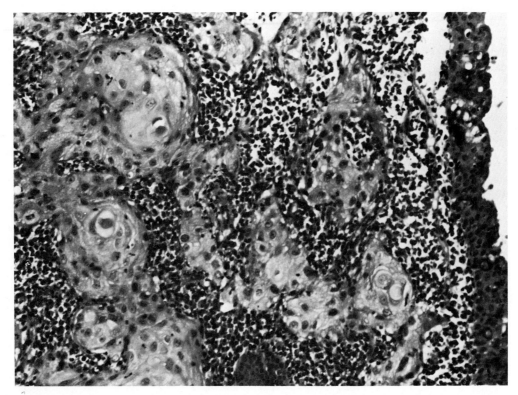

Fig. 13.2 Squamous carcinoma of the maxillary sinus in an 82 year-old male. Carcinoma in a 'nasal polyp'. M ×208

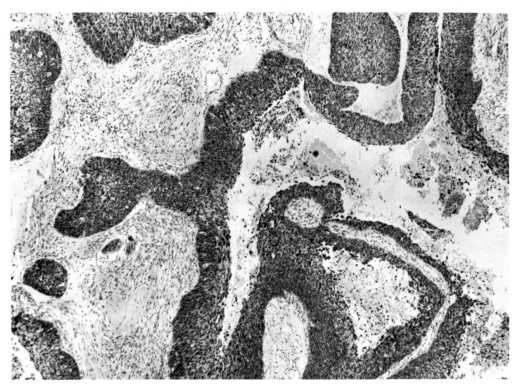

Fig. 13.3 Transitional carcinoma of the maxillary sinus in a 75 year-old female, showing infolding and persistence of the basement membrane. M ×56

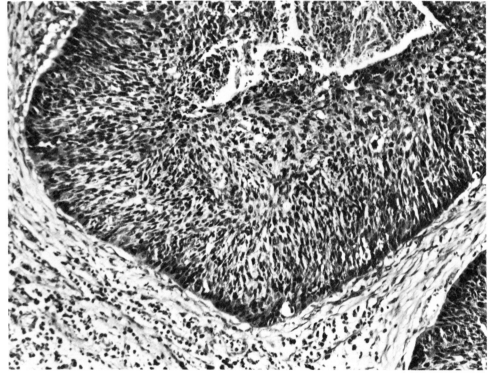

Fig. 13.4 Transitional carcinoma of the nose in a 71 year-old male, showing the transitional structure with disturbed polarity of the cells. M ×154

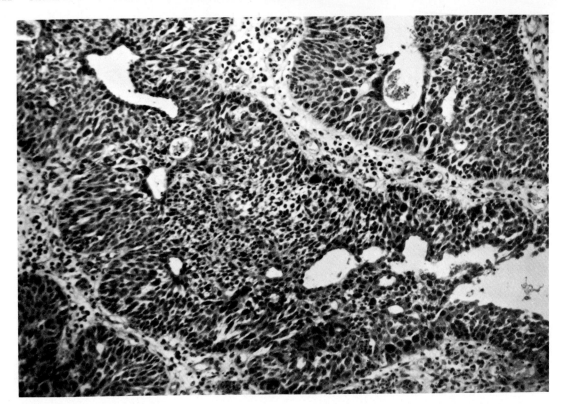

Fig. 13.5 Transitional carcinoma of the nose in a 74 year-old male, showing persistence of the basement membrane and intraepithelial malignancy. M × 170

a prognostic point of view. In fact, the prime justification for delineating this type of carcinoma from the squamous type, to which many pathologists have consigned it, is related to its behaviour.

Anaplastic carcinomas account for approximately 20 per cent of paranasal carcinomas but less than 10 per cent of those arising in the nasal cavity. Ethmoidal carcinomas are more likely to be of this type. Microscopically, the pattern is that of formless sheets of irregular or spheroidal cells (Fig. 13.7) and admixture with lymphocytes sometimes presents the picture of the so-called lympho-epithelioma. The bronchogenic 'oat cell' variety is not seen in this region but spindle cell (pseudosarcoma) types are not uncommon (Figs. 13.8 & 13.9).

Summarizing the histological distribution, the squamous type is the commonest in the nasal and antral cavities, whereas in the ethmoid sinuses, the transitional and anaplastic types are more frequent. The simple adenocarcinoma is found more frequently in the nasal and ethmoidal cavities, being a reflection of the relation to occupational hazard (see Chapter 14).

Aetiology and pathogenesis

Squamous carcinoma has been produced experimentally in the nasal cavity of rats following the intraperitoneal injection of 3,4,5 :trimethoxy cinnamaldehyde which is chemically related to lignin derivatives (Schoental and Gibbard, 1972). Although of interest in the context of woodworkers' adenocarcinoma (see Chapter 14) the observation does not appear to have any immediate relevance to human squamous carcinoma of the nose and sinuses.

The former high incidence of nasal and paranasal carcinoma amongst nickel workers in South Wales (Morgan, 1958; Doll, 1958) and in Sudbury, Ontario (Mastromatteo, 1967) appears to have been related to exposure to flue dusts produced by extraction processes and, although certain nickel compounds are known to be oncogenic, improvement in the working environment has apparently eliminated the risk. Chromium is also known to have a carcinogenic potential and chrome workers have long been known to be at risk to pulmonary cancer (Bidstrup and Case, 1956). For an even longer period of time it has been known that such workers may suffer from ulceration and perforation of the nasal septum but there is no evidence that these lesions become malignant (Kazantzis, 1972).

The increased frequency of carcinoma of the nose and sinuses in the South African Bantu race has been shown

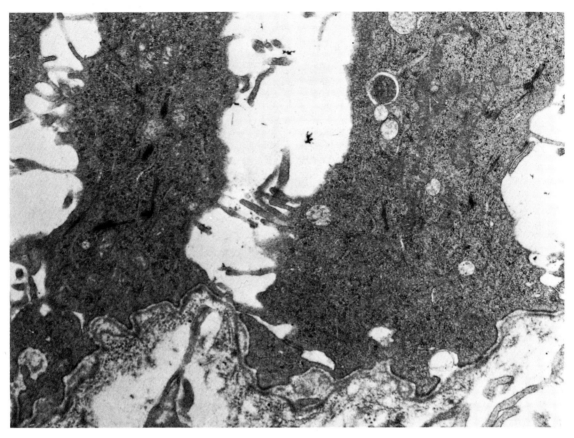

Fig. 13.6 Transitional carcinoma of the ethmoid sinus in a 52 year-old male showing persistence of the basal lamina. M × 17 500

by Keen et al. (1955) to be related to the habit of taking snuff, some forms of which they have shown to contain significant amounts of carcinogenic hydrocarbons, such as 3:4 benzpyrene.

Evidence of surface origin is sometimes found in squamous carcinoma but derivation from metaplastic squamous epithelium is unlikely in most cases since squamous metaplasia is uncommon in the maxillary sinus in the absence of neoplasia. An interesting association, albeit of limited significance, has been observed in connection with carcinoma of the frontal sinus. There have been several reports of carcinoma of this cavity being preceded by the development of an epidermoid cholesteatoma (Spencer, 1930; Osborn and Wallace, 1967; Maniglia and Villa, 1977). The combination of two rare events in this location suggests the possibility of a significant relationship; it calls to mind the association between chronic otitis media on the one hand with epidermoid cholesteatoma and on the other with carcinoma of the middle ear (Friedmann, 1974).

The morphological similarity between the transitional carcinoma and the transitional type papilloma raises the question as to whether the former is derived from the latter. A number of facts militate against this view; the male predominance in the papilloma is not found in the carcinoma, the papilloma is more common in the nose whereas the carcinoma is more frequent in the paranasal region and many papillomas show repeated recurrence without malignant change. Reference has already been made to the low incidence of malignant change in the papilloma (Chapter 12) and one has to conclude that most transitional carcinomas arise *de novo*.

The various aetiological factors so far mentioned clearly have limited relevance and, with the exception of the adenocarcinoma, no other external agents have been identified nor is there any evidence that chronic rhinitis or sinusitis have any role in carcinogenesis.

Behaviour

The local spread of intranasal carcinoma is largely confined to the nasal cavity; extension to the maxillary and ethmoid sinuses occurs in five to ten per cent of cases. Vestibular carcinomas of long standing may spread externally leading to destruction of the tip of the nose

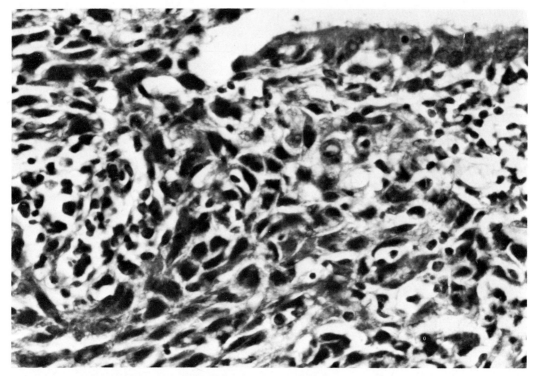

Fig. 13.7 Anaplastic carcinoma of the maxillary sinus in a 58 year-old male. M ×536

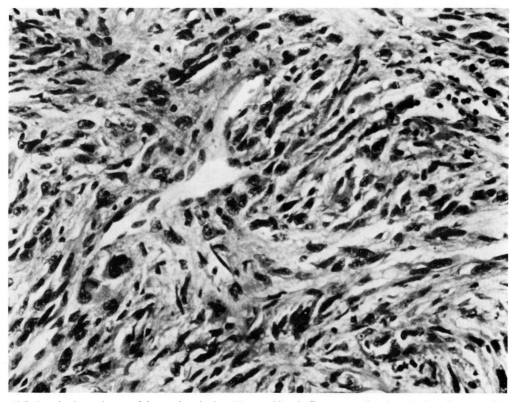

Fig. 13.8 Anaplastic carcinoma of the nasal cavity in a 77 year-old male. Recurrence showing spindle cell pattern. M ×325

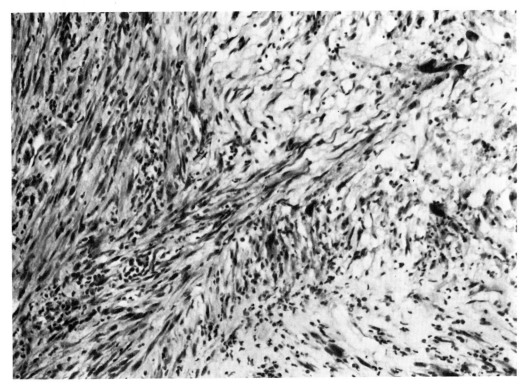

Fig. 13.9 Anaplastic carcinoma of the maxillary sinus in a 40 year-old male, simulating fibrosarcoma. M × 205

and infiltration of the upper lip though most cases are seen and treated before this stage is reached. In paranasal carcinoma, spread to adjacent structures is seen more frequently and this probably reflects in some degree the relative delay in diagnosis of a less conspicuous tumour whose early clinical manifestations are indistinguishable from those of chronic sinusitis. Extension to the nasal cavity results from involvement of the antronasal wall which, in the I.L.O. material, had occurred in nearly 50 per cent of cases. For this reason the primary diagnosis may sometimes be made on the histological examination of a nasal polyp (Osborn and Winston, 1961). Next in order of frequency are involvement of the roof and anterior wall of the antrum which may result in invasion of the orbit and the soft tissues of the cheek (Fig. 13.1). The approximate frequency of involvement of various sites are summarized in Table 13.1. Occasionally, invading paranasal carcinoma may involve the postnasal space.

Regional lymphadenopathy is observed clinically in both nasal and paranasal carcinoma in about 14 per cent of cases but, in the I.L.O. material, histological confirmation was found in only about three per cent which included no cases of transitional carcinoma. Systemic spread is relatively uncommon in intranasal carcinoma (less than four per cent) but is somewhat more frequent

in paranasal tumours, reaching a level of about ten per cent. The principal site of metastasis is the lung followed by the brain, chest wall, bone, liver and kidney.

Table 13.1 Paranasal Carcinoma: Frequency of local involvement

Site	%	Site	%
Main cavities:			
Antrum	68	Frontal Sinus	1.5
Ethmoid	30	Sphenoid Sinus	0.5
Detailed involvement:			
Antronasal wall	48	Cheek, soft tissues	15
Antral roof	30	Post-antral wall	9
Orbital cavity	30	Pterygoid region	5
Anterior antral wall	28	Cranial cavity	5
Antral floor, palate	19	Brain	3.5
Lateral antral wall	16		

It is noteworthy that in all these modes of spread, there are differences related to the histological type of carcinoma. In particular, the transitional carcinoma shows a lesser tendency to spread via the lymphatics or the bloodstream whilst analysis of local spread often reflects a relative reluctance to invade extensively as compared with the squamous type. Furthermore, there is a notable correlation with clinical behaviour.

The recurrence rate of paranasal carcinoma is of the order of 40 per cent whereas that of primary nasal carcinoma is less than 20 per cent. In spite of its less aggressive behaviour in other ways, transitional carcinoma exhibits a greater tendency to local recurrence as compared with the squamous and anaplastic types, a fact which may reflect its more widespread intra-epithelial change. Adenocarcinomas show a much higher recurrence rate (see Chapter 14).

As would be expected, the prognosis is much better in nasal than in paranasal carcinoma. Goepfert et al. (1974) found a five year survival rate of 78 per cent in vestibular carcinoma whilst Bosch, Vallecillo and Fries (1976) reported a five year survival rate of 56 per cent in carcinomas of the nasal cavity. In the I.L.O. material a five year rate of 60 per cent was found, including vestibular tumours. The five year survival rate in paranasal carcinoma ranges between 21 and 25 per cent (Fitzhugh and Gorman, 1960; Frazell and Lewis, 1963, Lederman, 1970). In the I.L.O. material, the rate was 23 per cent. Analysis according to histological type has shown that in both nasal and paranasal regions the transitional carcinoma emerges in a more favourable position (Table 13.2). Repeated attention has been drawn to the prognostic implication of this histological type of carcinoma (Ringertz, 1938; Larsson and Mar-

Table 13.2 Carcinoma of nose and sinuses. Five year survival rate (%) related to histology

Region	Total	Squam.	Trans.	Anapl.	Adenocarc.
Nose	54	53	60	40	57
Sinuses	24	14	40	14.5	43
'Cures'	18	10	37.5	14.5	12.5

tensson, 1954; Osborn and Winston, 1961; Lederman, 1970; Osborn, 1970) but this particular tumour still remains an unrecognized entity in many analyses. Prognostication based on the T.N.M. classification (Sakai and Hamasaki, 1967, Bosch et al. 1976) will have limited significance unless the histological type is taken into consideration. Sisson, Johnson and Amiri (1963) emphasized the importance of histology in relation to the T.N.M. system but clearly they did not recognize the entity of transitional carcinoma.

BIBLIOGRAPHY

Bidstrup P L, Case R A M 1956 Carcinoma of lung in workmen bichromates-producing industry in Great Britain. British Journal of Industrial Medicine 13: 260–264

Bosch A, Vallecillo L, Fries Z 1976 Cancer of the nasal cavity. Cancer 37: 1458–1463

Bosworth F H 1889 Carcinoma of the nasal passages. Diseases of the nose and throat, W Wood & Co, Ch 37, p 453

Citelli S, Calamida U 1903 Beiträge zu Lehre von den Epitheliomen der Nasenschleimhaut. Archiv für Laryngologie 13: 273–287

Cornil V, Ranvier L 1869 Manuel d'Histologie Pathologique. Paris, p 656

Deutsch H J 1966 Carcinoma of the nasal septum: report of a case and review of the literature. Annals of Otology, Rhinology and Laryngology 75: 1049–1057

Doll R 1958 Cancer of the lung and nose in nickel workers. British Journal of Industrial Medicine 15: 217–223

Ewing J 1927 Some phases of intraoral tumors. Radiology 9: 359–365

Fitz-Hugh G S, Gorman J B (1960) Cancer of the nasal accessory sinuses. Southern Medical Journal 53: 155–

Frazell E L, Lewis J S 1963 Cancer of the nasal cavity and accessory sinuses. Cancer 16: 1293–1301

Goepfert H, Guillamondegui O M, Jesse R H, Lindberg R D 1974 Squamous cell carcinoma of the nasal vestibule. Archives of Otolaryngology 100: 8–10

Harmer L, Glas E 1907 Die malignen Tumoren der inneren Nase. Deutsche Zeitschrift Chirurgie 89: 433–539

Hautant A, Monod O, Klotz A 1933 Les épithéliomes ethmoido-orbitaires. Annales d'Otolaryngologie 1933: 385–421

Hendrick J W 1958 Treatment of cancer of the paranasal sinuses and nasal fossa. Archives of Otolaryngology 68: 604–616

Kazantzis G 1972 Chromium and nickel. Annals of Occupational Hygiene 15: 25–29

Keen P, De Moor N G, Shapiro M P, Cohen L, Cooper R L, Campbell J M 1955 The aetiology of respiratory tract cancer in the South African Bantu. British Journal of Cancer 9: 528–538

Kümmel W 1900 Die bösartigen Geschwülste der Nase. In: Heymann P, (ed), Holder A, Handbuch der Laryngologie und Rhinologie, Wien

Larsson L G, Martensson G 1954 Carcinoma of paranasal sinuses and the nasal cavities. Acta Radiologica 42: 149–172

Lawrence 1856 Non-malignant tumour of six months' growth developed within the cavity of the left nostril. Lancet 1: 455–456

Lederman M 1970 Tumours of the upper jaw – natural history and treatment. Journal of Laryngology and Otology 84: 369–401

Lewis J S, Castro E B 1972 Cancer of the nasal cavity and paranasal sinuses. Journal of Laryngology and Otology 86: 255–262

Maniglia A J, Villa L 1977 Epidermoid carcinoma of the frontal sinus secondary to cholesteatoma. Transactions of the American Academy of Ophthalmology and Otolaryngology 84: 112–115

Mastromatteo E 1967 Nickel: a review of its occupational health hazards. Journal of Occupational Medicine 9: 127–136

Morgan J G 1958 Some observations on the incidence of respiratory cancer in nickel workers. British Journal of Industrial Medicine 15: 224–234

Osborn D A 1970 Nature and behaviour of transitional tumours of the upper respiratory tract. Cancer 25: 50–60

Osborn D A, Wallace M 1967 Carcinoma of the frontal sinus associated with epidermoid cholesteatoma. Journal of Laryngology and Otology 81: 1021–1032

Osborn D A, Winston P 1961 Carcinoma of the paranasal sinuses. Journal of Laryngology and Otology 75: 387–405

Quick D, Cutler M 1927 Transitional cell epidermoid carcinoma. Surgery, Gynecology and Obstetrics 45: 320–331

Registrar General's statistical review of England and Wales for the year 1973, Part I(B)

Ringertz N 1938 Pathology of malignant tumours arising in the nasal and paranasal cavities and maxilla. Acta Otolaryngologica, supplement 27, chapter 7

Sakai S, Hamasaki Y 1967 Proposal for the classification of carcinoma of the paranasal sinuses. Acta Otolaryngologica 63: 42–48

Schoental R, Gibbard S 1972 Nasal and other tumours in rats given 3,4,5,-Trimethoxy-cinnamaldehyde. British Journal of Cancer 26: 504–505

Sisson G A, Johnson N E, Amiri C S 1963 Cancer of the maxillary sinus. Annals of Otology, Rhinology and Laryngology 72: 1050–1059

Spencer F R 1930 Primary cholesteatoma of the sinuses and orbit; report of a case of many years' duration followed by carcinoma and death. Archives of Otolaryngology 12: 44–48

Additional references

Buchanan G, Slavin G 1972 Tumours of the nose and sinuses: a clinico-pathological survey. Journal of Laryngology and Otology 86: 685–696

Clemmesen J 1951 On cancer incidence in Denmark and other countries. Unio Internationalis contra cancrum Acta 7: 24–38

Fitz-Hugh G S, Gorman J B 1960 Cancer of the nasal accessory sinuses. Southern Medical Journal 53: 155–161

Frew I 1969 Frontal sinus carcinoma. Journal of Laryngology and Otology 83: 393–396

Friedmann I 1974 Pathology of the ear. Blackwell, Oxford

Harrison D F N 1964 Snuff – its use and abuse. British Medical Journal 2: 1649–1651

Keen P 1963 The management of jaw tumours in the South African Bantu. Clinical Radiology 14: 250–254

Shapiro M P, Keen P, Cohen L, De Moor N G 1955 Malignant disease in the Transvaal. III cancer of the respiratory tract. South African Medical Journal 29: 95–101

AMELOBLASTOMA IN THE NOSE AND SINUSES

Introduction

One of the earliest tumours of this type was reported by Falkson (1879) who described and illustrated a tumour in the mandible of a 40 year-old woman. Malassez (1885) recognized its origin from remnants of dental epithelium, using the term 'tumeur adamantine' from which the name 'adamantinoma' was derived. The more modern expression 'ameloblastoma' was introduced by Churchill (1934). The majority of these tumours occur in the lower jaw but between 16 and 20 per cent arise in the maxilla (Robinson, 1937; Small and Waldron, 1955; Masson, McDonald and Figi, 1959) where they may present as an antral or even nasal tumour. Involvement of the maxillary sinus has been reported by a number of workers (Bump, 1927; Simmonds, 1928; Vorzimer and Perla, 1932: McGregor, 1935; Kyriazis, Karkazis and Kyriazis, 1971; Shaw and Katsikas, 1973; Porter, Miller and Stratigos, 1977; Baker and Matukas, 1977).

Incidence

Ameloblastoma is the commonest of the odontogenic tumours although it only represents about one per cent of all odontogenic lesions. In the I.L.O. material, there were three cases representing less than 0.3 per cent of all tumours of the nose and sinuses and approximately two per cent of all antral tumours.

Clinical features

The age distribution is broadly based, ranging from the second to the ninth decade with a slight predominance of males. The common form of presentation is painless swelling of the cheek which usually develops slowly and may ultimately lead to proptosis. Involvement of the nasal cavity may cause longstanding nasal obstruction (Baker and Matukas, 1977). Multilocular shadows may be seen on X-ray but the appearances are not diagnostic whilst the naked eye features may include both solid and cystic elements.

Histopathology

Although a wide variety of histological patterns have been described (Aisenberg, 1953), the two main forms are designated follicular and plexiform, many of the variants now being regarded as separate entities. The follicular pattern is the commonest and mimics the enamel organ in the developing tooth. It consists of sharply circumscribed epithelial islands with a palisaded border of tall columnar cells (ameloblasts) which enclose a more loosely arranged cellular component, resembling the stellate reticulum (Figs. 13.10 & 13.11). Squamous metaplasia may occur in the central areas, sometimes proceding to the formation of epithelial pearls (the so-called acanthomatous ameloblastoma. Aisenberg (1953) believed that tumours exhibiting this feature were more aggressive but the claim has not been substantiated, although occasionally areas of frankly squamous carcinoma may be seen. The plexiform type consists of thin branching epithelial cords enclosing numerous spaces and presenting a cribriform pattern which may be confused with the cribriform adenocarcinoma (Fig. 13.12). Some of the cords may be expanded to contain stellate cells and a mixture of plexiform and follicular pattern may occur. The connective tissue stroma is of a loose character and often relatively acellular.

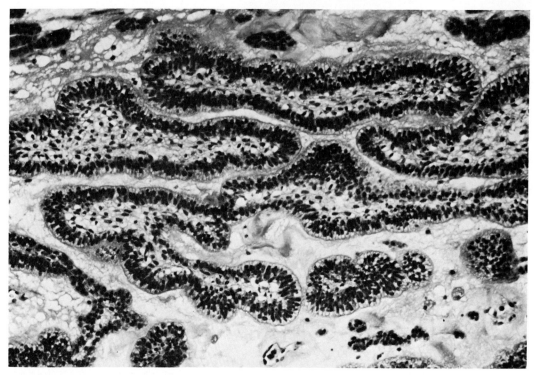

Fig. 13.10 Ameloblastoma of the maxilla involving the antrum in an 81 year-old male, showing the follicular pattern. M × 215

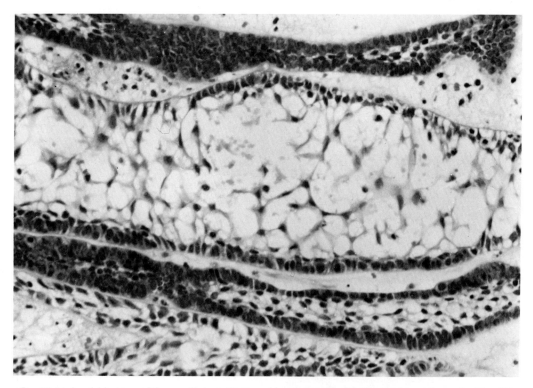

Fig. 13.11 Ameloblastoma of the maxilla in an 81 year-old male (see Fig. 13.10) showing stellate cells. M × 340

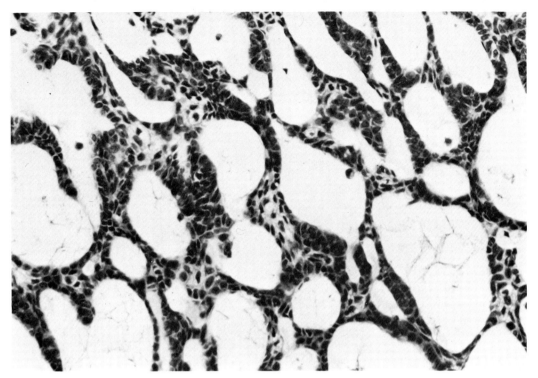

Fig. 13.12 Ameloblastoma involving the maxillary sinus in a 65 year-old male, showing the plexiform pattern. M × 335

In addition to the follicular and plexiform patterns, Small and Waldron (1955) included a primitive type, composed of small branching cords in a fibrous stroma. On the basis of age incidence and more benign behaviour, the last mentioned authors suggested that it might be a separate entity and this 'variant' is now classified as ameloblastic fibroma (Gorlin, Chaudhry and Pindborg, 1961). Small epithelial islands of follicular type may be present but the stroma is highly cellular being composed of spindle and stellate cells of fibroblastic type (Fig. 13.13). One such case, involving the maxillary sinus was found in the I.L.O. material, having been initially diagnosed as ameloblastoma. Ameloblastic fibroma tends to occur at an earlier age (mainly in the first two decades) and its behaviour is far less aggressive. Gorlin et al. (1961) reported 23 cases of which only five occurred in the maxilla.

A variant of the ameloblastoma may show granular cells (Figs. 13.14 & 13.15), Hoke and Harrelson (1967) suggested that this feature mimics the behaviour of ameloblasts in normal tooth development.

Aetiology and pathogenesis
The ameloblastoma has long been known to be associated with remnants of the dental epithelium (Malassez, 1885) and such tumours may be derived from remains of the

dental lamina, the enamel organ, the basal layer of the surface oral epithelium and occasionally from the epithelium lining a dentigerous cyst.

Behaviour
The ameloblastoma was originally regarded as being a benign tumour, an attitude which was probably influenced by histological confusion with the various benign entities showing similar features. Subsequently many cases were recognized as being at least locally invasive and reports of metastasis to lymphnodes and the lungs began to appear in the literature. Not all such accounts are acceptable but a small number of well authenticated cases are regarded as being genuine (Simmonds, 1928; Vorzimer and Perla, 1932; Schweitzer and Barnfield, 1943; Lee, White and Totten, 1959; Pennisi, Young, Anlyan and Grisez, 1966). Pulmonary secondaries are found in the lower lobes and there is always a history of repeated surgical intervention. These facts provide a strong basis for the belief that pulmonary spread is the result of aspiration rather than systemic involvement.

Published maxillary tumours have shown very variable behaviour. Approximately 40 per cent of patients have died of their tumour after periods ranging from less than one year to more than twenty years. Survival for five

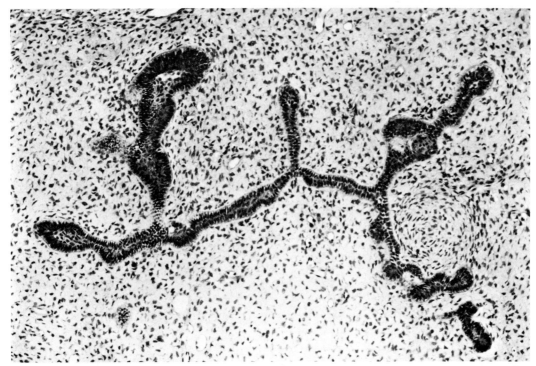

Fig. 13.13 Ameloblastic fibroma of the maxillary sinus in a 9 year-old boy, showing the 'primitive' epithelial pattern in a highly cellular stroma. No recurrence after 18 years. M ×134

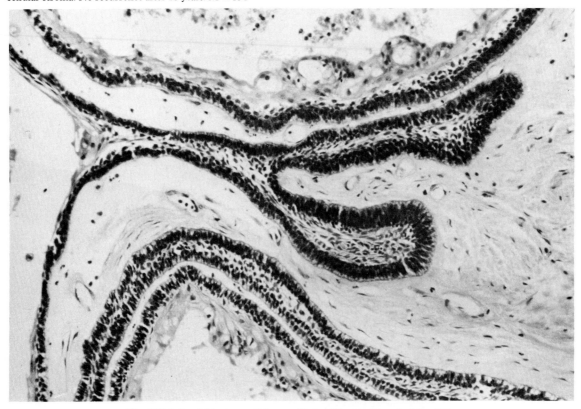

Fig. 13.14 Ameloblastoma of the maxilla in a 55 year-old male. M ×225

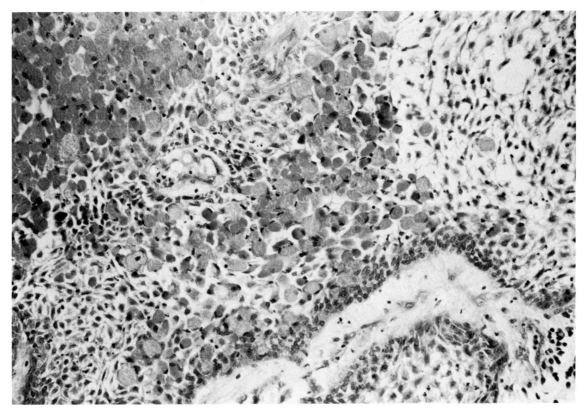

Fig. 13.15 Ameloblastoma of the maxilla in a 55 year-old male (see Fig. 13.14), showing the granular cell pattern. M × 225

years or more without recurrence is not uncommon (McGregor, 1935; Shaw and Katsikas, 1973). In the I.L.O. material, one case died after three years with extensive local disease but no remote spread, one was lost to follow-up and the other has survived without recurrence for 13 years. The case of the ameloblastic fibroma is known to have survived without recurrence for 18 years.

BIBLIOGRAPHY

Aisenberg M S 1953 Histopathology of ameloblastoma. Oral Surgery, Oral Medicine & Oral Pathology 6: 1111–1128

Baker B B, Matukas V J 1977 Ameloblastoma presenting as an intranasal mass. Laryngoscope 87: 1367–1372

Bump W S 1927 Adamantine epithelioma. Surgery, Gynecology and Obstetrics 44: 173–180

Churchill H R 1934 Histological differentiation between certain dentigerous cysts and ameloblastoma. Dental Cosmos 76: 1173–1178

Falkson R 1879 Zur Kenntniss der Kiefercysten. Virchows Archiv für pathologische Anatomie 76: 504–510

Gorlin R J, Chaudhry A P, Pindborg J J 1961 Odontogenic tumors. Cancer 14: 73–101

Hoke H F, Harrelson A B 1967 Granular cell ameloblastoma with metastasis to the cervical vertebrae. Cancer 20: 991–999

Kyriazis A P, Karkasis G G, Kyriazis A A 1971 Maxillary ameloblastoma with intracerebral extension. Oral Surgery, Oral Medicine & Oral Pathology 32: 582–587

Lee R E, White W L, Totten R S 1959 Ameloblastoma with distant metastases. Archives of Pathology 68: 23–29

McGregor L 1935 A report of eleven instances of Adamantinoma with a review of the malignant cases in the literature. Acta Radiologica 16: 254–274

Malassez L 1885 Sur le rôle des debris épithéliaux paradentaires. Archives de Physiologie normale et pathologique, 3me. série, 6, 379–449

Masson J K, McDonald J R, Figi F A 1959 Adamantinoma of the jaws. Plastic and Reconstructive Surgery 23: 510–525

Pennisi V R, Young A, Anlyan J, Grisez J I 1966 Ameloblastoma with longstanding pulmonary metastases. Plastic and Reconstructive Surgery 28: 534–540

Porter J, Miller R, Stratigos G T 1977 Ameloblastoma of the maxilla. Oral Surgery, Oral Medicine and Oral Pathology 44: 34–38

Robinson H B G 1937 Ameloblastoma. Archives of Pathology 23: 831–843

Schweitzer F C, Barnfield W F 1943 Ameloblastoma of the mandible with metastasis to the lungs. Journal of Oral Surgery 1: 287–295

Shaw H J, Katsikas D K 1973 Ameloblastoma of the maxilla. Journal of Laryngology and Otology 87: 873–884

Simmonds C C 1928 Adamantinoma. Annals of Surgery 88: 693–704

Small I A, Waldron C A 1955 Ameloblastoma of the jaws. Oral Surgery, Oral Medicine and Oral Pathology 8: 281–297

Vorzimer J, Perla D 1932 An instance of adamantinoma of the jaw with metastases in the right lung. American Journal of Pathology 8: 445–453

14

Tumours of mucosal glands

MUCOSAL GLAND TUMOURS OF THE NOSE AND SINUSES

The lining membrane of the nose and sinuses contains numerous mucosal glands from which may arise a wide variety of tumours. Many of these tumours have their counterparts in the major salivary glands but, although the range of histological pattern is similar, the relative frequency of the various types shows significant differences. It should be emphasized that the mucosal glands are a normal feature of the part hence, in the context of tumours derived therefrom, the term 'ectopic' should not be used. Compared with the major salivary gland sites, the mucosal group contains a much higher proportion of malignant tumours, amounting to over 60 per cent. The various types of mucosal gland tumour, which differ greatly in incidence and importance, are considered under the following headings:

1. Tubulo-cystic adenoma
2. Microcystic papillary adenoma
3. Eosinophilic granular cell tumour (oncocytoma)
4. Simple adenocarcinoma
5. Acinic cell tumour
6. Muco-epidermoid tumour
7. Pleomorphic (mixed) tumour
8. Cribriform adenocarcinoma (adenoid cystic carcinoma)
9. Basal cell tumour

TUBULO-CYSTIC ADENOMA OF THE NOSE AND SINUSES

This type of tumour is not very common in this region. It consists of simple tubules and cysts lined by cubical or columnar epithelium which may sometimes be mucus-secreting (Fig. 14.1) but frequently exhibits the intense eosinophilic granularity seen in 'oncocytes' (Hamperl. 1931). This striking appearance (Fig. 14.2) is the result of packing of the cytoplasm with swollen mitochondria. Sometimes the epithelium forms papillary structures to which the term 'papillary cystadenoma' has been applied

and may sometimes be confused with metastatic renal carcinoma. Difficulty may sometimes be encountered in distinguishing between adenoma and well differentiated adenocarcinoma.

MICROCYSTIC PAPILLARY ADENOMA

Introduction
The restriction of these tumours to the upper respiratory tract has undoubtedly delayed their more general recognition. The bizarre microcystic appearance of the epithelial component has resulted in erroneous diagnoses such as rhinosporidiosis whilst the columnar papillary structure has prompted an equally incorrect suggestion that they represent a variant of the transitional type papilloma. The case described by Johns, Batsakis and Short (1973) under the title of oncocytoid cylindrical cell papilloma would appear to have been an example of this type of tumour. The light and electron microscopical appearances have promoted the present authors to adopt the epithet 'microcystic' as an informative label.

Incidence
Although more common than the tubulo-cystic type, they are still relatively rare. In the I.L.O. material they represent 1.6 per cent of all tumours of the nose and sinuses and 2.4 per cent of all benign tumours in the region.

Clinical features
Characteristically, the peak age distribution is in the seventh decade and there is no significant sex difference. The usual form of presentation is that of nasal obstruction due to the presence of polypoid swellings whose solid consistency may well raise suspicions of neoplasia rather than simple polyposis (Fig. 14.3).

Anatomical site of origin
These tumours have not been encountered outside the upper respiratory tract, about three-quarters of them occurring in the nasal cavity whilst the remainder involved the maxillary and ethmoid sinuses.

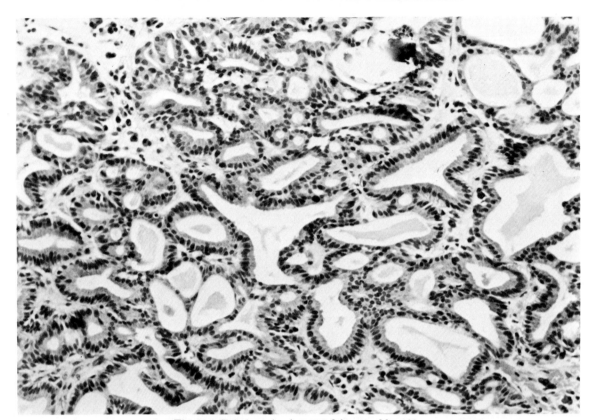

Fig. 14.1 Tubulocystic adenoma of the nose. M × 180

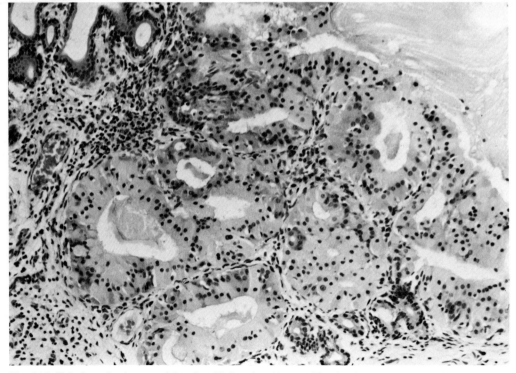

Fig. 14.2 Tubulocystic adenoma of the ethmoid sinus in a 52 year-old male, showing oncocytic change. M × 208

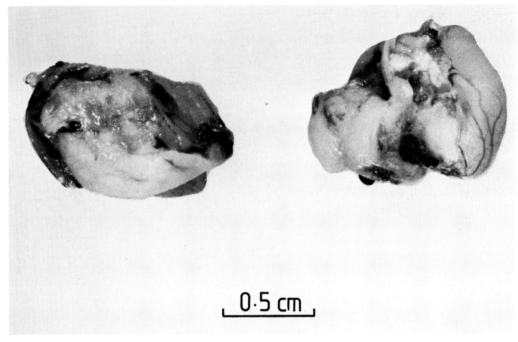

Fig. 14.3 Microcystic papillary adenoma of the nose in a 60 year-old male.

Histopathology

The microscopical picture is a very striking one. Papillary structures project into cystic spaces which often contain mucous secretion (Figs. 14.4 & 14.5). The constituent cells vary in size but are often tall and cylindrical with abundant eosinophilic granular cytoplasm resembling Hamperl's oncocytes. The free border may sometimes display cilia, giving an impression of overgrown respiratory type epithelium with pseudostratification though multiple layers may develop. A prominent feature is the presence of numerous intra-epithelial microcysts (Figs. 14.6 & 14.7) which often contain epithelial type mucin, giving a diastase-fast Periodic acid Schiff reaction (Fig. 14.8). Under the electron microscope, many of the cells are seen to contain either greatly enlarged mitochondria or mucous secretory granules or a mixture of both (Fig. 14.9) whilst the microcysts are seen to be true cysts with a well developed microvillous margin and a variegated content of secretory product (Fig. 14.10).

Aetiology and pathogenesis

No causal agent has been identified but the presence of ciliated cells would suggest the possibility of surface origin and certainly some of the secretory cells are consistent with goblet cells. Nevertheless, the occurrence of oncocytic change, the tendency to form cystic structures and the marked mucous secretory activity would seem to justify retention of this tumour in the glandular group.

Behaviour

Local recurrence is not uncommon and may sometimes be multiple but malignant transformation has never been encountered.

EOSINOPHILIC GRANULAR CELL TUMOUR

Introduction

This tumour was first described by Gruenfeld and Jorsted (1936) in the parotid gland and, because of the resemblance of the cells to Hamperl's oncocytes, they labelled it 'oncocytoma'. Later, Meza-Chavez (1949) reported five tumours of parotid origin under the name of 'oxyphilic granular cell adenoma'. In view of subsequent observations on the behaviour of these tumours, the term adenoma is no longer specified.

Incidence

The tumour is rare in any location but has been reported more frequently in the major salivary glands (Blanck, Eneroth and Jakobsen, 1970). As far as the nasal region is concerned, a small number of cases have been reported by Hamperl (1962), Cohen and Batsakis (1968) and by

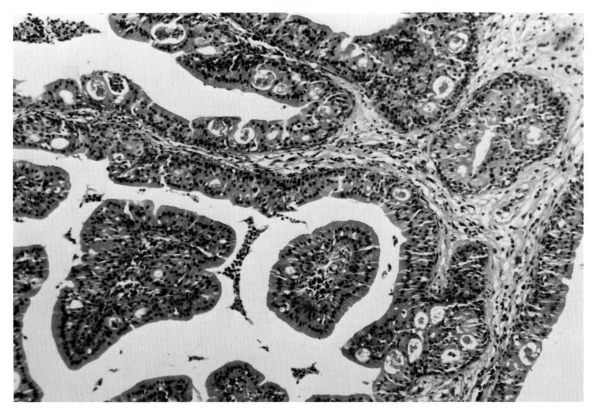

Fig. 14.4 Microcystic papillary adenoma of the nose in a 47 year-old male. Note papillary pattern with pseudostratified columnar epithelium containing microcysts filled with mucous secretion or pus cells. M × 135

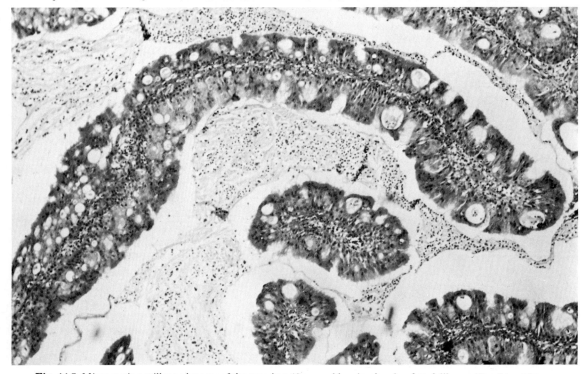

Fig. 14.5 Microcystic papillary adenoma of the nose in a 48 year-old male, showing frond-like papillae. M × 90

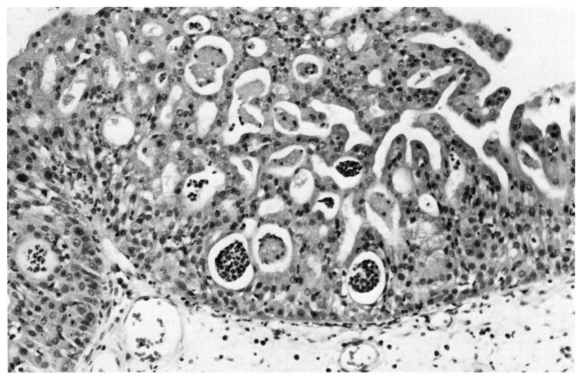

Fig. 14.6 Microcystic papillary adenoma of the nose in a 48 year-old male (see Fig. 14.5), showing numerous microcysts, many containing polymorphonuclear leucocytes. M × 225

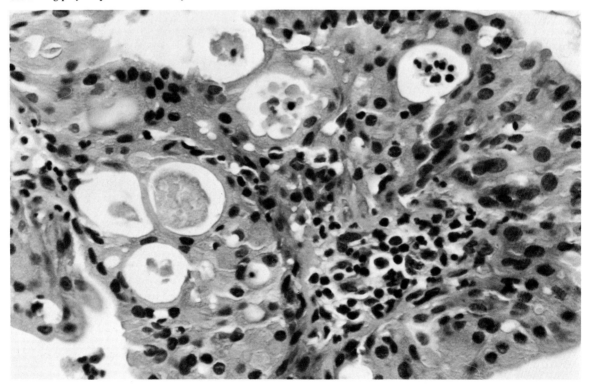

Fig. 14.7 Microcystic papillary adenoma of the nose in a 47 year-old male (see Fig. 14.4), showing microcysts within the epithelium. M × 595

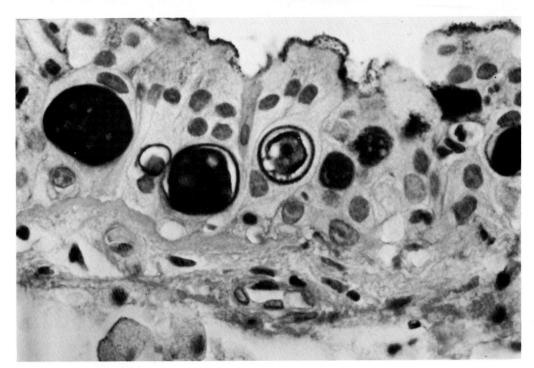

Fig. 14.8 Microcystic papillary adenoma of the nose in a 60 year-old male, showing microcysts filled with epithelial type mucin. Periodic acid-Schiff reaction. M ×820

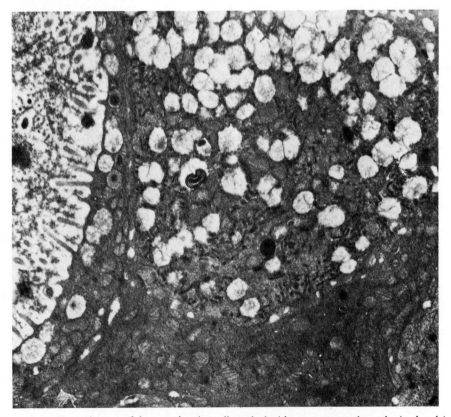

Fig. 14.9 Microcystic papillary adenoma of the nose showing cells packed with mucous granules and mitochondria. M ×12 000

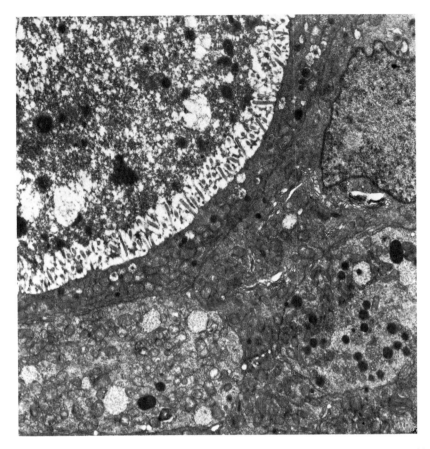

Fig. 14.10 Microcystic papillary adenoma of the nose showing microvillous border of a microcyst. M ×8000

Spiro, Koss, Hajdu and Strong (1973), giving a total of four nasal tumours. No example was found in the I.L.O. material but the present authors were able to study a biopsy from an extramural case.

Clinical features

The tumour appears to occur only in the older age groups, all the nasal cases being over sixty years old. By contrast, the age distribution in those of major salivary gland origin is more broadly based. There is no evidence of sex predilection. Nasal obstruction, epistaxis or discharge constitute the expected mode of presentation.

Anatomical site of origin

In the present context, all the tumours so far observed appear to have arisen primarily in the nasal cavity, only secondary involvement of the paranasal region having been encountered.

Histopathology

Although no gross characteristics have been noted, the microscopical picture is instantly recognizable. Rela-

tively large, closely packed cells of varying shape are interspersed with obvious attempts to form tubular structures (Fig. 14.11). The abundant cytoplasm is coarsely granular and predominantly intensely eosinophilic though some palely staining cells may be observed. Nuclei are usually rounded and well stained with fairly abundant heterochromatin but irregularity and hyperchromatism may occur, raising the question of behavioural interpretation. Mitoses are infrequent. The attempt to form tubular structures gives the clue to its glandular origin whilst the intense eosinophilic staining and the relative size of the nuclei serve to distinguish it from granular cell myoblastoma which, in any case, has not been reported in the nasal cavity. The stromal component is minimal being represented largely by small blood vessels and the close arrangement of the cells accounts for the fleshy consistency of the tumour observed at naked eye level.

Ultrastructural studies on extranasal tumours of this type have been reported by Tandler, Hutter and Erlandson (1970) and by Fechner and Bentinck (1973). The common finding was packing of the cells with

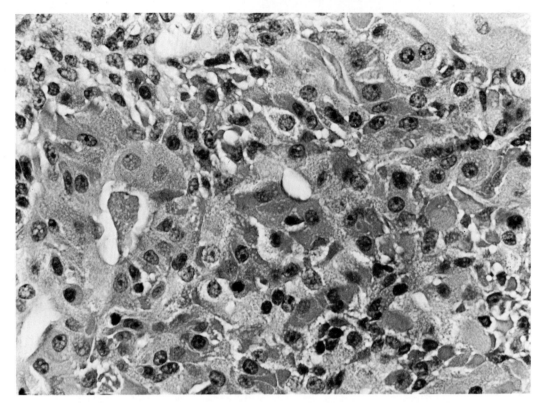

Fig. 14.11 Eosinophilic granular cell tumour of the nose in a 74 year-old female, showing formation of tubular structures. M × 600

enlarged mitochondria which varied in shape though the majority tended to be spherical. Glycogen particles were observed both in the cytoplasm and within the mitochondria.

Aetiology and pathogenesis

'Oncocytes' have a widespread distribution, particularly in exocrine and endocrine glands but also in other epithelial structures such as the gall bladder and Fallopian tube (Hamperl, 1950). The last mentioned author maintained that they represented some form of degenerative process related to age. Apart from the eosinophilic granular cell tumour, cells with similar characteristics tend to predominate in the tubulo-cystic and microcystic papillary adenomas and also in the so-called adenolymphoma or Warthin' tumour. Relevant to Hamperl's observations is the fact that the age distribution in all these lesions is similar. Clearly, the oncocytic change does not necessarily interfere with the capacity for multiplication but, on the other hand, the presence of such cells so transformed does not necessarily imply neoplasia. Oncocytic change could be merely a coincidental phenomenon. This could accord with the high frequency of oncocytes and the low incidence of 'Oncocytoma'.

Behaviour

Although originally regarded as a benign tumour, it has now become apparent that some examples in both the major salivary glands and the mucosal glands are capable of malignant behaviour, giving rise to remote spread. Metastasis from malignant variants in the parotid gland have been reported by Bauer and Bauer (1953) and by Bazaz-Malik and Gupta (1968) whilst three of the four published nasal tumours (Hamperl, 1962; Cohen and Batsakis, 1968) also exhibited malignant features.

SIMPLE ADENOCARCINOMA

Introduction

The early literature was somewhat deficient in reports of this type of adenocarcinoma in the nasal region although such tumours were recognized (Citelli and Calamida, 1903; Harma and Glas, 1907). It was only following the classical study by Ahlbom (1935) on mucous and salivary gland tumours that interest in adenocarcinomas of the upper respiratory tract became manifest. Ahlbom found five examples out of nine glandular tumours of the nose and sinuses.

Terminology

In so far as the label adenocarcinoma has been applied to another histological type of malignant glandular tumour, the present authors have added the epithet simple in order to eliminate any possible confusion.

Incidence

Simple adenocarcinoma is not a common type of tumour in this region. Ringertz (1938) found ten out of 31 glandular tumours involving the nose and sinuses, representing less than four per cent of all carcinomas in the region. McDonald and Havens (1948) reported 57 out of 95 glandular tumours of the nose and sinuses whilst Spiro, Koss, Hajdu and Strong (1973) found 49 out of 122 glandular tumours. In the I.L.O. material, there were 15 cases out of a total of 60 glandular tumours, representing six per cent of all carcinomas in the nose and sinuses and 1.4 per cent of all tumours in the region.

Clinical features

The age distribution shows a peak occurrence in the sixth to seventh decades with a marked predominance of males (Gamez-Araujo, Ayala and Guillamondegui, 1975; Ironside and Matthews, 1975). In the I.L.O. material the peak was in the sixth decade with only two females out of 15 cases.

Patients suffering from this condition may present with nasal obstruction, epistaxis, pain or local swelling whilst extension of the growth may lead to epiphora, proptosis and disturbance of vision.

Anatomical site of origin

In the greater proportion of cases adenocarcinoma has involved primarily the nasal cavity or the ethmoid region (McDonald and Havens, 1948; Batsakis, Holz and Sueper, 1963; Ironside and Matthews, 1975). In the I.L.O. material, the ethmoid sinuses were involved in eight cases, the nasal cavity in four and the antrum in three. On the other hand, there have been reports of higher frequency in the antrum: 22 out of 49 by Spiro et al. (1973), 10 out of 18 by Gamez-Araujo et al. (1975). These differing proportions are difficult to explain although histological interpretation may have played a part.

Gross appearances

The macroscopical features are often unremarkable, the tumours presenting as polypoid mucosal masses which, inevitably, have been removed piecemeal and presented to the pathologist as multiple irregular fragments.

Histopathology

Tubulo-cystic structures lined by cubical or columnar epithelium are usually well differentiated with varying numbers of interspersed mucus-secreting cells (Figs. 14.12 & 14.13). Papillary processes may be present, sometimes projecting into cyst-like spaces and a high degree of differentiation may prompt an initial diagnosis of 'papillary cystadenoma'. Evidence of invasion may be found in irregular clumps of cells lying in the stroma though in many areas the basement membrane appears to be intact. A not uncommon appearance in a biopsy is that of multiple fragments of apparently detached columnar epithelium lying in a sea of blood and mucus (Fig. 14.14). Close examination of such a pattern is essential in order to avoid the erroneous interpretation of desquamated normal epithelium. Rupture of mucous secretory components results in mucous pervasion of the stroma, thus adding to the complexity of the picture. A more solid type of structure containing small lumina may present a difficulty in distinguishing simple adenocarcinoma from the acinic cell tumour but sometimes ultrastructural studies may be of help in elucidating the problem.

Under the electron microscope, mucous secretory granules can be identified as either discrete or semi-confluent structures after the manner of normal mucous glands. Less specific features include accumulations of glycogen, swollen mitochondria and lipochondria which should not be confused with secretory granules such as one might find in an acinic cell tumour. Occasionally, basally located cells may be found showing myo-epithelial differentiation (Fig. 14.15).

Aetiology and pathogenesis

The particular interest in this tumour is centred on location in relation to occupation. At least six out of the 15 cases in the I.L.O. material were known to have been employed as woodworkers. The relationship between nasal adenocarcinoma and the furniture industry was first established by Hadfield and her colleagues (Macbeth, 1965; Acheson, Hadfield and Macbeth, 1967; Hadfield, Acheson, Cowdell and Macbeth, 1968; Hadfield, 1970; Hadfield and Macbeth, 1971). Their observations were based on a geographical area in southern England, covering the adjacent parts of the counties of Buckingham and Oxford. This region, with High Wycombe as its principal focus, has been the centre of the furniture industry for about 200 years. It was noted that the incidence of adenocarcinoma in the nose and sinuses was much higher relative to both other histological types and to the general expectation of nasal carcinoma. Furthermore, it was found that a high proportion of the sufferers had been employed in furniture making for many years. Subsequently, confirmation of this hazard appeared in reports from France

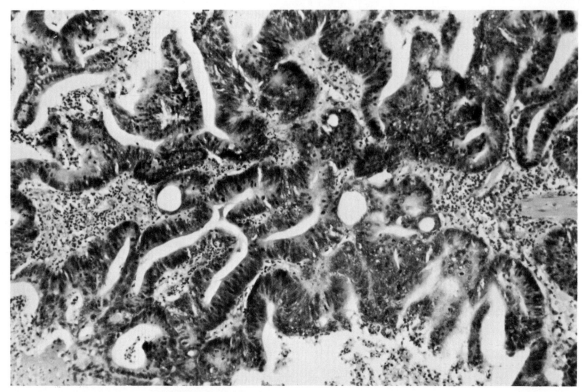

Fig. 14.12 Simple adenocarcinoma of the nose in a 69 year-old male woodworker, showing well differentiated tumour. M × 135

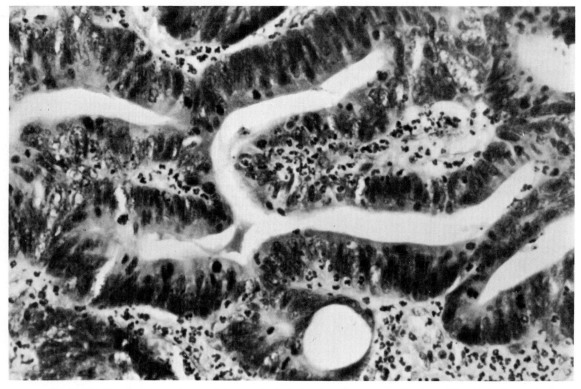

Fig. 14.13 Simple adenocarcinoma of the nose in a woodworker. Higher magnification of Fig. 14.12. M × 360

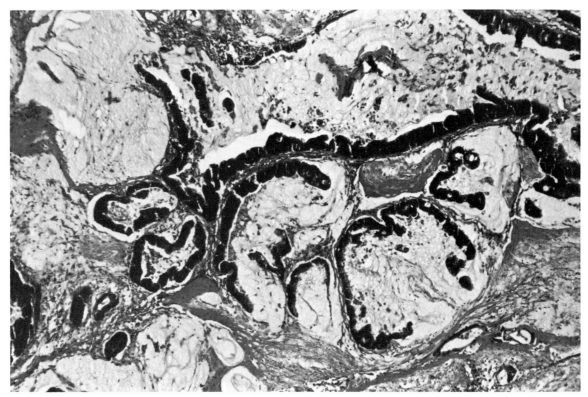

Fig. 14.14 Simple adenocarcinoma of the nose in a 49 year-old male woodworker, showing fragments of epithelium lying in a sea of mucus and blood. M × 60

(Gignoux and Bernard, 1969), Belgium (Debois, 1969), Denmark (Mosbech and Acheson, 1971), Australia (Ironside and Matthews, 1975) and finally from the United States (Brinton, Blot, Stone and Fraumeni, 1977). In the United Kingdom, nasal adenocarcinoma has now been prescribed as an industrial disease. In the course of the investigation in southern England, it was found that there was also a high incidence in the neighbouring county. of Northampton, relating to the boot and shoe industry (Acheson, Cowdell and Jolles, 1970) and it would appear that the frequency of nasal and paranasal adenocarcinoma was 20 to 50 times the expected value. The suggestion that workers in the bakery trade might also be at risk has not been confirmed.

Investigation of woodworkers has shown that there is, in those so employed for ten years or more, an impairment of muco-ciliary clearance which is probably related to the development of squamous metaplasia at the site of deposition of wood dust (Black, Evans, Hadfield and Macbeth, 1974). It is suspected that the influence might be chemical rather than mechanical though the effect of simple drying of respiratory type epithelium cannot be entirely excluded. No carcinogenic agent has been specifically identified although it seems clear that it is present in the dust of the fine woods used in furniture making and it may be that the high temperatures attained in cutting and sanding have a modifying influence on the basic chemical components of the wood. Reference has already been made in Chapter 13 to the observations of Schoental and Gibbard (1972) in connection with the experimental production of nasal carcinoma in rats following the administration of a lignin derivative. These workers suggested a possible relevance to woodworkers' adenocarcinoma but this would be more acceptable if their derivative had been introduced intranasally and had produced an adenocarcinoma instead of a squamous type. Nevertheless, it does serve to underline the potential hazard of wood dust and it should be emphasized that even non-woodworkers are at risk if continually exposed to such an atmosphere, as occurred in one of the I.L.O. cases.

Hadfield (1970) expressed the belief that woodworkers' adenocarcinoma probably arose primarily in the middle turbinate on the anterior end of which the wood

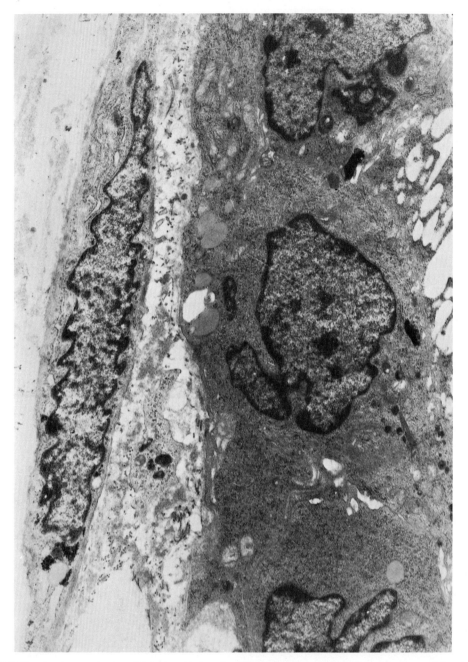

Fig. 14.15 Simple adenocarcinoma of the ethmoid sinus in a 55 year-old male woodworker, showing peripherally located myoepithelial cell on a luminal structure. M × 12 000

dust is found to be deposited. Spread to the paranasal region would be a subsequent event. One unresolved issue in adenocarcinoma of this region is the tissue of origin. Järvi (1945) was so impressed with the similarity to colonic carcinoma that he suggested origin from ectopic remnants but such a concept has found little support. The main argument revolves round origin from surface or glandular epithelium. Sanchez-Casis, Devine and Weiland (1971) believed that the tumour arose from tissue of common origin with the gastro-intestinal tract, on which basis they concluded that the tumour could arise from either surface epithelium or from mucosal glands. Batsakis, Holz and Sueper (1963) maintained that mucus producing adenocarcinomas arose from mucosal glands whilst the predominantly papillary type was derived from the surface epithelium or the glandular ducts. In so far as there is frequently a lack of differentiation between ductular and secretory components in mucosal glands, distinction may be difficult and not necessarily valid. Furthermore, origin from non-glandular surface epithelium is more likely to produce a cylindrical or transitional type of carcinoma thus calling to mind the earlier confusion between the two types of carcinoma which Hautant, Monod and Klotz (1933) found difficult to resolve.

Behaviour

Local spread between the nasal and paranasal cavities is an almost invariable event but dissemination *via* the lymphatics or bloodstream is less frequent, occurring in under a quarter of the cases. Local recurrence is encountered in about 50 per cent of cases and is frequently multiple. More than half the cases die ultimately from their disease but in the I.L.O. material, five have survived for at least five years (35 per cent). Two of these cases died subsequently, one from his disease and the other from an unrelated cause whilst two of the three survivors have had many local recurrences. In the series reported by Gamez-Araujo et al. (1975), one-third survived without recurrence for periods ranging from two to eleven years but several of their cases had features resembling acinic cell tumours.

ACINIC CELL TUMOURS OF THE NOSE AND SINUSES

In 1892, Nasse reported and illustrated an adenoma of the parotid which showed an acinar structure. Since then the occurrence of acinic cell tumours has become well recognized in the major salivary glands (Godwin,

Foote and Frazell, 1954) but such tumours are extremely rare in the nose and sinuses. Only one case was reported in the largest published series of mucosal gland tumours (Spiro, Koss, Hajdu and Strong, 1973) although Kleinsasser (1970) presented three mucus producing nasal tumours which he classified as acinic cell type, whilst Manace and Goldman (1971) described such a tumour arising in the antro-ethmoidal region and resembling histologically serous secretory units. The present authors have seen one acinic cell tumour in the nasal cavity of an East African. It is possible, however, that some cases may have been overlooked owing to misinterpretation of the histological picture.

On the basis of those arising in major salivary glands, acinic cell tumours tend to occur in early or middle adult life. Two of Kleinsasser's mucous tumours occurred in the seventh decade but the other cases referred to above fit into the general pattern.

The microscopical picture may show a wide range of variation (Abrams, Cornyn, Scofield and Hansen, 1965). The most readily recognizable examples are those which reproduce the typical acinar structure showing small lumina surrounded by wedge-shaped cells with peripherally located nuclei (Figs. 14.16 & 14.17). Sometimes the lumina are a little larger and the cells more cuboidal or columnar (Fig. 14.18) and in such cases the tumour is likely to be classified as merely adenocarcinoma but electron microscopy may reveal all the paraphernalia of secretory activity. Solid masses of cells, completely lacking in any identifiable structure, are not uncommon and a particular variant is the presence of sheets of clear cells (Fig. 14.19), some of which may exhibit acinar formation. Such areas, if exclusive, could resemble metastatic renal carcinoma.

In this group of neoplasms there is no sharp distinction between the benign and the malignant. Local recurrence and metastasis via lymphatics or bloodstream are not unknown in tumours of mucosal gland origin in which malignant behaviour is at least as common as in those arising in major salivary glands. Kleinsasser's cases were unquestionably malignant and the tumour reported by Manace and Goldman (1971) was at least locally invasive.

MUCO-EPIDERMOID TUMOURS

Introduction

Although more commonly found in the parotid where it was first described by Masson and Berger (1924), the muco-epidermoid tumour is now recognized as occurring in a variety of mucosal sites. Stewart, Foote and Becker (1945) reported 45 tumours which they desig-

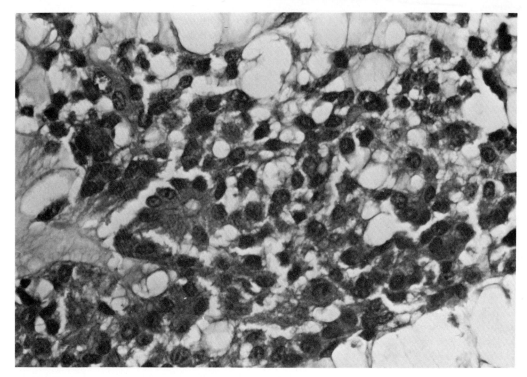

Fig. 14.16 Acinic cell tumour involving the palate in a 59 year-old female, showing acinic differentiation. M × 520

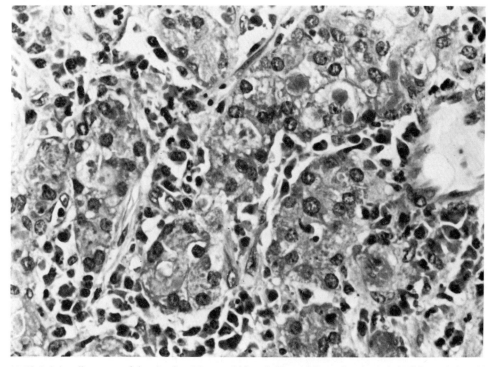

Fig. 14.17 Acinic cell tumour of the nose in a 34 year-old female East African, showing acinic differentiation. M × 488

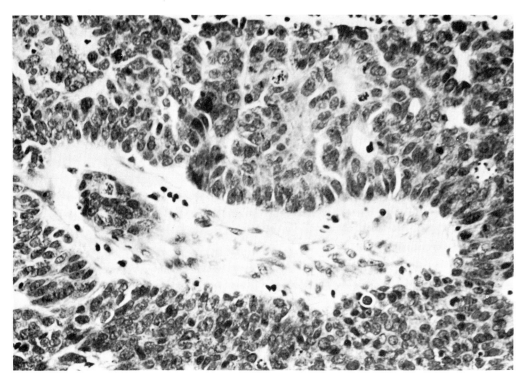

Fig. 14.18 Acinic cell tumour of the maxillary sinus in a 60 year-old male. M × 325

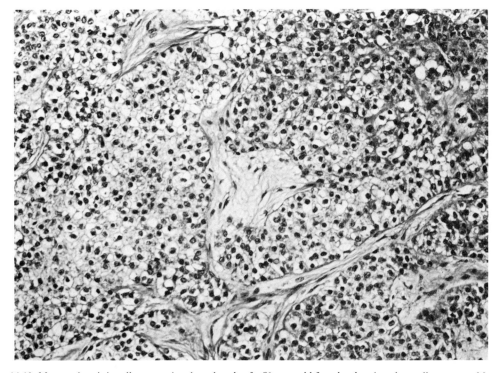

Fig. 14.19 Metastatic acinic cell tumour in a lymphnode of a 59 year-old female, showing clear cell structure. M × 195

nated 'muco-epidermoid'. Fourteen of their series originated in mucosal glands of which four arose in the nose or sinuses. Under the title 'adeno-squamous carcinoma', Gerughty, Henninger and Brown (1968) reported ten such tumours of mucosal origin, two involving the nasal cavity.

Incidence

These tumours comprise one of the less common groups of glandular neoplasms in any location. Bergman (1969) found two such tumours in the nasal region amongst 46 mucosal gland neoplasms. Spiro et al. (1973) reported 20 out of 122 glandular tumours of the nose and sinuses (16 per cent). In the I.L.O. material, tumours of this type represented about 12 per cent of all glandular neoplasms in the region and about 0.6 per cent of all tumours of the nose and sinuses.

Clinical features

Age distribution is broadly based irrespective of the location of the tumour and there is no significant sex difference. In the I.L.O. cases, ages ranged from 26 to 71 years. Patients commonly present with local swelling and nasal obstruction whilst epistaxis may also occur.

Invading tumours may give rise to epiphora, proptosis and disturbance of vision, whilst local pain is not uncommon.

Anatomical site of origin

In reported series, the maxillary sinus has been the main site of election. Healey, Perzin and Smith (1970) found seven maxillary tumours (though only one was specified as antral) and one in the nasal cavity. Spiro et al. (1973) reported 13 tumours in the antrum and seven in the nasal cavity. In the I.L.O. material, four tumours involved the ethmoid region, two the nasal cavity and one the frontal sinus.

Gross appearances

Excised tumour is invariably fragmented, presenting a solid appearance in which cystic spaces may sometimes be seen. The translucent appearance of the pleomorphic tumour is notably absent.

Histopathology

The microscopical picture is characterized by greatly varying combinations of solid cellular masses and tubulo-cystic structures. (Fig. 14.20). The latter vary consid-

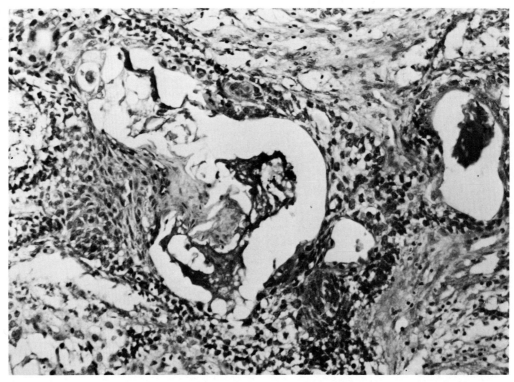

Fig. 14.20 Muco-epidermoid tumour of the ethmoid sinus in a 41 year-old male, showing solid squamoid areas and tubulocystic structures. M × 208

erably in size and may be lined by cubical, columnar, mucus-secreting or even squamous cells whilst the lumina usually contain mucous secretion of epithelial type and occasionally the lining squamous cells may produce keratin. Blending in with the cystic structures are solid areas composed of a multiplicity of cell types which are packed closely together. Frequently present are nondescript irregularly polyhedral cells (intermediate cells) which may be transformed into squamous cells whilst interspersed may be found mucus-secreting elements and clear cells resembling those seen in renal carcinoma (Fig. 14.21). Sometimes, solid areas may show a palisaded border of basal cells, suggesting either a basal cell tumour or even transitional carcinoma (Fig. 14.22).

Biopsies may not always be representative with the result that cystic areas may be diagnosed as adenocarcinoma whilst predominance of a squamoid element may be interpreted as squamous carcinoma. At ultrastructural level, a variety of cytoplasmic organelles are to be found including mucous secretory granules, bundles of tonofibrils, swollen degenerate mitochondria and an abundance of glycogen particles.

Histological distinction between benign and malignant varieties is no longer attempted. Healey et al. (1970)

subdivided muco-epidermoid tumours into low grade, intermediate and high grade malignancy. This was based on the relative proportions of cystic structures and solid cellular areas and the degree of anaplasia.

Aetiology and pathogenesis

No causal agent has yet been identified in respect of this type of glandular tumour, occupations appearing too diverse to suggest any potential hazard in that context. Muco-epidermoid tumours are generally regarded as being of ductal origin (Stewart et al., 1945; Foote and Frazell, 1954). Hamperl and Helweg (1957) believed that such tumours reflected the divergent differentiation of ductal cells. Whilst cells in mucosal gland 'ducts' certainly exhibit flexibility, they do not usually follow that pattern of differentiation, a fact which would accord with the relatively low frequency of this type of glandular tumour.

Behaviour

Stewart et al. (1945) noted that muco-epidermoid tumours of mucosal glands were more likely to be malignant. Furthermore, Healey et al. (1970) found no muco-epidermoid tumours of mucosal origin in their

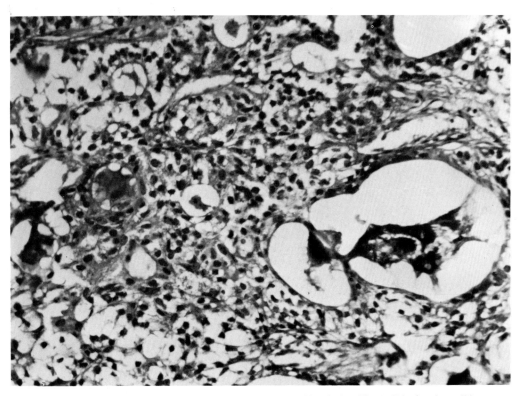

Fig. 14.21 Muco-epidermoid tumour of the ethmoid sinus in a 41 year-old male (see Fig. 14.20), showing solid areas containing clear cells (lower left) and cysts containing mucous secretion. M × 260

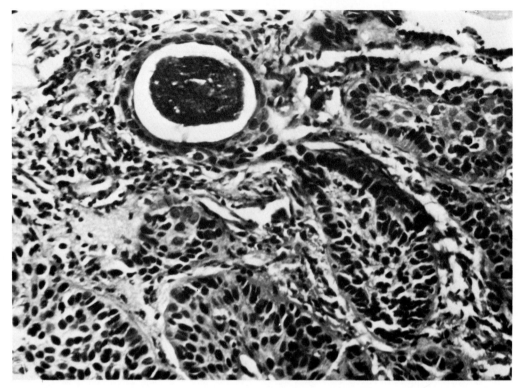

Fig. 14.22 Muco-epidermoid tumour of the nose in a 42 year-old female, showing a small cyst containing epithelial type mucin and peripheral palisading of solid cell masses. Periodic acid-Schiff reaction. M × 325

lowest grade of malignancy and the mucosal series reported by Gerughty et al. (1968) all showed a high malignant potential with seven out of ten (including the two nasal tumours) metastasizing to regional lymphnodes. Three of their cases also showed systemic spread. In the I.L.O. material, recurrence was frequent and often multiple whilst lymphatic and systemic metastasis occurred respectively in two cases. All the paranasal tumours have died over a period ranging from six months to five years and only the two nasal cases have survived for eight and twelve years, apparently free from disease.

PLEOMORPHIC TUMOURS

Introduction

These neoplasms have long been known to arise in mucosal glands, especially in the palate but they also occur less frequently in the nasal region although the much higher incidence in the parotid gland has tended to overshadow all other locations. One of the earliest reports of nasal tumours of this type was by Ahlbom (1935) who found two cases.

Terminology

The epithet 'mixed' was first introduced by Paget in 1853 and, notwithstanding the protracted argument over its significance in relation to pathogenesis, the expression 'mixed parotid tumour' became hallowed by time. Ultimately, the opponents of the dualist theory of origin adopted the term 'pleomorphic tumour' which has gained widespread acceptance though, in the light of modern views, the former label was not so very far short of the mark.

Incidence

Pleomorphic tumours are not so very common in the nose and sinuses and comprise less than ten per cent of all glandular tumours in the region. McDonald and Havens (1948) found 7 per cent whilst Spiro et al (1973) reported only 3 per cent. In the I.L.O. material, pleomorphic tumours constituted less than 7 per cent of all glandular neoplasms and about 0.4 per cent of all tumours in the region.

Clinical features

The age distribution is broadly based and in the published cases has ranged from the second to the eighth decade without any significant sex difference. Local swelling leads to nasal obstruction which may be present for many years before the patient seeks advice. In two of the I.L.O. cases, symptoms had been present for more than ten years, the third patient presented with recent epistaxis whilst in the remaining case, the tumour was an incidental finding.

Anatomical site of origin

The commonest location is in the nasal cavity. Paranasal tumours of this type are rare although antral tumours have been reported by McDonald and Havens (1948), Russell (1955), Potdar and Paymaster (1969), Martis and Karakasis (1971), Spiro et al. (1973).

Gross appearances

To the naked eye such tumours appear as firm sessile slightly lobulated masses that appear sharply circumscribed. The cut surface contains opaque whitish areas but the presence of translucent zones indicates the existence of a myxoid component.

Histopathology

The microscopical picture is no different from that of the major salivary gland tumours of this type. The proportion of epithelial and stromal components varies greatly and bears no relationship to behaviour. Solid cellular areas or tubulo-glandular structures alternate with myxoid or chondroid zones (Fig. 14.23). Solid areas often consist of nondescript cells in varying degrees of compactness. Under the light microscope, obvious squamous metaplasia may be apparent but at ultrastructural level the cells often show divergent differentiation with orientation either to squamous or myoepithelial types. Tubules are usually lined by cuboidal epithelium forming true lumina which often contain epithelial type mucin (diastase-fast P.A.S. positive). The peripheral cells of the epithelial component tend to form a ragged margin from which they straggle out into the stroma. Peripheral palisading of tubular structures (Fig. 14.24) underlines the derivation of the connective tissue component from the 'myothelium'. The myxo-chondroid areas are P.A.S. negative but exhibit hyaluronidase-labile metachromasia with Toluidine Blue, thus characterizing the mucin of connective tissue origin. The 'stromal cells' may sometimes show the presence of glycogen (diastase-labile P.A.S. reaction) or of 'myofibrils' (P.T.A.H. staining) but these reactions are very inconsistent indicating the variability of differentiation which is also demonstrable by electron microscopy. The two main components may be so intimately mixed that pseudo-lumina are formed (often containing connective

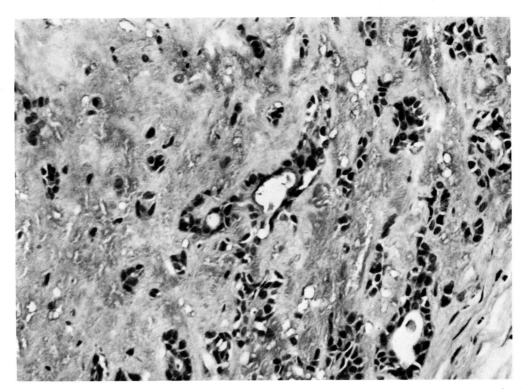

Fig. 14.23 Pleomorphic tumour of the nasal cavity in a 57 year-old female, showing epithelial component in a myxo-chondroid background. M × 330

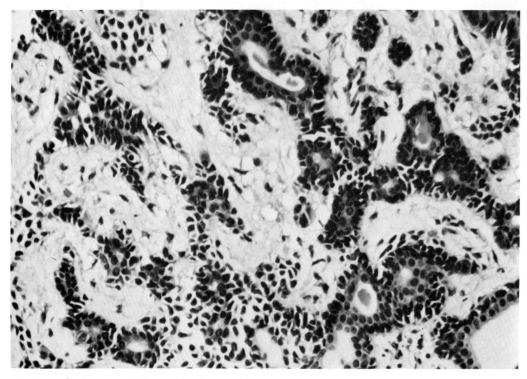

Fig. 14.24 Pleomorphic tumour of the nasal cavity in a 41 year-old female, showing tubular structures with a layer of outer cells tending to become detached and lying free in the myxoid stroma. M × 337

tissue mucin) and may produce a superficial impression of a cribriform pattern (Fig. 14.25) which must not be confused with the cribriform adenocarcinoma. Any of the common variants of this tumour, such as epidermoid cysts or basaloid structures may be encountered.

Aetiology and pathogenesis

The cause of these tumours is unknown but for more than a century there has been continuing speculation on their pathogenesis. Following the observations of a number of workers, including Sheldon (1943), Bauer and Bauer (1953), it has become generally accepted that pleomorphic or 'mixed' tumours are basically ectodermal in origin, being derived from epithelial and myo-epithelial cells. The progeny from the latter cell type does not necessarily retain myo-epithelial characteristics, many of the cells becoming fibroblasts or even chondroblasts, being responsible for the mucopolysaccharide content of the stroma.

Behaviour

Recurrence has not been reported in the majority of published cases occurring in the nasal region and no such event was noted in the four I.L.O. cases. Two cases have so far survived 10 and 13 years whilst two have died of unrelated causes after 6 and 16 years. Recurrence in

a nasal tumour was reported by Miller (1967), a diagnosis of malignancy having been made on the original biopsy. Malignant pleomorphic tumours in the nasal cavity and maxillary sinus were included in the series respectively reported Bergman (1969) and Spiro et al. (1973). The question of malignancy in pleomorphic tumours is still an unresolved problem. Over the years, there has been a very wide spectrum of opinion, the major difficulty being that there are no generally accepted histological criteria. Primary malignant pleomorphic tumour is extremely rare, if it ever occurs. When malignancy supervenes, it affects a particular component, presenting and behaving as a pure tumour of that type of tissue. Thus the original tumour may be overgrown and obscured by a squamous or adenocarcinoma. Eneroth (1964) estimated an incidence of malignant change in about two per cent of major salivary gland pleomorphic tumours.

CRIBRIFORM ADENOCARCINOMA

Introduction

This well-known glandular tumour was first described by Billroth in 1856. A 22 year-old painter presented with a tumour involving the orbit. In a microscopical

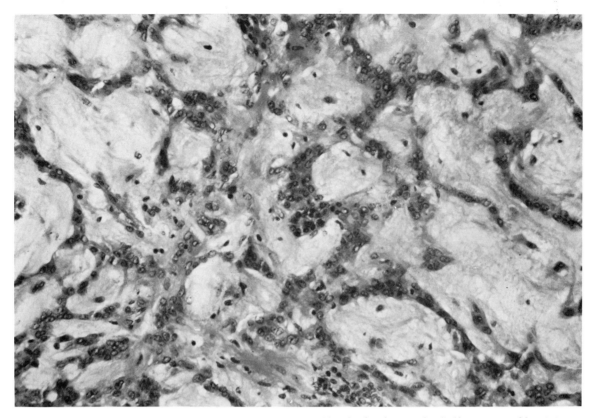

Fig. 14.25 Pleomorphic tumour of the nasal cavity in a 24 year-old male, showing pseudocribriform pattern. M × 585

examination, Billroth noted the surrounding of tumour cells by hyaline material giving the impression of cylindrical structures cut in cross section and it was on the basis of this appearance that he used the term 'Zylindrome'. The precise origin of the tumour was not clear but in 1859 Billroth briefly reported a similar tumour occurring in the maxillary sinus.

Terminology

The label 'Cylindroma' was widely adopted and is still used by some workers although there are cogent histological reasons why it should be abandoned. A vast number of alternative names have been suggested including Basalioma, Pseudoadenomatous basal cell carcinoma, Adenomyoepithelioma and Cystic adenocarcinoma. In 1952, Reid proposed the term 'Adenoid Cystic Carcinoma' and recently the WHO Sub-committee on the classification of tumours recommended its adoption. However, in 1966, Friedmann and Osborn introduced the expression 'Cribriform Adenocarcinoma' as being more appropriate to its character.

Incidence

This neoplasm is one of the more common glandular tumours and in the ear, nose and throat region it occurs at least as frequently as the pleomorphic type. It occurs more frequently in mucosal than in major salivary glands, the ratio probably being of the order of 4:1 (Russell, 1955). A review of published series (Osborn, 1977) showed that cribriform adenocarcinoma represented 32.5 per cent of all types of mucosal gland tumours and about one-third of all glandular tumours of the nose and sinuses are of this type. In the I.L.O. material, the tumour comprised 1.3 per cent of all tumours of the nose and sinuses, 4 per cent of all malignant tumours and 5.6 per cent of all carcinomas.

Clinical features

The age distribution is broadly based but calculation of age incidence reveals a peak in the fourth decade (Osborn, 1977). There is no significant sex difference. The common forms of presentation are local swelling and pain whilst epistaxis is not uncommon. Orbital involvement results in proptosis and disturbance of vision.

Anatomical site of origin

The commonest sites of election are the maxillary sinus and the nasal cavity. McDonald and Havens (1948) found their 31 cases almost equally divided between the two sites but Spiro et al. (1973) reported 29 tumours in the antrum and 14 in the nasal cavity. In the I.L.O. material, 11 tumours arose in the antrum, 2 in the ethmoid region and one in the nasal cavity.

Gross appearances

These tumours present a firm, opaque whitish mass of tissue indistinguishable from other forms of carcinoma and never exhibiting the semi-translucent areas which characterize the pleomorphic tumour (Fig. 14.26).

Histopathology

The microscopical appearances are well-known (Thackray and Lucas, 1960). They may be summarized in four patterns of growth:

1. Areas of cribriform pattern
2. Tubulo-glandular structures
3. Solid cellular areas
4. Cylindromatous pattern

The classical cribriform pattern (Fig. 14.27) is pathognomonic of this neoplasm and must be distinguished from the tubulo-glandular appearance and also from the pseudocribriform pattern sometimes seen in the pleomorphic tumours. Rounded intercellular spaces often contain secretory material which exhibits the staining reactions of connective tissue type mucin (P.A.S. negative and hyaluronidase-labile metachromasia with Toluidine Blue). The lining cells are characteristically flattened and blend with the closely packed cells in the intervals between spaces. The cells are usually small with darkly staining nuclei though very occasionally they may assume a squamoid appearance. The microcystic spaces are sometimes separated from the bordering cells by basement membrane-like material which has been identified by both light and electron microscopy. In view of these observations, the spaces in cribriform areas are designated pseudolumina.

By contrast, the tubulo-glandular structures are lined by cuboidal cells and contain epithelial type mucin (diastase-fast P.A.S. positive reaction). They are appropriately called true lumina and may vary greatly in size and number (Fig. 14.28). The tubules are usually surrounded by a compact outer layer of cells which may appear to exhibit a clear cytoplasm but electron microscopy shows that this may often be an artefact due to shrinkage.

Solid areas composed of the same small darkly staining cells are variable in extent but rarely very large and never exclusive (Fig. 14.29). In the absence of cribriform areas, an alternative diagnosis of basal cell tumour would have to be considered. A higher proportion of solid areas

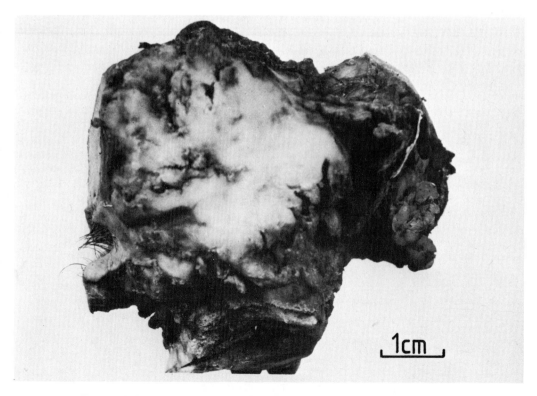

Fig. 14.26 Cribriform adenocarcinoma of the maxillary sinus in a 36 year-old male.

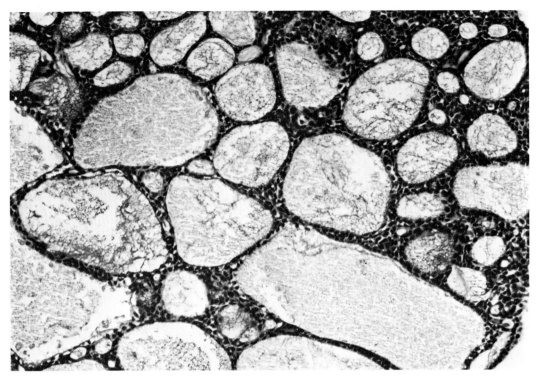

Fig. 14.27 Cribriform adenocarcinoma of the maxillary sinus in a 64 year-old female, showing the classical cribriform pattern with pseudolumina containing connective tissue type mucin. M × 214

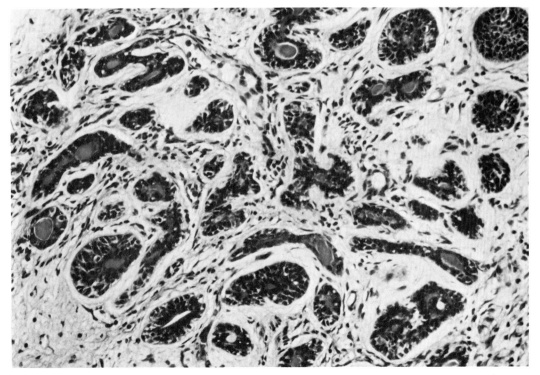

Fig. 14.28 Cribriform adenocarcinoma of the maxillary sinus in a 36 year-old male (see Fig. 14.26), showing tubular pattern with true lumina containing epithelial type mucin. M × 268

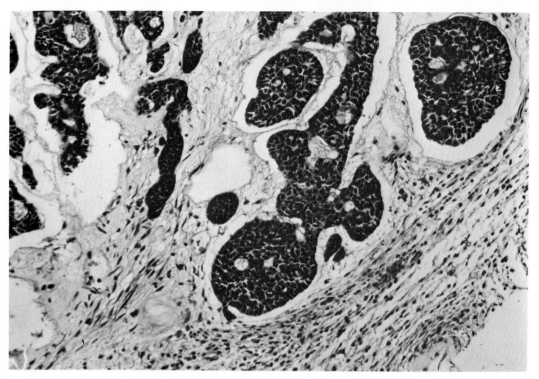

Fig. 14.29 Cribriform adenocarcinoma of the maxillary sinus in a 64 year-old female (see Fig. 14.27), showing solid cellular areas. M × 214

relative to the cribriform pattern was thought by Eneroth, Hjertman and Moberger (1967) to indicate a worse prognosis but this has not been confirmed in the I.L.O. material.

The stroma is characteristically sharply delineated from the epithelial component, in contrast with the appearances found in the pleomorphic tumour. The stroma itself is often unremarkable, consisting of loose connective tissue and occasional vessels. A notable but inconstant feature is the presence of thickened hyaline material, sometimes surrounding groups of tumour cells and sometimes forming irregular projections into epithelial masses (Fig. 14.30). This pattern constitutes the 'Glashelle Zylinder mit kolbigen Auswüchsen' of Billroth (1856). The hyaline material often takes up the Van Gieson stain, indicating its collagen content but it may also exhibit a P.A.S. positive reaction suggesting the presence of basement membrane material. Not only is this pattern frequently absent from such tumours but a similar appearance may be found occasionally in a pleomorphic tumour. Hence, it is not a pathognomonic feature, which fact invalidates the use of the term cylindroma.

The essential histological feature is the cribriform pattern, without which the diagnosis cannot be established. Appearances that may mimic this pattern are found in ameloblastoma and occasionally in pleomorphic tumours. Tauxe, McDonald and Devine (1962) noted five instances of antral tumours being incorrectly diagnosed as ameloblastomas. The pseudocribriform areas in the pleomorphic tumour are usually distinguishable on the basis that the cells are generally larger and less tightly packed whilst the pseudolumina are less sharply rounded.

Ultrastructural studies on these tumours (Friborsky, 1965; Eneroth, Hjertman, Moberger and Wersäll, 1968; Tandler, 1971; Osborn, 1977) have shown the presence of fine filaments of smooth muscle type in cells lining both true and pseudolumina whilst many cells exhibit desmosomal attachments. In the pseudolumina basement membrane material and even collagen have been demonstrated.

Aetiology and pathogenesis

No cause has so far been identified but one curious fact would appear to have a profound relevance to pathogenesis. The cribriform adenocarcinoma and the pleomorphic tumour are apparently mutually exclusive, suggesting a predetermined line of differentiation at the inception of neoplasia. In both tumours, cells display both epithelial and connective tissue characteristic but in true cribriform areas the cells have retained the

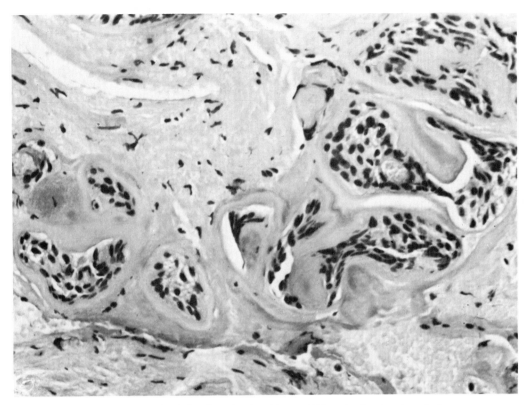

Fig. 14.30 Cribriform adenocarcinoma involving the palate in a 46 year-old female, showing the cylindromatous pattern. Periodic acid-Schiff reaction. M × 325

epithelial characteristic of firm attachment with the result that the secretion they have produced remains confined within distended intercellular spaces. The induction of basement membrane material and the formation of collagen in pseudolumina is a further example of the dual role of these cells.

Behaviour

Local invasion is invariable and in the I.L.O. material over 60 per cent of the paranasal tumours invaded the orbit. The reported incidence of regional lymphnode metastasis has varied greatly. Many observers have found no lymphatic involvement, whilst others have reported varying frequencies reaching as high as 32 per cent in tumours of major salivary gland origin (Eneroth et al., 1967). Spiro et al. (1973) found less than 14 per cent amongst those of mucosal origin. Systemic spread is much more common, Spiro et al., reporting an incidence of nearly 40 per cent. In the I.L.O. material there was no lymphatic spread and a systemic dissemination of 20 per cent was probably an underestimate.

Recurrence is frequent, ranging from 50 per cent (Osborn, 1977) to 100 per cent (Tauxe et al., 1962). A particular feature of this tumour is its propensity to infiltrate perineural spaces (Fig. 14.31). This was first observed by Leroux and Leroux–Robert (1934) whilst Smout and French (1961) found this mode of spread in over 40 per cent of their cases.

Ultimately, most cases die of their disease and Eneroth et al. (1967) stated that five year survival rates were somewhat optimistic. Nevertheless, it is of interest to compare such figures with those for other types of carcinoma in the same regions. The five year survival rate in the I.L.O. material was 53 per cent which is substantially better than even the transitional carcinoma (40 per cent) but the frequency of recurrence creates a high morbidity rate and in less than ten years the survival rate had dropped to less than 15 per cent.

This tumour is clearly an unusual form of carcinoma in which, microscopically, the cells are seen to assume certain mesenchymal characteristics and this would appear to be reflected in the age incidence and the predilection for systemic spread.

BASAL CELL TUMOURS

Under the title of 'basal cell adenoma' Kleinsasser and Klein (1967) described what they believed to be a new entity, representing about two per cent of their collection

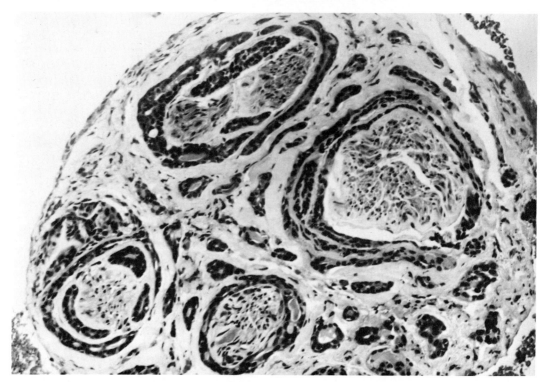

Fig. 14.31 Cribriform adenocarcinoma of the maxillary sinus in a 36 year-old male, showing perineural infiltration. M × 260

of salivary gland tumours. They also used the term 'Monomorphic' and, subsequently, reports of such lesions have appeared in the literature under these labels (Christ and Crocker, 1972; Nelson and Jacoway, 1973) or as 'canalicular adenoma' (Davis and Davis, 1971). More common in the parotid gland, it has also been described in mucosal glands, especially in the lip but no reports of occurrence in the nasal region have so far appeared.

The histological appearance has been extensively described and illustrated by Evans and Cruickshank (1970). The tumour consists of compact epithelial masses sharply demarcated from the stroma which contains no myxoid element. The appearance is not unlike the solid areas seen occasionally in the cribriform adenocarcinoma but frequently there are small tubular structures lying within the cell masses whilst a palisaded border of basal cells is not uncommon. Evans and Cruickshank also described a malignant variant and, in

the I.L.O. material there was one antral tumour which showed solid cellular areas resembling the basal cell adenoma and no evidence of cribriform pattern (Fig. 14.32). The tumour proved to be extremely aggressive, invading the cheek, orbit and pterygoid region, with ultimate death of the patient after 14 months.

A crucial issue for many years was the possible relationship of 'cylindromatous tumours' to basal cell carcinoma. In 1918, Krompecher described a series of basal cell carcinomas of the upper respiratory tract, dividing them into 'cylindromatous' and 'solid' types. It is interesting to note that he regarded the former group as being relatively benign and it is probable that the solid type represented malignant basal cell tumours. In 1972, Koss, Spiro and Hajdu described another group of mucosal gland tumours which they designated 'oat cell carcinomas'. These tumours were highly malignant and it is likely that they too belonged to the malignant basal cell group.

BIBLIOGRAPHY

Abrams A M, Cornyn J, Scofield H H, Hanse L S 1965 Acinic cell adenocarcinoma of the major salivary glands. Cancer 18: 1145–1162

Acheson E D, Cowdell R H, Hadfield E H, Macbeth R G 1968 Nasal cancer in woodworkers in the furniture industry. British Medical Journal 2: 587–596

Acheson E D, Cowdell R H, Jolles B 1970 Nasal cancer in the Northamptonshire boot and shoe industry. British Medical Journal 1: 385–393

Acheson E D, Hadfield E H, Macbeth R G 1967 Carcinoma of the nasal cavity and accessory sinuses in woodworkers. Lancet 1: 311–312

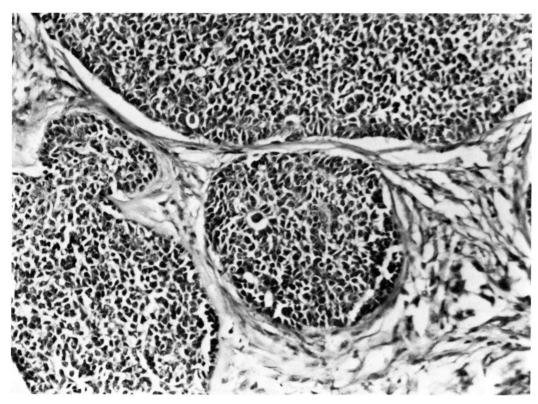

Fig. 14.32 Malignant basal cell tumour of maxillary sinus in a 62 year-old female, showing peripheral palisading and tendency to form tubular structures within the cell masses. Note absence of cribriform pattern. M × 300

Ahlbom H E 1935 Mucous and salivary gland tumours. Acta Radiologica, Supplement 23

Batsakis J G, Holz F, Sueper R H 1963 Adenocarcinoma of nasal and paranasal cavities. Archives of Otolaryngology 77: 625–633

Bauer W H, Bauer J D 1953 Classification of glandular tumours of salivary glands. Archives of Pathology 55: 328–346

Bazaz-Malik G, Gupta D N 1968 Metastasizing (malignant) oncocytoma of the parotid gland. Zeitschrift für Krebsforschung 70: 193–197

Bergman F 1969 Tumors of the minor salivary glands. Cancer 23–5381543

Billroth T 1856 Untersuchungen über die Entwicklung der Blutgefässe. Dissertation, Georg Reimer

Billroth T 1859 Beobachtungen über Geschwülste der Speicheldrüsen. Virchows Archiv für pathologische Anatomie 17: 357–375

Black A, Evans J C, Hadfield E H, Macbeth R G 1974 Impairment of nasal muco-ciliary clearance in woodworkers in the furniture industry. British Journal of Industrial Medicine 31: 10–17

Blanck C, Eneroth C M, Jakobsen P A 1970 Oncocytoma of the parotid gland. Cancer 25: 919–925

Brinton L A, Blot W J, Stone B J, Fraumeni J F 1977 A death certificate analysis of nasal cancer among furniture workers in North Carolina. Cancer Research 37: 3473–3474

Christ T F, Crocker D 1972 Basal cell adenoma of minor salivary gland origin. Cancer 30: 214–219

Citelli S, Calamida U 1903 Beiträge zu Lehre von dem Epitheliomen der Nasenschleimhaut. Archiv für Laryngologie 13: 273–287

Cohen M A, Batsakis J G 1968 Oncocytic tumour of minor salivary glands. Archives of Otolaryngology 88: 71–73

Davis W M, Davis W 1971 Canalicular adenoma. Journal of Oral Surgery 29: 500–501

Debois J M 1969 Tumoren van de neusholte bij houtbewerkers. Tijdschrift Geneeskunde 25: 92–93

Eneroth C M 1964 Histological and clinical aspects of parotid tumours. Acta Otolaryngologica, Supplement 191, 1–94

Eneroth C M, Hjertman L, Moberger G 1967 Malignant tumours of submandibular gland. Acta Otolaryngologica 64: 514–536

Eneroth C M, Hjertman L, Moberger G, Wersäll J 1968 Ultrastructural characteristics of adenoid cystic carcinoma of salivary glands. Archiv klinische und experimentelle Ohren-, Nasen- und Kehlkopfheilkunde 192: 356–368

Evans R W, Cruickshank A H 1970 Basal cell adenoma in epithelial tumours of the salivary glands. Saunders W B ch 5, pp 58–76

Fechner R E, Bentinck B R 1973 Ultrastructure of bronchial oncocytoma. Cancer 31: 1451–1457

Foote F W, Frazell E L 1954 Muco-epidermoid tumors in atlas of tumour pathology. Armed Forces Institute of Pathology, Fascicle 11, Section IV, 79–100

Friborsky V 1965 The submicroscopical structure of adenoid cystic carcinoma of salivary glands. Acta Morphologica (Academy of Sciences, Hungary) 14: 105–116

Friedmann I, Osborn D A 1966 In: Wright G P, Symmers W St C (eds) Malignant tumours of the nasopharynx in Systemic Pathology, 1st ed. Longmans, London

Gamez-Araujo J J, Ayala A G, Guillamondegui O 1975 Mucinous adenocarcinomas of the nose and paranasal sinuses. Cancer 36: 1100–1105

Gerughty R M, Henniger G R, Brown F M 1968 Adeno-squamous carcinoma of the nasal, oral and laryngeal cavities. Cancer 22: 1140–1155

Gignoux M, Bernard P 1969 Tumeurs malignes de l'ethmoide chez les travailleurs du bois. Journal médical de Lyon 50: 731–736

Godwin J T, Foote F W, Frazell E L 1954 Acinic cell adenocarcinoma of the parotid gland. American Journal of Pathology 30: 465–477

Gruenfeld G E, Jorsted L H 1936 Adenoma of the parotid salivary gland: oncocyte tumor. American Journal of Cancer 26: 571–575

Hadfield E H 1970 A study of adenocarcinoma of the paranasal sinuses in woodworkers in the furniture industry. Annals of the Royal College of Surgeons of England 46: 301–319

Hadfield E H, Macbeth R G 1971 Adenocarcinoma of ethmoids in furniture workers. Annals of Otology, Rhinology and Laryngology 80: 699–703

Hamperl H 1931 Beiträge zur normalen und pathologischen Histologie menschlicher Speicheldrüsen. Zeitschrift für mikroskopische und anatomische Forschung 27: 1–55

Hamperl H 1950 Onkocytes and the so-called Hurthle cell tumor. Archives of Pathology 563–567

Hamperl H 1962 Onkocytom der Speicheldrüsen. Zeitschrift für Krebsforschung 64: 427–440

Hamperl H, Hellweg G 1957 Muco-epidermoid tumors of different sites. Cancer 10: 1187–1192

Harmer L, Glas E 1907 Die malignen Tumoren der inneren Nase. Deutsche Zeitschrift Chirurgie 89: 433–539

Hautant A, Monod D, Klotz A 1933 Les épithéliomes ethmoido-orbitaires. Annals d'Otolaryngologie 1933: 385–421

Healey W V, Perzin K H, Smith L 1970 Muco-epidermoid carcinoma of salivary gland origin. Cancer 26: 368–388

Ironside P, Matthews J 1975 Adenocarcinoma of the nose and paranasal sinuses in woodworkers in the State of Victoria, Australia. Cancer 36: 1115–1121

Järvi O 1945 Heterotopic tumours with intestinal mucous membrane structure in the nasal cavity. Acta Otolaryngologica 33: 471–485

Johns M E, Batsakis J G, Short C D 1973 Oncocytic and oncocytoid tumours of the salivary glands. Laryngoscope 83: 1940–1952

Kleinsasser O 1970 Acinuszelltumoren der Schleimdrüsen. Archiv für klinische und experimentelle Ohren-, Nasen- und Kehlkopfheilkunde 195: 345–354

Kleinsasser O, Klein H J 1967 Basalzelladenome der Speicheldrüsen. Archiv für klinische und experimentelle Ohren-, Nasen- und kehlkopfheilkunde 189: 302–316

Koss L G, Spiro R H, Hajdu S 1972 Small cell (oat cell) carcinoma of minor salivary gland origin. Cancer 30: 737–741

Krompecher E 1918 Zur Kenntniss der Basalzellenkrebse der Nase, der Nebenhöhlen, des Kehlkopfes under der Trachea. Archiv für Laryngologie 31: 443–460

Leroux R, Leroux-Robert J 1934 Essai de classification architecturale des tumeurs des glandes salivaires. Bulletin de l'Association Francaise pour l'étude du cancer 23: 304–340

Macbeth R G 1965 Malignant disease of the paranasal sinuses. Journal of Laryngology and Otology 79: 592–612

McDonald J R, Havens F Z 1948 A study of malignant tumors of glandular nature in the nose, throat and mouth. Surgical Clinics of North America 28: 1087–1106

Manace E D, Goldman J L 1971 Acinic cell carcinoma of paranasal sinuses. Laryngoscope 81: 1074–1082

Martis C S, Karakasis D T 1971 Pleomorphic adenoma arising in the maxillary sinus. Plastic and Reconstructive Surgery 47: 290–292

Masson P, Berger L 1924 Épithéliomes à double metaplasie de la parotide. Bulletin de l'Association Francaise pour l'étude du cancer 13: 366–375

Meza-Chavez L 1949 Oxyphilic granular cell adenoma of the parotid gland (oncocytoma). American Journal of Pathology 25: 523–548

Miller H 1967 Mixed salivary tumour of the nasal septum. Australian & New Zealand Journal of Surgery 36: 249–251

Mosbech J, Acheson E D 1971 Nasal cancer in furniture makers in Denmark. Danish Medical Bulletin 18: 34–35

Nasse D 1892 Die Geschwülste der Speicheldrüsen und verwandte Tumoren des Kopfes. Archiv klinische Chirurgie 44: 233–302

Nelson J F, Jacoway J R 1973 Monomorphic adenoma (canalicular type). Cancer 31: 1511–1513

Osborn D A 1977 Morphology and the natural history of cribriform adenocarcinoma (adenoid cystic carcinoma). Journal of Clinical Pathology 30: 195–205

Paget J 1853 Cartilaginous tumours, lecture VII in lectures on surgical pathology, vol 2. Longmans, pp 201–205

Potdar G G, Paymaster J C 1969 Tumors of minor salivary glands. Oral Surgery, Oral Medicine and Oral Pathology 28: 310–319

Reid J D 1952 Adenoid cystic carcinoma (cylindroma) of the bronchial tree. Cancer 5: 685–694

Ringertz N 1938 Pathology of malignant tumours arising in the nasal and paranasal cavities and maxilla. Acta Otolaryngologica, Supplement 27, Chapter 7

Russell H 1955 Adenomatous tumours of the anterior foregut region showing the cylindroma pattern. British Journal of Surgery 43: 248–254

Sanchez-Casis G, Devine K D, Weiland L H 1971 Nasal adenocarcinomas that closely resemble colonic carcinomas. Cancer 28: 714–720

Schoental R, Gibbard S 1972 Nasal and other tumours in rats given 3,4,5-Trimethoxy-cinnamaldehyde. British Journal of Cancer 26: 504–505

Sheldon W H 1943 So-called mixed tumours of the salivary glands. Archives of Pathology 35: 1–20

Smout M S, French A J 1961 Prognosis of pseudo-adenomatous basal cell carcinoma: cylindroma, adenocystic carcinoma. Archives of Pathology 72: 107–112

Spiro R H, Koss L G, Hajdu S I, Strong E W 1973 Tumors of minor salivary origin. Cancer 31: 117–129

Stewart F W, Foote F W, Becker W F 1945 Muco-epidermoid tumors of salivary glands. Annals of Surgery 122: 820–844

Tandler B 1971 Ultrastructure of adenoid cystic carcinoma of salivary gland origin. Laboratory Investigation 24: 504–512

Tandler B, Hutter R V P, Erlandson R A 1970 Ultrastructure of oncocytoma. Laboratory Investigation 23: 567–580

Tauxe W N, McDonald J R, Devine K D 1962 A century of cylindromas. Archives of Otolaryngology 75: 364–376

Thackray A C, Lucas R B 1960 The histology of cylindroma of mucous gland origin. British Journal of Cancer 14: 612–619

Additional reference

Seifert G, Rieb H, Donath K 1980 Klassifikation der Tumoren der kleinen Speicheldrüsen. Zeitschrift für Laryngologie und Rhinologie 59: 379–400

NECROTIZING SIALOMETAPLASIA

This condition was first reported by Abrams, Melrose and Howell in 1973 as a benign inflammatory process affecting the mucosal glands of the palate (Fig. 14.33). They characterized the lesion as having the following differentiating features: (a) lobular infarction or necrosis, (b) maintenance of the general lobular pattern, (c) simultaneous squamous metaplasia of mucous acini and ductal structures, (d) bland appearance of the squamous metaplastic cells and (e) considerable acute and chronic inflammatory infiltration around the affected glands. These authors presented seven cases to which Dunlap and Barker (1974) added a further five cases (all involving the palate) whilst Myers, Bankaci and Barnes (1975) published a solitary case and Fechner (1977) reported two palatal cases.

The above mentioned authors appear to have established evidence of an entity, in the palatal location, which could be confused with a muco-epidermoid tumour. Maisel, Johnston, Anderson and Cantrell (1977) reported two cases of alleged necrotizing sialometaplasia occurring in the nasal region. Neither of these cases are acceptable because both had unquestionable carcinoma. Nor is the solitary case published by Johnston (1977) any more convincing since the squamous metaplasia probably resulted from the inevitable exposure following maxillectomy.

To date, therefore, acceptable cases of this condition have not been found in the nose or sinuses.

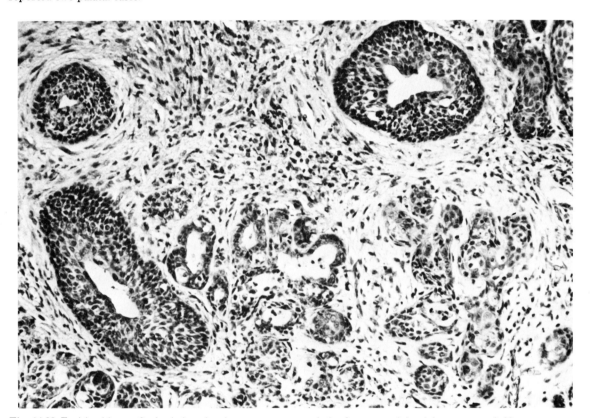

Fig. 14.33 Excision biopsy of palatal ulcer showing squamous metaplasia of mucous acini and ducts surrounded by inflammatory granulation tissue M × 144 (By courtesy of Dr M H Bennet)

BIBLIOGRAPHY

Abrams A M, Melrose R J, Howell F V 1973 Necrotizing sialometaplasia. Cancer 32: 130–135

Dunlap C L, Barker B F 1974 Necrotizing sialometaplasia. Oral Surgery, Oral Medicine and Oral Pathology 37: 722–727

Fechner R E 1977 Necrotizing sialometaplasia. American Journal of Clinical Pathology 67: 315–317

Johnston W H 1977 Necrotizing sialometaplasia involving the mucous glands of the nasal cavity. Human Pathology 8: 589–592

Maisel R H, Johnston W H, Anderson H A, Cantrell A W 1977 Necrotizing sialometaplasia involving the nasal cavity. Laryngoscope 87: 429–434

Myers E N, Bankaci M, Barnes E L 1975 Necrotizing sialometaplasia. Archives of Otolaryngology 101: 628–629

15

Melanotic tumours of the nose and sinuses

MALIGNANT MELANOMA OF THE NOSE AND SINUSES

Introduction

This is an important tumour in the region, not so much on the grounds of its frequency but because poorly or non-pigmented varieties are liable to be confused with other neoplasms. The first mention of malignant melanoma of the nose was by Lücke in 1869 and, in 1872, Viennois reported an example in a 63 year-old woman who died following invasion of the orbit. Wilkinson (1912) reported the first case in the United Kingdom.

Terminology

These tumours have been variously known as melanomas, malignant melanomas, melanocarcinomas and melanosarcomas. The last mentioned term is now obsolete but the expression melanocarcinoma is still favoured by some writers whilst others retain the label melanoma even though confusion with benign pigmented lesions or naevi may occur.

Incidence

Malignant melanoma is generally regarded as a relatively rare tumour in the nose. Allen and Spitz (1953) found that just over one per cent of all malignant malanomas occurred in the nose and sinuses whilst Moore and Martin (1955), in their review of 1546 cases, found the nose and sinuses to be involved in 0.5 per cent. Holdcraft and Gallagher (1969) found malignant melanoma to represent 0.5 per cent of all nasal and paranasal tumours. In the I.L.O. material malignant melanoma represents about five per cent of all tumours in the nasal cavity and is the second commonest malignant neoplasm (23 per cent) in that region.

Clinical features

The age distribution reaches a peak in the seventh decade and there is no significant sex difference. Cases commonly present with nasal obstruction and epistaxis whilst intranasal swellings range widely in colour. Submucosal haemorrhage may sometimes simulate melanotic deposits and, occasionally, nasal polypi may be removed without suspicion of their true nature which is only revealed by histology.

Anatomical site of origin

The tumour commonly arises in the nasal cavity and paranasal origin is generally regarded as uncommon (Rigertz, 1938; Moore and Martin, 1955; Ravid and Estaves, 1960; Holdcraft and Gallagher, 1969). Freedman, Desanto, Devine and Weiland (1973) and also Eneroth and Lundberg (1975) have reported extensive paranasal involvement but it is obviously difficult in many cases to exclude secondary extension from the nose. Ringertz (1938) considered that primary origin was probably nasal in all cases, a view reflected in the experience of the present authors in whose material only one case was possibly of paranasal origin. Within the nasal cavity, the common sites of origin are the septum, the lateral wall and inferior turbinate with less frequent involvement of the roof and floor. Multiple origin is a particular feature of this neoplasm though this may not be readily apparent in cases which present with the nasal cavity completely filled with newgrowth (Figs. 15.1 & 15.2).

Gross appearances

The naked eye appearance is variable, ranging from solid black masses to innocent-looking nasal polypi.

Histopathology

The light microscopical picture is characteristically variable, the common patterns being sheets of closely arranged spheroidal cells (Fig. 15.3) or spindle cells (Fig. 15.4). The picture may be largely monomorphic or pleomorphic (Fig. 15.5) whilst multinucleated giant cells may also be seen. Pigmentation is also extremely variable and when present it facilitates the diagnosis (Figs. 15.6, 15.7 & 15.8). Melanin stains (Masson-Fontana or Schmorl, combined with permanganate bleaching) may sometimes be of assistance in the detection of small amounts of pigment and, in any case, provide the essential confirmation of its nature. Pigment

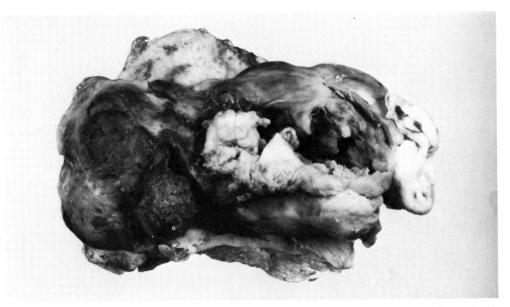

Fig. 15.1 Malignant melanoma of the nose in a 68 year-old male, showing extensive involvement of the nasal cavity.

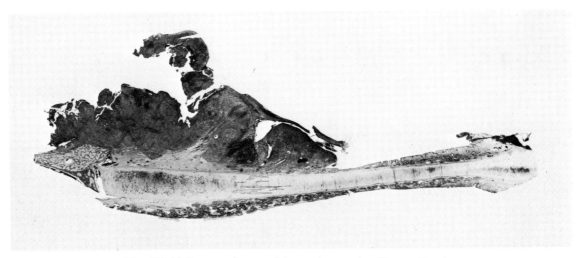

Fig. 15.2 Malignant melanoma of the nasal septum in a 55 year-old male.

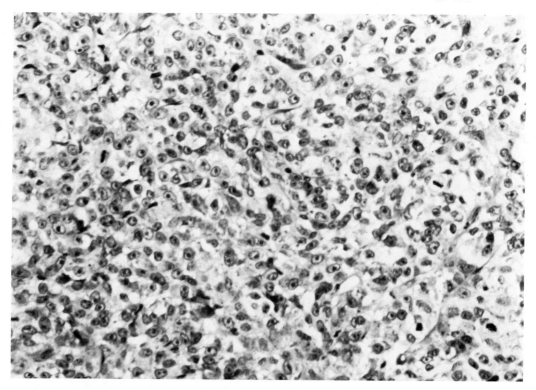

Fig. 15.3 Malignant melanoma of the nose in a 68 year-old male (see Fig. 15.1) showing polyhedral cell structure. M × 330

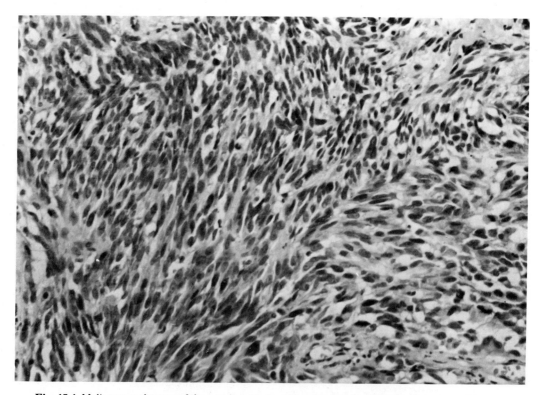

Fig. 15.4 Malignant melanoma of the nose in a 43 year-old male, showing spindle cell structure. M × 260

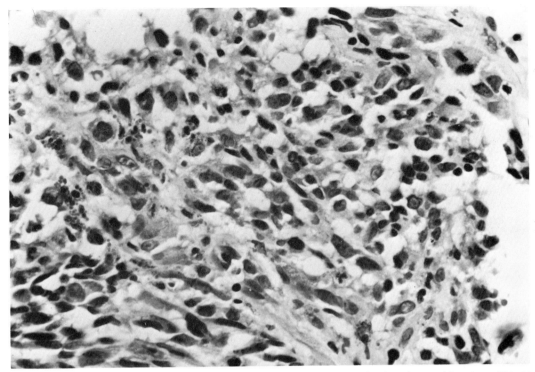

Fig. 15.5 Malignant melanoma of the nose in a 43 year-old male (see Fig. 15.4), showing pleomorphic pattern. M ×536

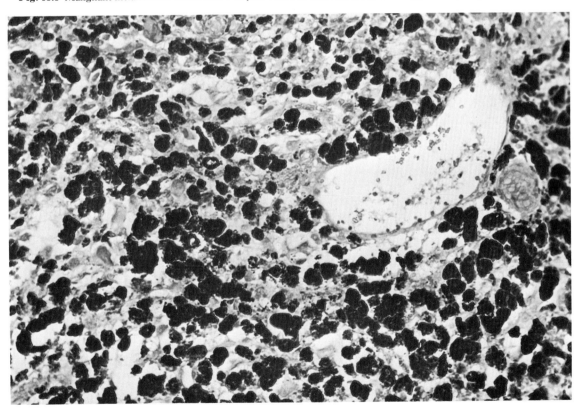

Fig. 15.6 Malignant melanoma of the nose in a 47 year-old male, showing heavily pigmented cells. M ×230

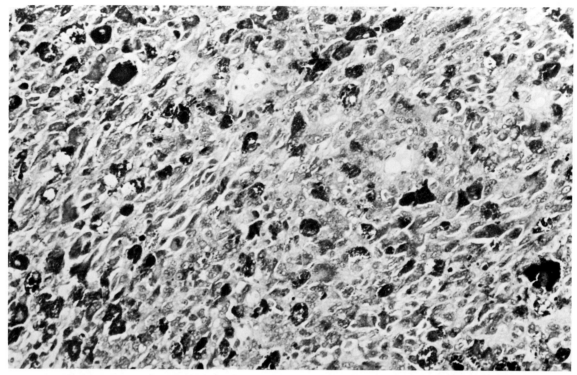

Fig. 15.7 Malignant melanoma of the nose in a 56 year-old female, showing moderate pigmentation. M ×225

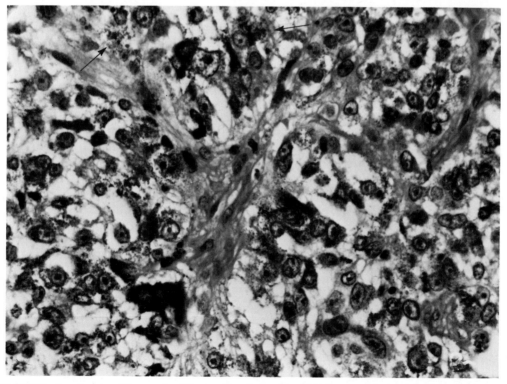

Fig. 15.8 Malignant melanoma of the nose in a 68 year-old male (see Fig. 15.1) showing a finely pigmented area (arrows).
M ×520

should be found in the tumour cells but when liberated it is frequently taken up by macrophages where its distinction from iron compounds is clearly necessary. The possibility of malignant melanoma must be borne in mind when confronted with primary biopsies composed of non-pigmented tumour tissue without recognizable structure (Fig. 15.9).

A problem of immediate practical importance is the confirmation of the presence of a local primary tumour and the significant feature is the presence of intra-epithelial (junctional) changes in persistent surface epithelium (Fig. 15.10). Although more commonly seen in metaplastic squamous epithelium, this change may sometimes be found in the columnar type.

Ultrastructural studies of malignant melanoma have been largely concerned with the cutaneous neoplasms (Currant and McCann, 1976) but Friedmann (1961) and Wright and Heenan (1975) reported electron microscopical observations in malignant melanoma of the nose. However, the fine structure is essentially the same irrespective of the origin of the tumour. Neoplastic melanocytes are characterized by the presence of varying numbers of pigmentary organelles (melanosomes) which

tend to be scattered diffusely throughout the cytoplasm. Golgi complexes and irregular profiles of rough endoplasmic reticulum are readily identified. Mitochondria vary in number and size and may appear degenerate. Desmosomes are absent but scattered bundles of fine filaments are not uncommon. The melanosomes present a pleomorphic pattern, ranging from elongated or cigar-shaped to short oval or rounded bodies (Fig. 15.11) whilst ring forms or irregular masses are not uncommon. When melanization is incomplete, the internal structure of the premelanosomes is visible in varying degree (Fig. 15.12). In the elongated type the crystal-like cross banding with a periodicity of about 9Å (thought to be due to the alignment of tyrosinase molecules) has superimposed on it a longitudinally disposed arrangement of fibrillar structures which become progressively thicker with increasing deposition of melanin. The more rounded type of organelle does not possess this type of internal structure but exhibits a finely granular matrix in which pigmented masses are embedded and may well represent lysosomal degradation which is believed to be a normal controlling mechanism of pigmentation.

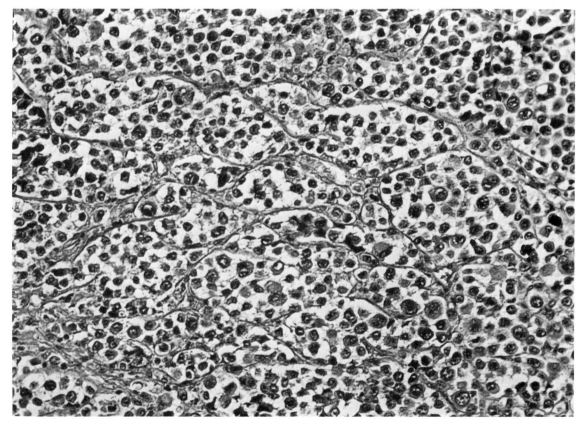

Fig. 15.9 Amelanotic malignant melanoma of the nose in a 51 year-old male. M × 240

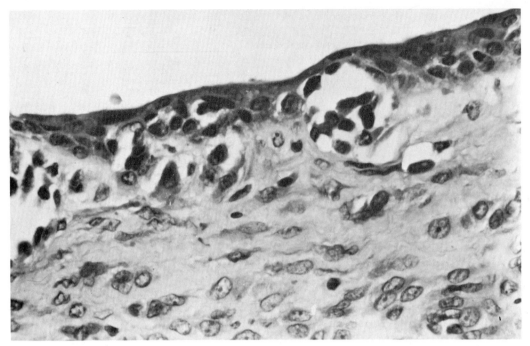

Fig. 15.10 Malignant melanoma of the nose in a 45 year-old male, showing junctional activity in metaplastic squamous epithelium. M ×528

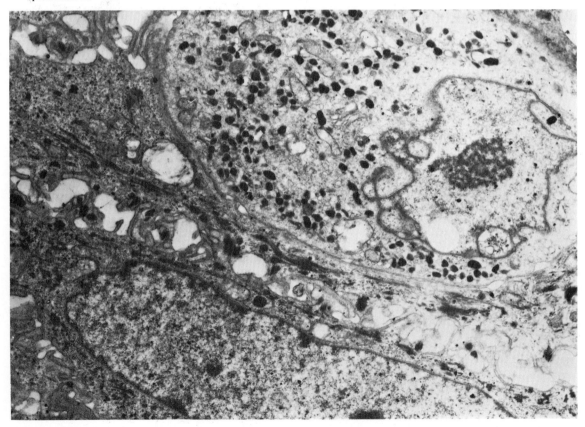

Fig. 15.11 Malignant melanoma of the nose in a 50 year-old male, showing numerous melanosomes. M ×14 000

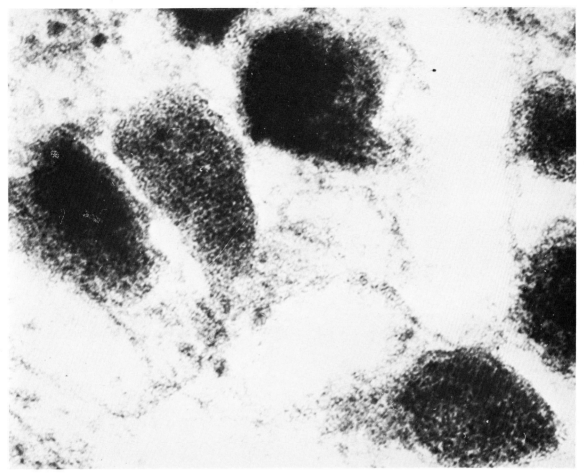

Fig. 15.12 Malignant melanoma of the nose in a 50 year-old male (see Fig. 15.12) showing partial pigmentation of premelanosomes. M × 240 000

Aetiology and pathogenesis

The origin of malignant melanoma in the nasal cavity has been the subject of considerable speculation. The early concept of origin from the mucocutaneous junction (Wilkinson, 1912) does not accord with the observed facts. Melanin pigment is not readily seen in the nasal cavity except in the olfactory area where it may be found in the supporting cells (Ringertz, 1938) but primary origin in this region is relatively uncommon (Grace, 1947).

It is generally accepted that malignant melanomas of the skin commonly arise from pre-existing pigmented lesions – either junctional naevi (Allen and Spitz, 1953) or the pre-cancerous melanosis of Dubreuilh (Mishima, 1967) but, in spite of the analogy drawn by Allen and Spitz regarding malignant melanomas of mucous membranes, there is no clinical or histological evidence for the occurrence of any benign pigmented lesion in the nasal cavity (Mayoux and Perron, 1939; Freedman et

al., 1973). However, careful examination of nasal mucosa in cases of malignant melanoma of this region reveals two interesting facts. Firstly, junctional activity comparable with that seen in skin lesions may be observed (Ravid and Estaves, 1960; Crone, 1966; Holdcraft and Gallagher, 1969; Freedman et al., 1973). Secondly, melanin pigment may be found in the nasal epithelium with or without junctional activity. In the I.L.O. material, junctional activity was found in over 50 per cent of cases and the observation was of particular importance in two patients who had had a previous malignant melanoma of the skin, thus supporting the assertion of Allen and Spitz that patients with a malignant melanoma have an increased liability to develop a second primary tumour in another site.

Clearly, melanocytes must be present in the nasal epithelium but their identification requires more than the mere finding of intracellular pigment since this may have been transferred to ordinary epithelial cells (Borrel,

1913; Masson, 1948; Billingham, 1948). The claim of Zak and Lawson (1974) to have demonstrated melanocytes in the nasal mucosa by the Masson-Fontana staining technique still requires substantiation. The demonstration of DOPA oxidase activity in skin melanocytes is well established and Szabo (1959) used this technique to demonstrate the presence of such cells in the nasal vestibule but, so far, attempts to identify pigment producing cells in the nasal mucosa by this method have been unsuccessful. There may exist in the normal nasal mucosa a dormant, non-functional variant of the melanocyte which becomes activated only under conditions of neoplasia. The penultimate stage of activation is the development of junctional activity, the presence of which may be observed in material from recurrences as well as from primary biopsies, clearly indicating the multicentric origin of the tumour in a continuing state of activity.

The functional melanocyte produces the copper-containing enzyme Tyrosinase or DOPA oxidase which mediates the slow change from tyrosine into DOPA and the more rapid conversion of the latter into $5:6$ dihydroxyindole from which melanins are derived. The excess pigment production which may occur in malignant melanoma is believed to follow the same chemical pathway and gross excess, associated particularly with hepatic metastases, may result in the appearance of both DOPA (phenol) and indole melanogens in the urine where the latter give rise to the positive Thormalen test. Melanin production by these tumours would appear to be an incidental by-product and has no influence on the prognosis (Mason and Friedmann, 1955). On the other hand, dietary restriction of tyrosinase substrates in melanoma-bearing mice caused a four-fold reduction in the size of the tumours (Mitamura, Yuen, Duke and Demopoulos, 1966).

Inasmuch as occasional regression has been observed in these tumours (Bulkley, Cohen, Banks, Char and Ketcham, (1975), it has been suspected that there might be an immunological basis for the phenomenon. The sera of patients with malignant melanomas have been shown to contain antibodies which are cytotoxic to the tumour cells in tissue culture although there is no cross reaction with malignant melanoma cells from other patients (Lewis, 1967; Lewis, Ikonopisov, Nairn, Phillips, Hamilton Fairley, Bodenham and Alexander, 1969). Unfortunately, although a rise in antibody level has been produced by injecting patients with their own tumour cells, no regression of the primary tumour has been observed. Induction of non-specific immunity by the intralesional injection of vaccines such as vaccinia (Burdick, 1960) and B.C.G. (Morton, Eilber, Malmgren and Wood, 1970) had limited success, being confined to the lesions in which the vaccine was inserted. More recently, however, Mastrangelo, Bellet, Berkelhammer and Clark (1975) claimed more impressive results in which not only the injected but the non-injected lesions and even pulmonary metastases underwent regression. Tumour antigens have been located both within the cells and on the surface, the latter being of greater importance. Lewis et al. (1969) demonstrated specific antibodies in about 30 per cent of patients with malignant melanomas and found that they were more likely to be present in patients with solitary, slowly growing tumours.

Behaviour

Malignant melanomas of the nose tend to follow the familiar pattern well known in their cutaneous and ocular counterparts. Recurrence is frequent. Conley and Pack (1974) reported a local recurrence rate of 40 per cent but in the I.L.O. material the frequency was nearly 70 per cent. In the same series, regional lymphnode metastasis was observed in about 36 per cent whilst systemic spread is known to have occurred in more than a quarter of the cases. The five year crude survival rate was of the order of 20 per cent and Harrison (1976), reporting on the clinical aspects of much of the same material, noted the unfavourable comparison with the behaviour of cutaneous tumours.

JUVENILE MELANOMA OF THE NOSE

The occurrence of this type of melanotic tumour and the problems of histological diagnosis are well recognized in the context of cutaneous lesions (Spitz, 1948) but its existence as a tumour of mucosal origin is less well established. Ravid and Estaves (1960) reported an example in an eight month old coloured girl but the tumour was vestibular in origin and therefore of cutaneous type.

Amongst the I.L.O. material was a melanotic tumour arising from the nasal mucosa of a fifteen year-old boy. Histologically, it showed all the features which have been described in the cutaneous juvenile melanoma – junctional change, dominant spindle cell growth (Fig. 15.13) angiectasia and giant cells (Fig. 15.14). Following incomplete excision, the patient was alive and well nine years later with no evidence of intranasal disease.

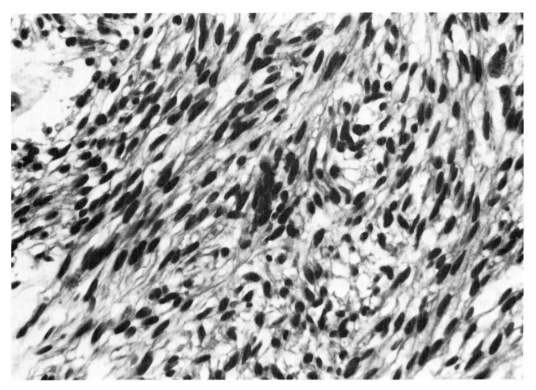

Fig. 15.13 Juvenile melanoma of the nose in a 15 year-old boy, showing spindle cell structure. M ×528

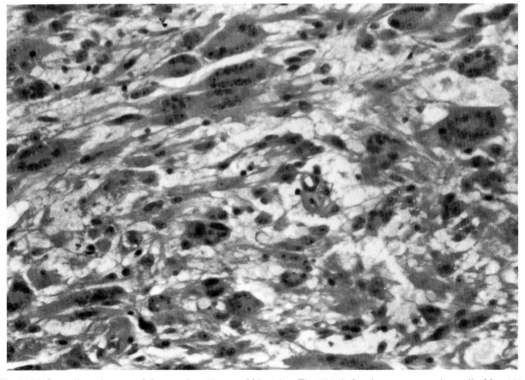

Fig. 15.14 Juvenile melanoma of the nose in a 15 year-old boy (see Fig. 15.14) showing numerous giant cells. M ×330

BIBLIOGRAPHY

Allen A C, Spitz S 1953 Malignant melanoma. A clinico-pathological analysis of the criteria for diagnosis and prognosis. Cancer 6: 1–45

Billingham R E 1948 Dendritic cells. Journal of Anatomy 82: 93–109

Borrel A 1913 Cellules pigmentaires et associations cellulaires. Comptes Rendus de Societé de Biologie 74: 1215–1218

Bulkley G B, Cohen M H, Banks P M, Char D H, Ketcham A S 1975 Long-term spontaneous regression of malignant melanoma with visceral metastases. Cancer 36: 485–494

Burdick K H 1960 Malignant melanoma treated with vaccinia injection. Archives of Dermatology 82: 438

Conley J, Pack G T 1974 Melanoma of the mucous membranes of the head and neck. Archives of Otolaryngology 99: 315–319

Crone R P 1966 Malignant amelanotic melanomas of the nasal septum and maxillary sinus. Laryngoscope 76: 1826

Curran R C, McCann B G 1976 The ultrastructure of benign pigmented naevi and melanocarcinomas in man. Journal of Pathology 119: 135–146

Eneroth C M, Lundberg C 1975 Mucosal malignant melanomas of the head and neck. Acta Otolaryngologica (Stockholm) 80: 452–458

Freedman H M, Desanto L W, Devine K D, Weiland L H 1973 Malignant melanomas of the nasal cavity and paranasal sinuses. Archives of Otolaryngology 97: 322–325

Friedmann I 1961 Electron microscopy of human biopsy material. Proceedings of the Royal Society of Medicine 54: 1064–1071

Grace C C 1947 Malignant melanoma of the nasal mucosa. Archives of Otolaryngology 46: 195–210

Harrison D F N 1976 Malignant melanoma arising in the nasal mucous membrane. Journal of Laryngology and Otology 90: 993–1005

Holdcraft J, Gallagher J C 1969 Malignant melanomas of the nasal and paranasal sinus mucosa. Annals of Otology, Rhinology and Laryngology 78: 1–20

Lewis M G 1967 Possible immunological factors in human malignant melanoma in Uganda. Lancet 2: 921–922

Lewis M G, Ikonopisov R L, Nairn R C, Phillips T M, Fairley G H, Bodenham D C, Alexander P 1969 Tumour-specific antibodies in human malignant melanoma and their relationship to the extent of the disease. British Medical Journal 2: 547–552

Lücke A 1869 Die melanotischen Geschwülste. Die Lehre von den Geschwülsten in anatomischer und klinische Beziehung. Handbuch der allgemeinen und speziellen Chirurgie, (Pitha F, Billroth T), Erlangen, Band 2, Abteil 1, Seite 244

Mason M, Friedmann I 1955 Melanoma of the nose and ear. Journal of Laryngology and Otology 69: 98–107

Masson P 1948 Pigment cells in man. Biology of melanomas. S.P. New York Academy of Sciences 4: 15–51

Mastrangelo M J, Bellet R E, Berkelhammer J, Clark W H 1975 Regression of pulmonary metastatic disease associated with intralesional B.C.G. therapy of intracutaneous melanoma metastases. Cancer 36: 1305–1308

Mayoux R, Perron R 1939 Les tumeurs mélanique du nez. Revue de Laryngologie, Otologie et Rhinologie 60: 245–272

Mishima Y 1967 Melanocytic and nevocytic malignant melanomas. Cancer 20: 632–649

Mitamura A, Yuen T, Duke P S, Demopoulos H B 1966 Ultra-structure of S-91 mouse melanomas subjected to phenyl alanine and tyrosine restriction in vivo. American Journal of Pathology 49: 309–313

Moore E S, Martin H 1955 Melanoma of the upper respiratory tract and oral cavity. Cancer 8: 1167–1176

Morton D L, Eilber F R, Malmgren R A, Wood W C 1970 Immunological factors which influence response to immunotherapy in malignant melanoma. Surgery 68: 158–164

Ravid J M, Estaves J A 1960 Malignant melanoma of the nose and paranasal sinuses and juvenile melanoma of the nose. Archives of Otolaryngology 72: 431–444

Ringertz N 1938 Malignant melanoma. In malignant tumours arising in nasal and paranasal cavities and maxilla. Acta Otolaryngologica, Supplement 27, 250–267

Spitz S 1948 Melanomas of childhood. American Journal of Pathology 24: 591–609

Szabo G 1959 In: Gordon M (ed) Pigment cell biology, p 99

Viennois 1872 Polype mélanique du nez (Mélano-sarcome). Lyon Médicine 11: 8–12

Wilkinson G 1912 A case of melanotic sarcoma of the nose. Journal of Laryngology and Otology 27: 1–9

Wright J W L, Heenan P J 1975 Electron microscopy findings in malignant melanoma of the nose. Oto-Rhino-Laryngology 37: 233–236

Zak F G, Lawson W 1974 The presence of melanocytes in the nasal cavity. Annals of Otology, Rhinology and Laryngology 83: 515–519

Additional References

Cove H 1979 Melanosis, melanocytic hyperplasia, primary malignant melanoma of the nasal cavity. Cancer 44: 1424–1433

Mesara B W, Burton W D 1968 Primary malignant melanoma of the upper respiratory tract. Cancer 21: 217–225

16

Neurogenic tumours of the nose and sinuses

PERIPHERAL NERVE TUMOURS OF THE NOSE AND SINUSES

Introduction
One of the earliest references to such tumours in this location was by Weinhold in 1810 who briefly mentioned a nerve swelling which involved the maxillary sinus. There being no microscopical details, the precise nature of the lesion is uncertain but doubt and confusion have persisted for a long time. Although histological distinction between certain solitary peripheral nerve tumours and the multiple lesions described by Von Recklinghausen (1882) has long been established, the overlap between the two conditions is still not understood. Stout (1935) described a solitary type lesion in the maxillary sinus of a woman exhibiting the multiple manifestations of Von Recklinghausen's disease.

Terminology
A wide variety of labels have been applied to peripheral nerve tumours (neuroma, neurinoma, neurofibroma, neurilemmoma and Schwannoma). The modern trend is to reserve the term neurofibroma for the microscopical pattern presented by the multiple lesions of neurofibromatosis of Von Recklinghausen, the epithet 'plexiform' being sometimes added. The characteristic solitary lesion, described by Verocay (1910) under the title of 'neurinoma' is now commonly referred to as neurilemmoma or Schwannoma whilst the expression neuroma is usually applied to the traumatic lesion. Lassmann, Jurecka, Lassmann, Gebhart, Matras and Watzek (1977) reviewed the terminology used by various authors from the time of Virchow onwards.

Incidence
Peripheral nerve tumours are not very common in the nose and sinuses and they are almost invariably of the Schwannoma type. Stout (1935) found only one in a series of fifty cases. Kragh, Soule and Masson (1960) collected 143 cases of neurilemmomas involving the head and neck region, of which five arose in the nose or sinuses. Robitaille, Seemayer and El Deiry (1975), in a review of the literature, found 14 examples of peripheral nerve tumours in the paranasal sinuses and added one of their own. They were mostly Schwannomas but two were neurofibromas and two showed a mixed pattern. In the I.L.O. material, there were five neurilemmomas and one neurofibroma, representing approximately 0.5 per cent of all tumours of the region.

Clinical features
In the nose and sinuses the age distribution tends to be concentrated in early middle life, being maximal in the third and fourth decades. There is a slight predominance of males but the sex difference is not significant. The symptoms include pain, nasal obstruction, epistaxis and unilateral exophthalmos. Pain is common in tumours of the maxillary antrum and epistaxis occurs when the tumour is located in the nasal fossa or ethmoid air cells. Surgical removal may be accompanied by severe bleeding because of the rich vascularity of the Schwannomas.

Anatomical site of origin
Most of these tumours are found in the nasal cavity or the maxillary sinus in that order of precedence. Less commonly they are found in the ethmoid region although extension from the antrum may occur. Calcaterra, Rich and Ward (1974) reported two neurilemmomas involving the sphenoid sinus. In the nasal cavity, the tumour may involve the lateral wall and turbinates (Dutt, 1969; Kaufman and Conrad, 1976) or the septum (Bogdasarian and Stout, 1943; Thomas, 1977). In the I.L.O. cases there were one antral and four nasal tumours.

Gross appearances
The naked eye picture is characterized by firm circumscribed masses showing a yellowish grey cut surface sometimes mottled by haemorrhage. Schwannomas are usually single and encapsulated whilst neurofibromas may be solitary or multiple and are not encapsulated.

Histopathology
The light microscopical features of peripheral nerve tumours are somewhat variable and there has been a

tendency to treat them as a single group. However, distinction can usually be made between the neurilemmoma or Schwannoma and the plexiform neurofibroma, even though a mixed pattern is sometimes encountered. In the former type the essential cells are spindle-shaped and often arranged in compact bundles. The nuclei are usually tapered and may be arranged in palisades with a distinct space between rows (Fig. 16.1) forming the characteristic structures described by Verocay (1910). Single rows of nuclear palisading are not pathognomonic of neurilemmoma and may be found in other spindle celled tumours such as fibro- and leiomyosarcomas (Krumbein, 1925). This solid pattern (Fig. 16.2), which may be interspersed with round or oval foam cells, was designated by Antoni (1920) as type A whilst a looser arrangement with more cellular pleomorphism (Fig. 16.3) was referred to by the same author as type B. Kragh et al. (1960) suggested that this histological subdivision was of academic interest only but, in view of the obvious diagnostic confusion of various types of spindle celled tumours, the identification of the Antoni types A and B and especially of the Verocay bodies are particularly helpful in establishing the presence of a neurilemmoma. Nuclear irregularity may be encoun-

tered, especially in the type B areas but rarely has sinister significance.

The plexiform neurofibroma (originally described in detail by de Morgan in 1875) contains obvious bands of collagen and is distinguished from neurilemmoma by the presence of axons. Verocay bodies are not present and the picture is quite different from that of the neurilemmoma (Fig. 16.4). Distinction may have to be made from traumatic neuroma but this lesion has rarely been observed in the nasal region (Burtner and Goodman, 1977).

Melanin pigment is sometimes found in neurilemmomas (Mandybur, 1974) and has also been observed in tissue cultures. The so-called glandular differentiation (Woodruff, 1976) has not, so far, been observed in the nasal region.

Electron microscopical studies have been carried out by Luse (1960), Mandybur (1974) and Lassmann et al. (1977). The neurilemmomas are composed almost entirely of Schwann cells whilst neurofibromas contain, in addition, variable numbers of fibroblasts. The Schwann cells possess elongated cytoplasmic processes surrounded by a basal lamina in contradistinction to the fibroblasts where there is no such structure. The collagen

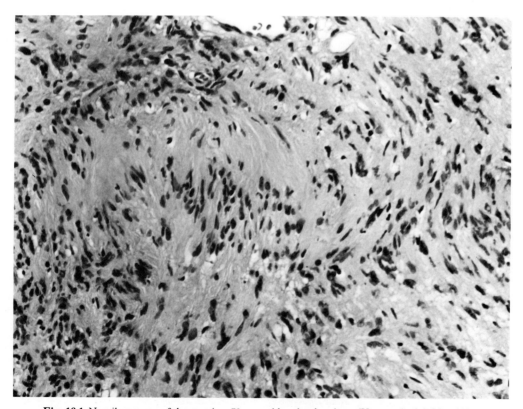

Fig. 16.1 Neurilemmoma of the nose in a 59 year-old male, showing a 'Verocay body'. M × 260

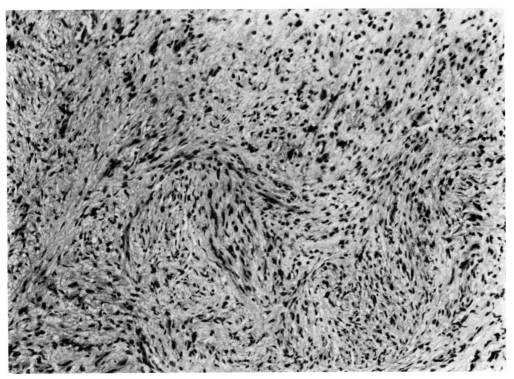

Fig. 16.2 Neurilemmoma of the nose in a 20 year-old male, showing 'Antoni type A' area. M ×208

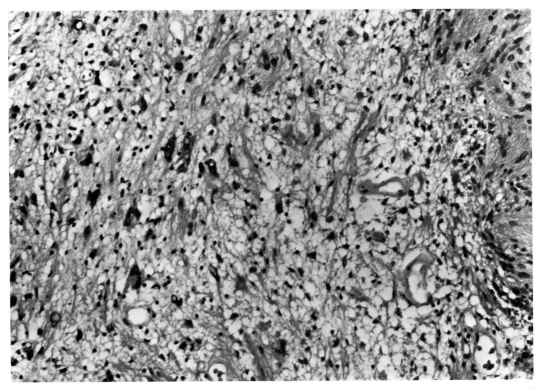

Fig. 16.3 Neurilemmoma of the nose in a 32 year-old male (see Fig. 16.2, recurrence after 12 years) showing 'Antoni type B' area. M ×224

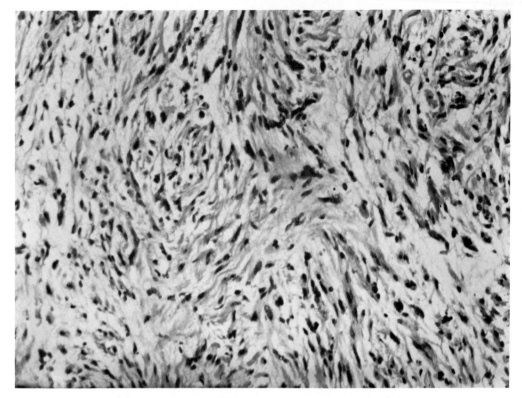

Fig. 16.4 Neurofibroma (solitary) of the nose in a 65 year-old female. M × 260

fibrils of neurofibromas have a normal periodicity of about 640 Å but the Schwannomas frequently contain banded fibrils with the periodicity of 1000 Å or more (Luse, 1960). These Luse bodies are almost certainly procollagen Fig. 16.5) and have been described as a type of long-spaced collagen (Friedmann, Cawthorne and Bird, 1965).

Aetiology and pathogenesis
No causal agent has been identified in human tumours but chemically induced neurilemmomas in rats have been reported by a number of workers using nitrosourea compounds administered orally and trans–placentally (Georgsson, Wessel and Thomas, 1969; Cravioto, Palekar, Weiss and Bennett, 1972; Rubinstein, Conley and Herman, 1976). The last mentioned authors took explants for tissue and organ cultures and in the latter procedure the tumour tissue showed resemblance to the neurilemmoma but also exhibited malignant characteristics. In the early part of the present century there was considerable debate regarding the origin of these tumours – whether they were derived from Schwann cells or arose from the endo- or perineural fibroblasts. Murray and Stout (1940) studied neurilem-momas in tissue culture and came to the conclusion that

the tumour cells resembled those of normal nerve sheaths (Schwann cells). They observed no fibroblasts but the Schwann cells appeared to be able to induce collagen and reticulin formation. Cravioto and Lockwood (1969) noted tropocollagen formation in tissue cultures of eighth nerve tumours. Shuangshoti, Netsky and Jane (1971) observed structural overlap between meningioma and neurilemmoma and concluded that meningocytes, fibroblasts and Schwann cells were all of mesenchymal origin. Nevertheless, whatever the origin of the Schwann cell, the concensus of opinion is that the neurilemmoma is derived from this cell.

Multiple neurofibromas (Von Recklinghausen's disease) have long been known to have a familial incidence, being transmitted through a Mendelian dominant gene (Preiser and Davenport, 1918). The tumours in this disease are not exclusively plexiform neurofibromas, occasional neurilemmomas also being found. Furthermore, the solitary neurofibroma is not necessarily related to multiple syndrome.

Behaviour
Incomplete removal of a neurilemmoma is liable to be followed by recurrence and the presence of nuclear irregularity has sometimes prompted a diagnosis of

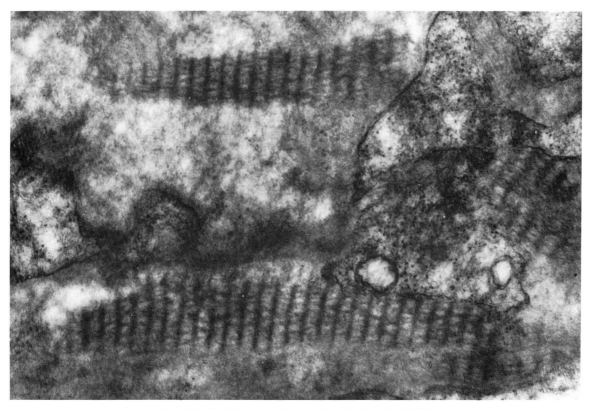

Fig. 16.5 Neurilemmoma showing Luse bodies. M × 38 500

malignant change. In fact, malignant change in a Schwannoma is probably an extremely rare event if it ever occurs (Stout, 1935; Kragh et al. 1960; Robitaille et al. 1975). Malignant change is more likely to occur in Von Recklinghausen's disease and is usually confined to a single tumour. Ghosh, Ghosh, Huvos and Fortner (1973) reviewed 115 cases of malignant peripheral nerve tumours and found that 30 per cent were associated with Von Recklinghausen's disease. Russell and Rubinstein (1977) distinguish malignant Schwannomas and malignant neurofibromas as seperate entities. In fact, it would appear that malignant Schwannomas are usually primary in nature and, in so far as they show few identifying features (D'Agostino, Soule and Miller, 1963), the diagnosis depends on establishing unequivocal connection with a peripheral nerve. Robitaille et al. (1975) pointed out that such a connection is difficult to identify

in tumours of the nose and sinuses. Neither of the two reports of malignant Schwannoma in the maxillary sinus (Leroux, 1952; Loiseau, Marchand and Vandenbrouck, 1963) are entirely convincing and, so far, no unequivocal example of a malignant peripheral nerve tumour in the nose or sinuses has been reported.

Recrudescence of a neurilemmoma after excision is not unknown. One of the nasal tumours in the I.L.O. material had to be excised again ten years after primary surgery but another fifteen years has now elapsed without further recurrence. The other three nasal neurilemmomas are known to have been without recurrence for periods ranging from two to nine years whilst the antral tumour did not recur and the patient died from an unrelated cause after 17 years. The patient with the solitary neurofibroma has survived five years without recurrence after total excision.

BIBLIOGRAPHY

Antoni N R E 1920 Über Rückenmarkstumoren und Neurofibrome. J F Bergmann, Verlag, München.
Bogdasarian R M, Stout A P 1943 Neurilemmoma of the nasal septum. Archives of Otolaryngology 38: 62–64
Burtner D, Goodman M 1977 Traumatic neuroma of the nose. Archives of Otolaryngology 103: 108–109

Calcaterra T C, Rich J R, Ward P W 1974 Neurilemmoma of the sphenoid sinus. Archives of Otolaryngology 100: 383–385
Cravioto H, Lockwood R 1969 The behaviour of acoustic neuroma in tissue culture. Acta Neuropathologica (Berlin) 12: 141–157

Cravioto H, Palekar L, Weiss E, Bennett K 1972 Experimental neurinoma in tissue culture. Acta Neuropathologica 21: 154–164

D'Agostino A N, Soule E H, Miller R H 1963 Primary malignant neoplasms of nerves (Malignant neurilemmomas) in patients without manifestations of multiple neurofibromatosis (Von Recklinghausen's disease). Cancer 16: 1003–1014

De Morgan C 1875 Case of multiple neuroma of the forearm. Transactions of the Pathological Society of London 26: 2–10

Dutt P K 1969 A case of nasal neurilemmoma. Journal of Laryngology and Otology 83: 1209–1213

Friedmann I, Cawthorne T, Bird E S 1965 The laminated cytoplasmic inclusions in the sensory epithelium of the human macula. Journal of Ultrastructure Research 12: 92–103

Georgsson G, Wessel W, Thomas C 1969 Zur Feinstruktur experimenteller Nerventumoren. Zeitschrift für Krebsforschung 72: 12–23

Ghosh B C, Ghosh L, Huvos A C, Fortner J G 1973 Malignant schwannoma, a clinicopathologic study. Cancer 31: 184–190

Kaufman S M, Conrad L P 1976 Schwannoma presenting as a nasal polyp. Laryngoscope 86: 595–597

Kragh L V, Soule E H, Masson J K 1960 Benign and malignant neurilemmomas of the head and neck. Surgery, Gynecology and Obstetrics 111: 211–218

Krumbein C 1925 Über die 'Band oder Pallisadenstellung' der Kerne, eine Wuchsform des feinfibrillären mesenchymalen Gewebes. Virchows Archiv für pathologische Anatomie 255: 309–331

Lassmann H, Jurecka W, Lassmann G, Gebhart W, Matras H, Watzek G 1977 Different types of benign nerve sheath tumours. Virchows Archiv für pathologische Anatomie 375: 197–210

Leroux M L 1952 Schwannome du maxillaire supérieur d'évolution maligne. Les Annales d'Otolaryngologie 69: 706–708

Loiseau G, Marchand J, Vandenbrouck C 1963 Schwannome malin du sinus maxillaire. Les Annals d'Otolaryngologie 80: 920–921

Luse S A 1960 Electron microscopic studies of brain tumours. Neurology 10: 881–905

Mandybur T I 1974 Melanotic nerve sheath tumors. Journal of Neurosurgery 41: 187–192

Murray M R, Stout A P 1940 Schwann cell versus fibroblast as the origin of the specific nerve sheath tumor. American Journal of Pathology 16: 41–60

Preiser S A, Davenport C B 1918 Multiple neurofibromatosis (Von Recklinghausen's disease) and its inheritance with description of a case. American Journal of Medical Sciences 156: 507–540

Robitaille Y, Seemayer T A, El Deiry A 1975 Peripheral nerve tumors involving the paranasal sinuses. Cancer 35: 1254–1258

Rubinstein L J, Conley F K, Herman M M 1976 Studies on experimental nerve sheath tumors maintained in tissue and organ culture systems. I light microscopy observations. Acta Neuropathologica 34: 277–291

Russell D S, Rubinstein L J 1977 Pathology of tumours of the nervous system, Williams & Wilkins, Baltimore, 4th ed, pp 282–304

Shuangshoti S, Netsky M G, Jane J A 1971 Neoplasms of mixed mesenchymal and neuroepithelial type; with consideration of the relationship between meningioma and neurilemmoma. Journal of the Neurological Sciences 14: 277–291

Stout A P 1935 The peripheral manifestation of the specific nerve sheath tumor (neurilemmoma). American Journal of Cancer 24: 751–796

Thomas J N 1977 Massive schwannoma arising from the nasal septum. Journal of Laryngology and Otology 91: 63–68

Verocay J 1910 Zur Kenntnis der Neurofibrome. Beiträge z. pathologische Anatomie und allgemeine Pathologie 48: 1–68

Von Recklinghausen F 1882 Über die multiplen Fibrome der Haut und ihre Beziehung zu den multiplen Neuromen. A Hirschwald, Berlin

Weinhold C A 1810 Ideen über die abnormen Metamorphosen der Hyghmorshöhle. Dritter Abschnitt, Seite 183–184. W. Rein, Leipzig

Woodruff J M 1976 Peripheral nerve tumors showing glandular differentiation (glandular schwannomas). Cancer 37: 2399–2413

Additional references

Arora M M L, Banerjee A K, Bhattacharya T K 1973 Neurilemmoma of the maxillary antrum. Journal of Laryngology and Otology 87: 405–407

Bird C C, Willis R A 1969 The histogenesis of pigmented neurofibromas. Journal of Pathology 97: 631–637

Gore D O, Rankow R, Hanford J M 1956 Parapharyngeal neurilemmoma. Surgery, Gynecology and Obstetrics 103: 193–201

Harkin J C, Reed R S 1969 Tumors of the peripheral nervous system. Atlas of Tumor Pathology, Armed Forces Institute of Pathology, Washington, fascicle 3: 2nd edition.

Johnson C I, Lineback M 1959 Intranasal ethmoidal schwannoma. Laryngoscope 69: 463–466

OLFACTORY NEUROBLASTOMA

Introduction

This relatively uncommon nasal tumour was first recognized and reported by Berger, Luc and Richard in 1924. Although its identity has now been established for more than fifty years, it is still noteworthy for errors in diagnosis owing to the unfamiliarity of the general pathologist with this type of neoplasm. In the 42 years following the first report over a hundred cases were published (Skolnik, Massari and Tenta, 1966).

Terminology

A variety of terms for the designation and subclassification of this tumour have been introduced but, unfortunately, their usage has been far from consistent. Berger et al. (1924) described the first case under the title of 'esthésioneuroépithéliome olfactif', indicating the presence of an epithelial component. Subsequently, Berger and Coutard (1926) found another case in which there did not appear to be any epithelial derivative and they labelled it 'esthésioneurocytome'. Furthermore, they suggested a generic term 'esthésioneurome olfactif'. These authors deserve full credit, not only for their priority in this field but also for their detailed description of the two main types which are accepted by many other authors. Later, the term neuroblastoma was introduced in the context of this tumour (Portmann, Bonnard and Moreau, 1929; Schall and Lineback, 1951) but was used with different connotations. Gerard-Marchant and Micheau (1964) applied the label to an undifferentiated form though subsequently they expressed doubts as to its entity. Lindstrom and Lindstrom (1975), while recognizing the Berger subtypes of neuroepithelioma and neurocytoma, have recommended the usage of the expression 'Olfactory Neuroblastoma' as a generic term.

Incidence

Notwithstanding the problems of diagnosis, this tumour is certainly uncommon and rarely appears in published series of nasal tumours. In the I.L.O material, two cases were collected over a period of 27 years representing about 0.25 per cent of all intranasal tumours. The present authors have also seen over ten other cases under the aegis of the Ear, Nose and Throat Tumour Panel.

Clinical features

The age distribution is broadly based with a maximal frequency in the second decade. The youngest reported case was a three year-old boy (Kadish, Goodman and Wang, 1976) whilst the oldest patient was a 79 year-old woman (Hutter, Lewis, Foote and Tollefsen, 1963). Occurrence in the first decade of life is uncommon and there is a slight predominance of males (about 1.3 : 1).

The usually presenting features are nasal obstruction and epistaxis. Local invasion may result in facial swelling, proptosis, pain and epiphora. Less commonly the patient may exhibit the picture of an intracranial neoplasm (Hamilton, Rubinstein and Poole, 1973).

Anatomical site of origin

The tumour usually arises in the upper part of the nasal cavity but other primary sites have been reported, including the nasopharynx (King, 1959; Castro, de la Pava and Webster, 1969) and the maxillary sinus (Mashberg, Thoma and Wasilewski, 1960).

Gross appearances

There are no characteristic naked eye features, the tumour usually being a firm pinkish mass. Sometimes, when in situ, the tumour may give a clinical impression of a simple nasal polyp.

Histopathology

Microscopically, the pattern varies considerably in detail but the general picture is characterized by compact cellular masses sharply separated by a highly vascular stroma which often appears angiomatoid (Figs. 16.6 & 16.7) and could lead to an erroneous diagnosis of a vascular tumour (Oberman and Rice, 1976). Typically, the nuclei are round or oval, sometimes giving a superficial impression of lymphoid tissue but the cytoplasm tends to be somewhat more abundant than in lymphocytes. Nucleoli may be observable but mitoses are infrequent. Often the cytoplasmic boundaries are poorly defined giving an appearance of naked nuclei in a background of fibrillary or granular material (Fig. 16.8). The cells may be aligned in rows with intervening fibrils producing geometric patterns (Fig. 16.9). The fibrils stain negatively for collagen and neuroglia but silver impregnation techniques may sometimes indicate the presence of axons (Fig. 16.10). Calcification (Fig. 16.11) has been reported by a number of authors (Martin, Dargent and Gignoux, 1949; Fitz-Hugh, Allen, Rucker and Sprinkle, 1965) and opacities due to this cause may sometimes be seen in radiographs.

A pathognomonic feature is the presence of rosettes. These may be either 'true rosettes' consisting of a circular arrangement of cylindrical cells about a central space, resembling a glandular structure which may be empty or contain eosinophilic material (Fig. 16.12) or 'pseudorosettes' characterized by a similar arrangement of less well defined cells enclosing fibrillary or granular material (Fig. 16.13). There has been some confusion over these structures which are encountered in a variety of neurogenic tumours. The situation was clearly outlined by Rubinstein in 1972. Bailey and Cushing (1926) restricted the term rosette (true rosette) to the structure originally described by Flexner (1891) in a retinoblastoma. He illustrated an arrangement of columnar cells about a central lumen and believed that they represented rods and cones. Such rosettes are also found in ependymomas and Bailey and Cushing considered that the constituent cells were derived from primitive spongioblasts. In 1910 Wright described 'ball-like' cellular masses surrounding central aggregations of fibrils in sympathicoblastomas. Such structures are also seen in medulloblastomas as well as in olfactory tumours (Fig. 16.14) and were designated by Bailey and Cushing as pseudo-rosettes. The cells do not surround a central lumen but include faintly staining fibrillated material occasionally having an affinity for silver preparations used for neurofibrils. The 'perivascular pseudorosette' of Bailey and Cushing, which is also found in olfactory tumours, is best designated as 'perivascular palisading' (Mendeloff, 1957).

True rosettes are rarely found in olfactory tumours but when present the lesion is often referred to as olfactory neuroepithelioma (see Fig. 16.12). Fruhling and Wild (1954) produced some very good illustrations of these structures. Pseudorosettes are a little more common but are not found in many of these tumours.

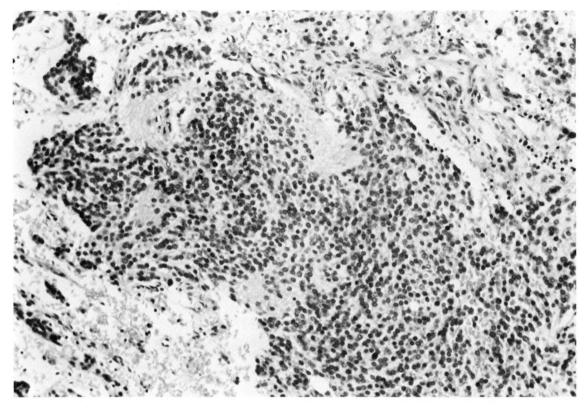

Fig. 16.6 Olfactory neuroblastoma in an elderly female showing angiomatoid stroma. M × 225

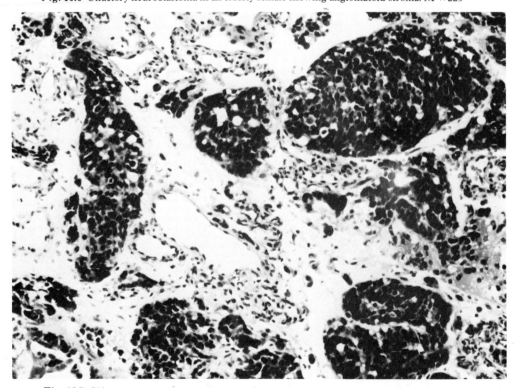

Fig. 16.7 Olfactory neurocytoma in a 63 year-old female showing angiomatoid stroma. M × 208

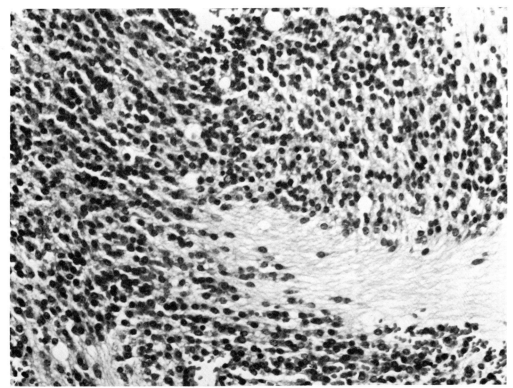

Fig. 16.8 Olfactory neurocytoma in a 20 year-old female showing naked nuclei in a fibrillary background. M × 260

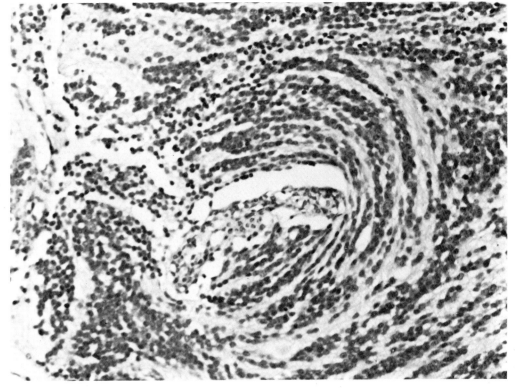

Fig. 16.9 Olfactory neurocytoma in an 11 year-old boy, showing a geometric pattern of the cells. M × 260

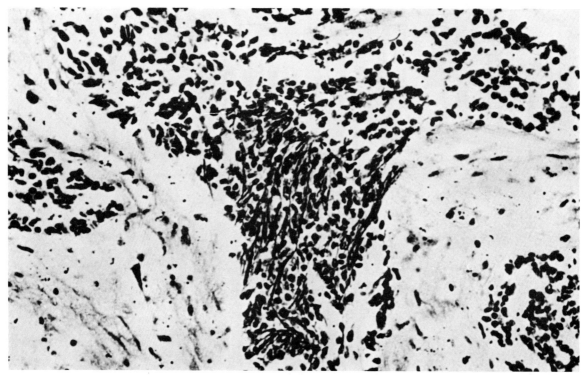

Fig. 16.10 Olfactory neurocytoma in a 17 year-old male showing neurofibrils. Glees stain on frozen section. M ×250

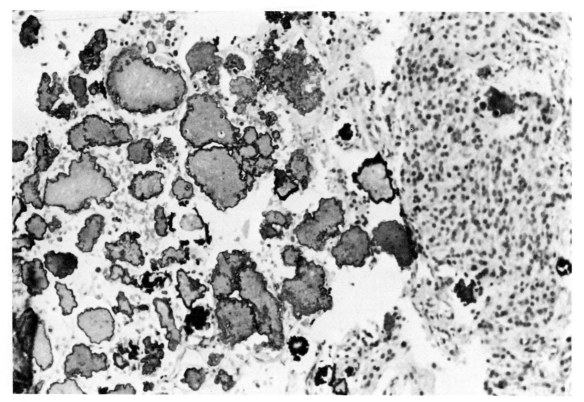

Fig. 16.11 Olfactory neuroblastoma in an elderly female, showing calcification. M ×225

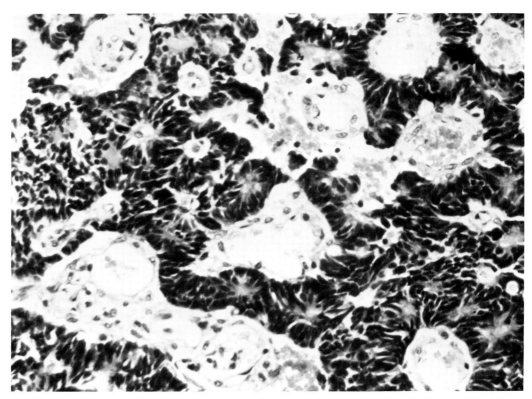

Fig. 16.12 Olfactory neuro-epithelioma in a 54 year-old male, showing true rosettes and vascular stroma. M × 325

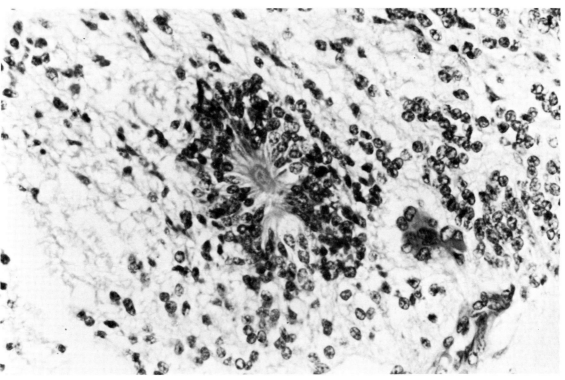

Fig. 16.13 Olfactory neurocytoma in a 5 year-old child, showing a pseudorosette. M × 585

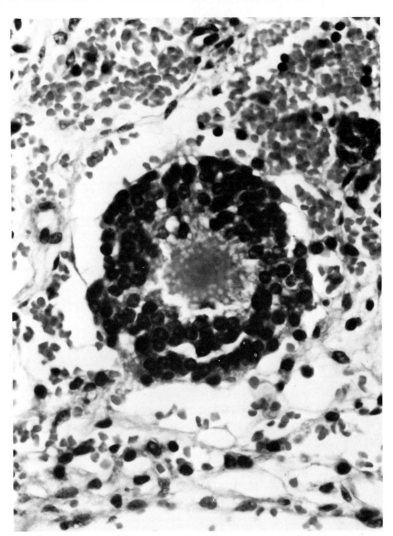

Fig. 16.14 Olfactory neurocytoma in a 20 year-old female showing a pseudorosette with the 'ball-like' appearance described by Wright in 1910. M × 520

The distinction between neurocytoma and neuroblastoma on the basis of the respective absence or presence of pseudorosettes (Fig. 16.15) is somewhat tenuous. Gerard-Marchant and Micheau (1965) had doubts regarding the entity of the neuroblastoma in this context whilst Lindstrom and Lindstrom (1975) considered the subdivision to be unjustifiable. Very occasionally, both types of rosette may be present (Skolnik et al., 1966; Friedmann and Osborn, 1974).

Ultrastructural studies have been reported by many workers (McGravran, 1970; Friedmann and Osborn, 1974; Kahn, 1974; Osamura and Fine, 1976; Mackay, Luna and Butler, 1976; Berard, Tripier, Choux Gambarelli, Grisoli and Toga, 1976; Taxy and Hidvegi,

1977; Wilander, Nordlinder, Grimelius, Larsson and Angelborg, 1977). The principal cells are polygonal or spherical, containing large rounded nuclei which often have finely distributed chromatin and variable occurrence of nucleoli. There is a profuse network of neurites attached to the cells and forming synaptic connections. Many of the cells contain neurosecretory granules characterized by dense centres separated from the limiting membrane by a narrow clear zone (Fig. 16.16). The granules range in size from about 100 to 200 nanometres in diameter and they may also be found in the neurites (Fig. 16.17). Similar granules have been observed in adrenal neuroblastomas (Tannenbaum, 1970) which are known to produce catecholamines.

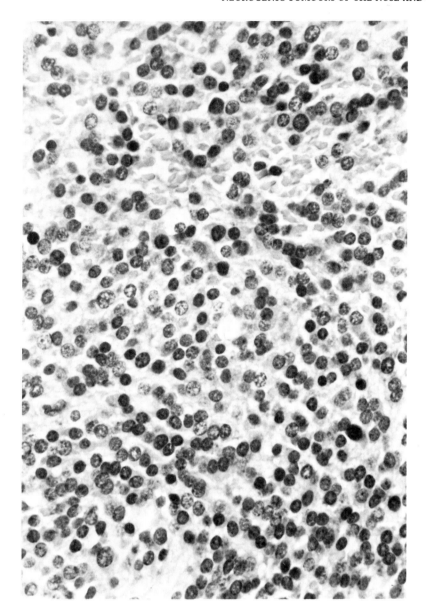

Fig. 16.15 Olfactory neurocytoma in an elderly female, showing predominance of rounded nuclei. M ×595

Falck (1962) showed that catecholamines and other biological amines form highly fluorescent condensation products with formaldehyde and the technique has been applied to the histological diagnosis of olfactory tumours (Judge, McGavran and Trepukdi, 1976).

The histological diagnosis of these tumours is not always easy. Neither true rosettes nor pseudorosettes are commonly present and care has to be taken not to confuse the former with true glandular structures which may have become infiltrated by tumour tissue. In some cases the neurofibrils are not very obvious so that diagnostic difficulties are greatly increased. Confusion with transitional or anaplastic carcinoma, malignant lymphoma or even plasmacytoma is not unknown.

Aetiology and pathogenesis

No clue to the causation of these tumours in the human species has so far emerged although Herrold (1964) produced olfactory tumours in Syrian hamsters following the injection of di-ethyl nitrosamine. The origin of

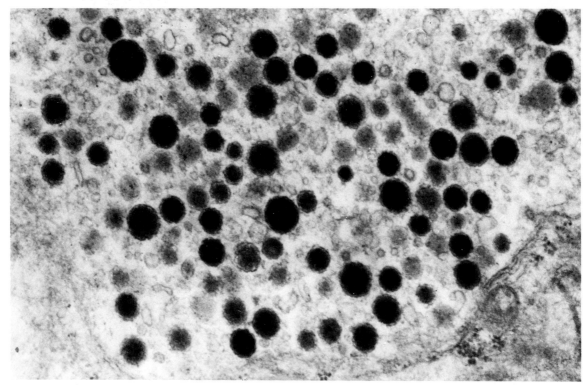

Fig. 16.16 Olfactory neuroblastoma in a 40 year-old female, showing catecholamine granules. M × 49 000

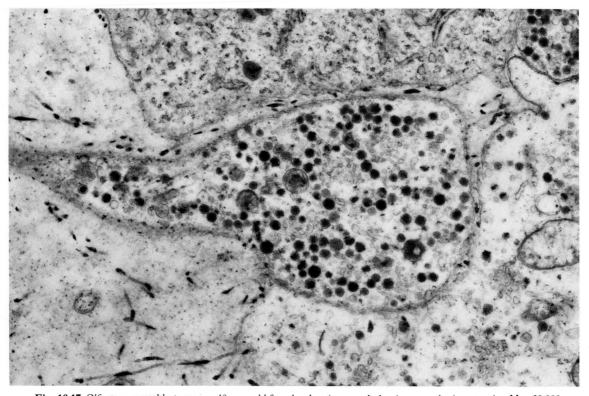

Fig. 16.17 Olfactory neuroblastoma in a 40 year-old female, showing catecholamine granules in a neurite. M × 28 000

the olfactory neuroblastoma has been variously ascribed to the olfactory placode, the Organ of Jacobson, the sphenopalatine ganglion, the olfactory bulb and the olfactory mucosa. The olfactory placode is an embryological entity which no longer exists at the time of inception of the tumour. The Organ of Jacobson is a vestigial structure in a small number of human subjects and, although it represents an isolated area of olfactory membrane, its location is inconsistent with the common site of origin of the tumour. The sphenopalatine ganglion lies outside the nasal cavity but might possibly account for the infrequent origin in the nasopharynx. There is now general acceptance of origin from the olfactory mucosa in the upper third of the nasal cavity although Schenk and Ogura (1972) suggested that the abundant nerve supply in the nasal cavity might provide alternative sources. The olfactory epithelium contains two principal types of cell, the sustentacular cell and the olfactory cell. The neuroepithelial type of tumour (esthésioneuroépithéliome) represents a mixed origin from both supporting (epithelial) and olfactory (nervous) cells. The neurocytoma (esthésioneurocytome) is of purely nervous origin, without any epithelial component (Gerard-Marchant and Micheau, 1964 and 1965). These authors do not consider that true rosettes contain nerve cells and Micheau, Guerinot and Bohuon (1975) were not able to detect dopamine-β-hydroxylase, which catalyses the conversion of dopamine to noradrenalin, in cells of rosettes.

Behaviour

In many cases the tumour is a slowly growing neoplasm which may recur after surgical removal or radiotherapy. Local spread to the paranasal sinuses, the palate and the orbit is a common event (Mendeloff, 1957; Fitz-Hugh et al., 1965; Castro et al., 1969; Schenk and Ogura, 1972; Joachims, Altman and Mayer, 1975; Lindström and Lindström, 1975) whilst intracranial involvement has been reported in a number of cases (Fisher, 1955; Gerard-Marchant and Micheau, 1965; Hamilton et al., 1973). Metastases occur in over 20 per cent of cases

(Bailey and Barton, 1975), the usual sites being lymphnodes (especially cervical), lungs and bones in that order of frequency. Other sites, such as skin, liver and spleen may occasionally be involved.

Hughes, Marsden and Palmer (1974) tried to correlate prognosis with the histological pattern of neuroblastomas in children. They found that those cases with tumours showing a high degree of differentiation appeared to fare better. On the other hand, some authors have found the relationship less convincing in respect of olfactory tumours (Hutter et al., 1963; Batsakis, 1974; Bailey and Barton, 1975) although there have been a number of reports of poor survival in cases with tumours containing true rosettes (McCormack and Harris, 1955; Mendeloff, 1957; Obert, Devine and McDonald, 1960; Lewis, Hutter, Tollefsen and Foote, 1965). The general view is that true or pseudorosettes indicate incomplete differentiation.

Voorhess, Pickett and Gardner (1963) showed that neuroblastomas of the adrenal medulla or sympathetic ganglia in children are associated with increased urinary excretion of catecholamines. This has also been observed in some cases of olfactory neuroblastoma, including one of the present authors' cases.

In contrast with adrenal neuroblastomas or retinoblastomas, survival rates are much better in the case of the olfactory tumour where they correspond more closely with other extra-adrenal tumours of this type. Five year survival rates (with or without residual tumour) have been reported as over 50 per cent (Lewis et al., 1965; Bailey and Barton, 1975). The last mentioned authors, in a review of fifty cases, found that 62 per cent died eventually of their disease and 18 per cent had a five year cure but it has to be borne in mind that late recurrences may take place. Of the material seen by the present authors, over 40 per cent of cases are known to have survived for five years or more, one patient being alive and well over twenty years after presentation. One case, whose tumour exhibited rosettes, died after four years with multiple metastases whilst another case (without rosettes) died after two years with pulmonary secondaries.

BIBLIOGRAPHY

Bailey B J, Barton S 1975 Olfactory neuroblastoma. Archives of Otolaryngology 101: 1–5

Bailey P, Cushing H 1926 A classification of the tumors of the glioma group on a histogenetic basis with a correlated study of prognosis. J. B. Lippincott & Co. Philadelphia

Batsakis J G 1974 Neuroblastoma. Tumors of the head and neck. Williams and Wilkins & Co. Baltimore

Berard M, Tripier M F, Choux R, Gambarelli D, Grisoli F, Toga M 1976 Esthésioneurocytome olfactif. Acta Neuropathologica (Berlin) 35: 139–150

Berger L, Coutard H 1926 L'Esthésioneurocytome olfactif.

Bulletin de l'Association francaise pour l'étude du cancer 15: 404–414

Berger L, Luc, Richard 1924 L'Esthésioneuroépithéliome olfactif. Bulletin de l'Association francaise pour l'étude du cancer 13: 410–421

Castro L, de la Pava S, Webster J H 1969 Esthesioneuroblastoma. American Journal of Roentgenology 105: 7–13

Falck B 1962 Observations on the possibilities of the cellular localization of monoamines by a fluorescence method. Acta Physiologica Scandinavica Supplement 197

Fisher E R 1955 Neuroblastomas of the nasal fossa. Archives of Pathology 60: 435–439

Fitz-Hugh G S, Allen M S, Rucker T N, Sprinkle P M 1965 Olfactory neuroblastoma. Archives of Otolaryngology 81: 161–168

Flexner S 1981 A peculiar glioma (neuroepithelioma?) of the retina. Johns Hopkins Hospital Bulletin 2: 115–119

Friedmann I, Osborn D A 1974 The ultrastructure of the olfactory neuroblastoma. Minerva Otorinolaringologica 24: 66–74

Fruhling L, Wild C 1954 Olfactory aesthesioneuroepitheliomas of Louis Berger. Archives of Otolaryngology 60: 37–48

Gerard-Marchant R, Micheau C 1964 Les esthésioneuromes olfactifs. Annales d'Anatomie pathologique 9: 239–251

Gerard-Marchant R, Micheau C 1965 Microscopical diagnosis of olfactory esthesioneuromas. Journal of the National Cancer Institute 35: 75–82

Hamilton A E, Rubinstein L J, Poole G J 1973 Primary intracranial esthesioneuroblastoma (olfactory neuroblastoma). Journal of Neurosurgery 38: 548–556

Herrold K M 1964 Induction of olfactory neuroepithelial tumors in Syrian hamsters by di-ethyl nitrosamine. Cancer 17: 114–121

Hughes M, Marsden H B, Palmer M K 1974 Histologic pattern of neuroblastoma related to prognosis and clinical staging. Cancer 34: 1706–1711

Hutter R V P, Lewis J S, Foote F W, Tollefsen H R 1963 Esthesioneuroblastoma. American Journal of Surgery 106: 748–753

Joachims H Z, Altman M M, Mayer S W 1975 Olfactory neuroblastoma. Journal of Laryngology and Otology 89: 335–343

Judge D M, McGavran M H, Trepukdi 1976 Fume-induced fluorescence in diagnosis of nasal neuroblastoma. Archives of Otolaryngology 102: 97–98

Kadish S, Goodman M, Wang C C 1976 Olfactory neuroblastoma. Cancer 37: 1571–1576

Kahn L B 1974 Esthesioneuroblastoma: a light and electron microscope study. Human Pathology 5: 364–371

King J T 1959 Olfactory neurocytoma (esthésioneuroépithéliome olfactif). Archives of Otolaryngology 69: 729

Lewis J S, Hutter R V P, Tollefsen H R, Foote F W 1965 Nasal tumors of olfactory origin. Archives of Otolaryngology 81: 169–173

Lindström C G, Lindström D W 1975 Olfactory neuroblastoma. Acta Otolaryngologica 80: 447–451

McCormack L J, Harris H E 1955 Neurogenic tumors of the nasal fossa. Journal of the American Medical Association 137: 318–321

McGavran M H 1970 Neurogenous nasal neoplasms. Annals of Otology, Rhinology and Laryngology 79: 547–550

Mackay B, Luna M A, Butler J J 1976 Adult neuroblastoma. Cancer 37: 1334–1351

Martin J F, Dargent M, Gignoux M 1949 Les tumeurs nerveuses des fosses nasales. Annales d'Otolaryngologie 66: 253–266

Mashberg A, Thoma K H, Wasilewski E J 1960 Olfactory neuroblastoma (esthesioneuroepithelioma) of the maxillary sinus. Oral Surgery, Oral Medicine and Oral Pathology 13: 908–912

Mendeloff J 1957 The olfactory neuroepithelial tumors. Cancer 10: 944–956

Micheau C, Guerinot F, Bohuon C 1975 Dopamine-β-hydroxylase and catecholamines in an olfactory esthesioneuroma. Cancer 35: 1309–1312

Oberman H A, Rice D H 1976 Olfactory neuroblastomas. Cancer 38: 2494–2502

Obert G J, Devine K D, McDonald J R 1960 Olfactory neuroblastoma. Cancer 13: 205–215

Osamura R Y, Fine G 1976 Ultrastructure of the esthesioneuroblastoma. Cancer 38: 173–179

Portmann M M, Bonnard, Moreau 1929 Sur un cas de tumeur nerveuse des fosses nasales (esthésioneuroblastome). Acta Otolaryngologica 13: 52–56

Rubinstein L J 1972 Tumors of the central nervous system. Atlas of Tumor Pathology, Armed Forces Institute of Pathology, Washington, 2nd series, Fascicle 6, pp 124–125

Schall L A, Lineback M 1951 Primary intranasal neuroblastoma. Annals of Otology, Rhinology and Laryngology 60: 221–229

Schenk N L, Ogura J H 1972 Esthesioneuroblastoma. Archives of Otolaryngology 96: 322–324

Skolnik E M, Massari F S, Tenta L T 1966 Olfactory neuroepithelioma. Archives of Otolaryngology 84: 644–653

Tannenbaum M 1970 Ultrastructural pathology of adrenal medullary tumours. In: Sommers S C (ed) Pathology Annual, p 45

Taxy J B, Hidvegi D F 1977 Olfactory neuroblastoma. Cancer 39: 131–138

Voorhess M L, Pickett L K, Gardner L I 1963 Functioning tumors of the neural crest origin in childhood. American Journal of Surgery 106: 33–35

Wilander E, Nordlinder H, Grimelius L, Larsson L–I, Angelborg C 1977 Esthesioneuroblastoma: histological, histochemical and electron microscopic studies of a case. Virchows Archiv für pathologische Anatomie 375: 123–128

Wright J H 1910 Neurocytoma or neuroblastoma, a kind of tumor not generally recognized. Journal of Experimental Medicine 12: 556–560

Additional references
Jung H, Gutjahr P 1974 Primäre und sekundäre Neuroblastome im HNO – Bereich. Laryngologie, Rhinologie und Otologie (Stuttgart) 53: 500–509

Robinson F, Solitare G B 1966 Olfactory neuroblastoma. Neurosurgical implications of an intranasal tumour. Journal of Neurosurgery 25: 133–139

NASAL GLIOMA

Introduction

Early reports of this uncommon nasal lesion were made by Ried (1852) and Hildebrand (1888). The latter illustrated his case, showing a large swelling over the root of the nose and the details were redescribed by Berger (1890). The first comprehensive account of the condition was given by Schmidt (1900) and in 1950 Black and Smith reviewed the literature, collecting 32 cases to which they added two of their own.

Terminology

A large number of terms have been used to describe this lesion, including glioma, astrocytoma, fibroglioma, encephaloma, encephalocele and choristoma. Such labels as glioma or astrocytoma are certainly open to serious criticism but the expression nasal glioma has become so deeply engrained that it would be difficult and perhaps pointless to abandon it.

Incidence

The condition is a rare one, reports of which are either solitary or in small series of six cases or less (Bratton and Robinson, 1946; Smith, Schwartz, Luse and Ogura, 1963; Katz and Lewis, 1971; Hirsh, Stool, Langfitt and Schut, 1977). In the I.L.O. material there were two cases representing approximately 0.25 per cent of all tumours in the nasal cavity.

Clinical features

The majority of cases present at or shortly after birth though a small number are encountered at later periods, occasionally extending into middle life (Smith et al., 1963; Blumenfeld and Skolnik, 1965). No significant sex difference has been observed.

External swelling on the root of the nose (Fig. 16.18) and nasal obstruction are common features. Intranasal lesions may occasionally present at the anterior nares (Deutsch, 1965).

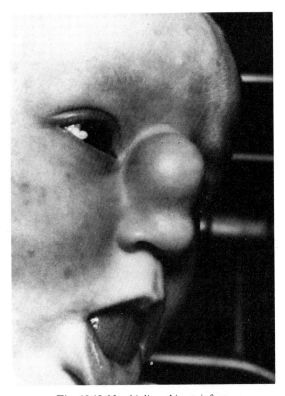

Fig. 16.18 Nasal 'glioma' in an infant.

Anatomical site of origin

The greater proportion of these lesions (about 60 per cent) are externally located producing a swelling beneath the skin on one side or the other of the bridge of the nose. About 30 per cent are intranasal whilst the remaining ten per cent exhibit a combination of the two locations.

Gross appearances

To the naked eye, the lesion presents as firm greyish tissue which is not obviously of neural origin. External lesions are often isolated from deeper structures but may be attached to the overlying skin. Sometimes a stalk may be found passing through a defect in the nasal wall or rarely into the cranium. Intranasal lesions may have the appearance of a pedunculated polyp with a pedicle which may extend through a bony defect in the roof of the nose, often involving the cribriform plate. Occasionally, there is attachment to the septum or the lateral wall of the nose.

Histopathology

In most cases the picture consists of glial tissue interspersed with fibrous tissue. The former contains largely astrocytes lying in a profusion of glial fibrils (Figs. 16.19, 16.20 & 16.21) and may show the normal characteristic disposition around blood vessels. The astrocytes may sometimes have a vesicular appearance and may contain multiple nuclei whilst, occasionally, they may be swollen presenting the gemistocytic appearance (Figs. 16.22 & 16.23). Very occasionally, nerve cells and their axons may be found (Musser and Campbell, 1961; Smith et al., 1963) and spaces lined by ependymal cells have also been reported (Bratton and Robinson, 1946; Hirsh et al., 1977). The tissue in these lesions is essentially non-neoplastic though it may show degenerative changes and distortion due to fibrosis. The infrequency of neurones is probably due to a relatively inadequate blood supply to sustain them.

Aetiology and pathogenesis

The common presentation in early life and the usually slow growth matching that of the body as a whole indicates a developmental anomaly rather than an autonomous tumour, although it is uncommon for the sufferers to exhibit any other defects. The fact that many of these lesions appeared to be completely isolated led to the view that they represented heterotopic brain tissue. Schmidt (1900) believed that they were all initially encephaloceles and this concept has now been generally accepted. The so-called nasal glioma represents an abnormal protrusion of brain substance which has lost its connection with the point of origin. The mechanism of development of these lesions has been outlined by

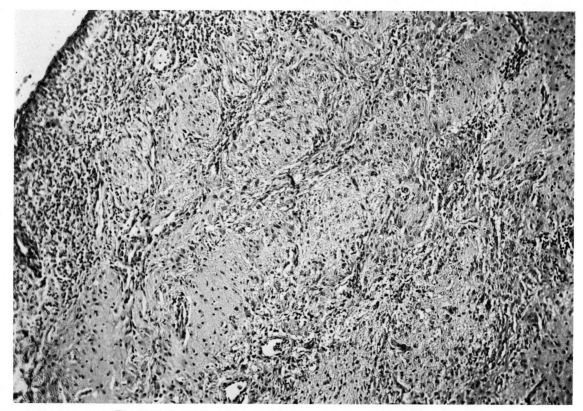

Fig. 16.19 Nasal 'glioma' in a 15 day-old boy, showing gliomatous tissue. M × 90

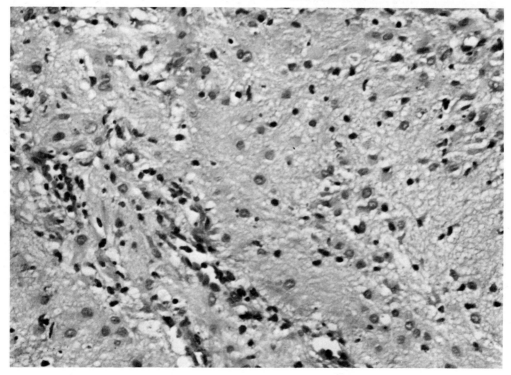

Fig. 16.20 Nasal 'glioma' in a 15 day-old boy. Higher magnification of Fig. 16.19. M × 325

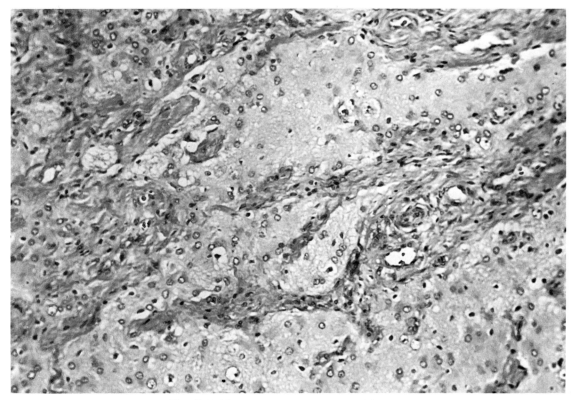

Fig. 16.21 Nasal 'glioma' (see Fig. 16.18). M ×200

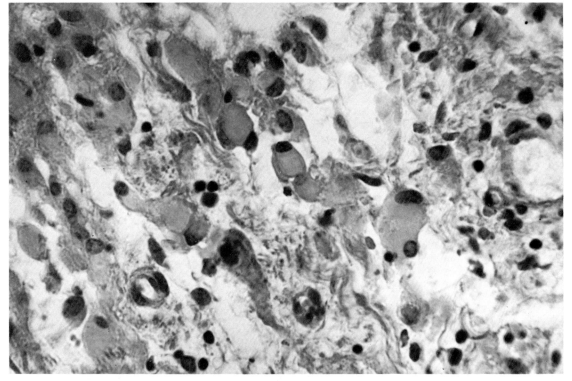

Fig. 16.22 Nasal 'glioma' showing gemistocytic astrocytes. M ×660

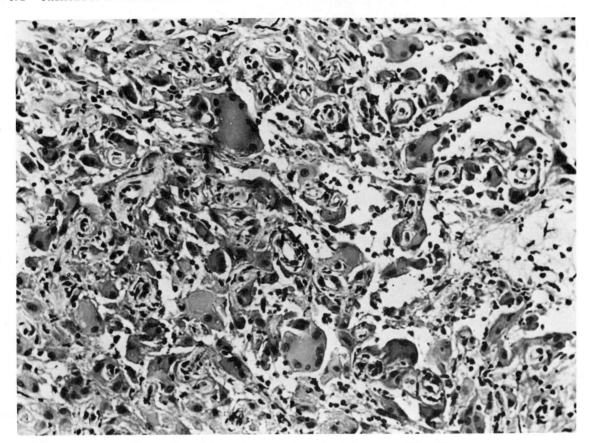

Fig. 16.23 Nasal 'glioma' showing gemistocytic astrocytes.M × 250

Katz and Lewis (1971) and by Hirsh et al. (1977). The last mentioned authors postulated that the external 'glioma' is the result of protrusion of brain through the fonticulus nasofrontalis, a membrane which covers the gap between the frontal and nasal bones in early embryonic life. Subsequent bony closure of this fontanelle obliterates the connection with the brain leaving an isolated mass of nervous tissue lying beneath the skin. Protrusion of brain substance through the foramen caecum gives rise to the intranasal lesion, in which the communication with the intracranial contents is less frequently obliterated. The lesion is essentially a developmental defect rather than a hereditary condition though the cause of the deviation from normal is not known.

Behaviour

Total excision of the lesion can be expected to effect a complete cure but where intracranial connection persists, simple intranasal removal may be followed by leakage of cerebrospinal fluid and the development of meningitis. Hence, frontal craniotomy may be necessary to deal with the dural or cerebral connection and to repair the bony defect. Recurrence due to residual tissue is not unknown but secondary excision usually results in permanent cure.

BIBLIOGRAPHY

Berger P 1890 Considérations sur l'origine, la mode de dévelopement et le traitement de certaines encéphalocèles. Revue de Chirurgie 10: 269–321

Black B K, Smith D E 1950 Nasal glioma. Archives of Neurology and Psychiatry 64: 614–630

Blumenfeld R, Skolnik E M 1965 Intranasal encephaloceles. Archives of Otolaryngology 82: 527–531

Bratton A B, Robinson S H G 1945 Gliomata of the nose and oral cavity. A report of two cases. Journal of Pathology and Bacteriology 58: 643–648

Deutsch H J 1965 Intranasal glioma. Annals of Otology, Rhinology and Laryngology 74: 637–644

Hildebrand 1888 Zur operativen Behandlung der Hirn und Rückenmarksbrüche. Deutsche Zeitschrift für Chirurgie 28: 438–457

Hirsh L F, Stool S E, Langfitt T W, Schut L 1977 Nasal glioma. Journal of Neurosurgery 46: 85–91

Katz A, Lewis J S 1971 Nasal gliomas. Archives of Otolaryngology 94: 351–355

Musser W A, Campbell R 1961 Nasal glioma. Archives of Otolaryngology 73: 732–736

Ried F 1852 Über angeborene Hirnbrüche in der Stirn- und Nasengegend. Illustrierte medizinische Zeitung 1: 133–141

Schmidt M B 1900 Über seltene Spaltbildungen in Bereiche des mittleren Stirnfortsatzes. Virchows Archiv für pathologische Anatomie 162: 340–370

Smith K R, Schwartz H G, Luse S A, Ogura J H 1963 Nasal gliomas; a report of five cases with electron microscopy of one. Journal of Neurosurgery 20: 968–982

Additional references

Del Villar R 1956 Astrocytoma of nose. Archives of Otolaryngology 63: 466–473

Morley G H, Cross R M 1958 Nasal glioma. Journal of Pathology and Bacteriology 76: 590–592

New G B, Devine K D 1947 Neurogenic tumors of the nose and throat. Archives of Otolaryngology 46: 163–179

Ross D E 1966 Nasal glioma. Laryngoscope 76: 1602–1611

Wadsworth P 1969 Nasal glioma. Journal of Laryngology and Otology 83: 87–88

Walker E A, Resler D R 1963 Nasal glioma. Laryngoscope 73: 93–107

MENINGIOMA OF THE NOSE AND SINUSES

Introduction

This uncommonly located tumour is remarkable for the associated errors in diagnosis. In so far as the possibility has frequently been overlooked, early reports of such tumours in this region may well have masqueraded under totally different labels. Thus, Schmidtmann 1928 discussed tumours which were undoubtedly of this type under the heading of 'endothelioma'. On the other hand, the 'psammoma' of the maxillary sinus reported by Shaheen (1931) was probably an example of ossifying fibroma.

Incidence

Meningioma is extremely uncommon in the nose and sinuses. Ash, Beck and Wilkes (1964) found seven cases amongst tumours of the upper respiratory tract. In the I.L.O. material, one case was encountered, representing less than 0.1 per cent of all tumours in the nose and sinuses.

Clinical features

The age distribution is broadly based, ranging from the second to the seventh decade with a slight male predominance. The common forms of presentation are nasal obstruction, proptosis, epiphora, pain and occasionally epistaxis.

Anatomical site of origin

The more common sites of involvement are the nasal cavity, maxillary, ethmoid and frontal sinuses. The sphenoid sinus is less frequently affected. The precise site of origin varies, many tumours taking origin in the orbit or intracranial cavity. Primary orbital tumours may extend into the antrum (Rosalki and McGee, 1962) or into the ethmoid sinuses (Gerth and Steps, 1968). Primary intracranial tumours may involve secondarily the nasal or paranasal region (Belal, 1955; Saksela,

Holmstrom and Grahne, 1972; Kjeldsberg and Minckler, 1972).

Tumours of primary origin in the nose have been reported (Lindström and Lindström, 1969; Kjeldsberg and Minckler, 1972), in the maxillary sinus (Hill, 1962; Ash et al., 1964) and in the frontal sinus (New and Devine, 1947; Majoros, 1970). An external nasal tumour was reported by Lopez, Silvers and Helwig (1974).

Gross appearances

The tumours are of rubbery consistency and, in the nasal cavity, may give the impression of simple polyps (Kjeldsberg and Minckler, 1972).

Histopathology

The microscopical picture is variable and has been the subject of many classifications. Russell and Rubinstein (1977) recommend four subdivisions: syncytial, transitional, fibroblastic and angioblastic. The syncytial type (Fig. 16.24) consists of polyhedral cells which, at light microscopical level, appear ill-defined giving an impression of either syncytial or epithelial structure, a pattern referred to by some workers as 'endotheliomatous' (Cervós-Navarro and Vazquez, 1969). The transitional form is characterized by the presence of tight whorls of fusiform or spindle cells surrounded by fibrous tissue or syncytial areas (Figs. 16.25 & 16.26). Some of the whorls are essentially cellular (Fig. 16.27), some have central vessels whilst others contain collagen which may become hyalinized or even calcified producing the psammoma bodies. The fibroblastic variety is composed of bundles of spindle cells with intervening collagen, whilst loosely arranged whorls and even psammoma bodies may be found. The angioblastic form is debatable, many examples closely resembling haemangiopericytoma and some workers (Popoff, Malinin and Rosomoff, 1974) have recommended that these be excluded from the menin-

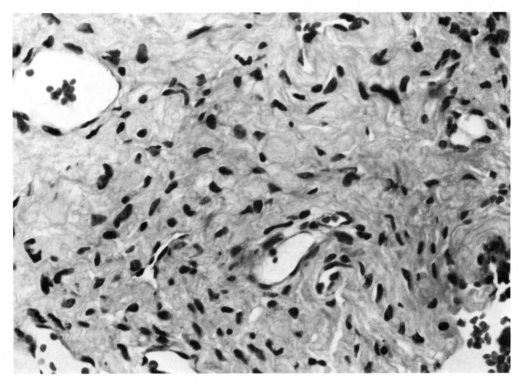

Fig. 16.24 Meningioma of the frontal sinus in a 28 year-old male, showing syncytial area. M ×520

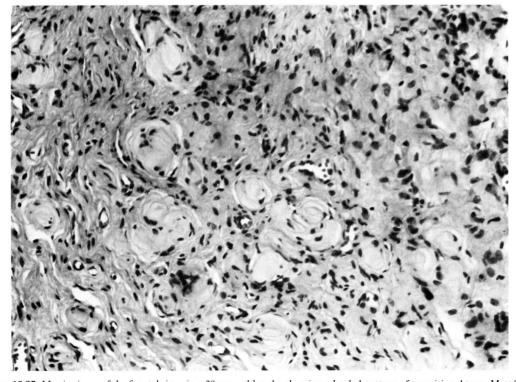

Fig. 16.25 Meningioma of the frontal sinus in a 28 year-old male, showing whorled pattern of transitional type. M ×260

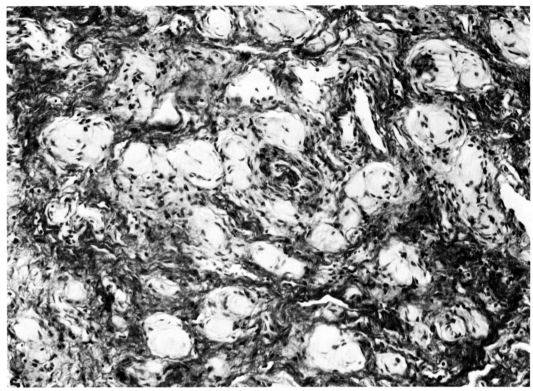

Fig. 16.26 Meningioma of the frontal sinus in a 28 year-old male, showing whorls surrounded by fibrous tissue. Van Gieson stain. M ×210

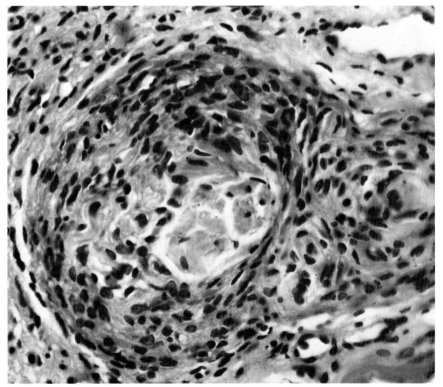

Fig. 16.27 Meningioma of the frontal sinus in a 28 year-old male, showing a cellular whorl. M ×520

gioma group. No angioblastic type has been reported as occurring in the nasal region although the existence of haemangiopericytomas in this location is now well established.

Essentially, the meningioma exhibits two types of cell, the polyhedral and spindle forms. The cytoplasm of both varieties shows a fibrillary appearance which, as a result of the poorly defined cell margins, gives an impression of being partly intercellular. These are the fibroglia fibrils originally described by Mallory (1920).

The ultrastructure of the meningiomas have been reported by many workers (Luse, 1960; Kepes, 1961; Neopolitano, Kyle and Fisher, 1964; Cervós-Navarro and Vazquez, 1969). The two principal types of cell are identifiable at electron microscopical level and both have been found to have a similar fine structure. A frequent feature is the complex interdigitation of plasma membranes. This occurs especially in the polyhedral type and numerous desmosomes are also found. The nuclei are generally rounded or oval but elongated in the spindle type, whilst indentations may produce the effect of pseudo-cytoplasmic inclusions. The cytoplasm contains variable numbers of mitochondria, prominent Golgi complexes and relatively small amounts of rough endoplasmic reticulum but a common cytoplasmic feature is the presence of fine filaments of the order of 10 nm. in diameter which may form whorl-like structures. Varying amounts of glycogen are also to be found.

Aetiology and pathogenesis

No particular cause of these tumours has been identified. There is an occasional association with Von Recklinghausen's disease or with gliomas but there are no reports of such a connection in the context of nasal or paranasal tumours, nor has trauma, meningitis or irradiation been shown to have any relevance. Ultrastructural studies have demonstrated the similarity between the so-called meningothelial cells and the normal arachnoid cells, thus confirming the concept of arachnoidal origin although possible endothelial origin was mooted by Schmidtmann (1928). The precise point of origin of nasal and paranasal tumours is variable and Kjeldsberg and Minckler (1972) have pointed out that intracranial origin with subsequent extension can frequently be demonstrated. On the other hand, primary meningiomas in the region are believed to arise from arachnoid cells which have migrated in the nerve sheaths and even become detached during development (Lopez et al. 1974). The main histological variants are explicable on the basis of origin from the multipotent meningothelial cell which not only retains both ectodermal and mesodermal characteristics but appears to be capable of producing collagen.

Behaviour

Most meningiomas are benign in so far as they do not metastasize but they often show a predilection for local permeation of crevices and foramina whilst pressure erosion may result in spread from one cavity to another. Recurrence is not uncommon, even after apparent total removal (Saksela et al., 1972). The last mentioned authors compared the clinical behaviour with the activity of such tumours in organ culture, observing an infiltration of the interstices of fibrin foam matrix and they suggested that the infiltrative capacity of these tumours was an inherent characteristic.

Cases have been reported as surviving for many years with or without recurrences. It is clearly important to watch for evidence of intracranial involvement which may cause epileptiform attacks. The solitary I.L.O. case has survived for nearly 30 years but more recently he has suffered from attacks of epilepsy. Malignant change in meningiomas is a rare event and reported deaths are usually the result of local effects rather than specific malignancy.

BIBLIOGRAPHY

Ash J E, Beck M R, Wilkes J D 1964 Tumours of the upper respiratory tract and ear. Atlas of Tumor Pathology, Armed Forces Institute of Pathology, Washington, Facsimile 12, p 96

Belal A 1955 Meningiomas infiltrating the nasal cavity, nasal sinuses and orbit. Journal of Laryngology and Otology 69: 59–69

Cervós-Navarro J, Vazquez J J 1969 An electron microscopic study of meningiomas. Acta Neuropathologica (Berlin) 13: 301–323

Gerth B, Steps H J 1968 Extradurale Meningeome. Zeitschrift für Laryngologie, Rhinologie und Otologie 47: 124–130

Hill C L 1962 Meningioma of the maxillary sinus. Archives of Otolaryngology 76: 547–549

Kepes J 1961 Electron microscopic studies of meningiomas. American Journal of Pathology 39: 499–510

Kjeldsberg C R, Minckler J 1972 Meningiomas presenting as nasal polyps. Cancer 29. 153–156

Lindström C G, Lindström D W 1969 On extracranial meningioma. A case of primary meningioma of the nasal cavity. Acta Otolaryngologica 68: 451–456

Lopez D A, Silvers D N, Helwig E B 1974 Cutaneous meningiomas – a clinicopathologic study. Cancer 34: 728–744

Luse S A 1960 Electron microscopic studies of brain tumors. Neurology 10: 881–905

Majoros M 1970 Meningioma of the paranasal sinuses. Laryngoscope 80: 640–645

Mallory F B 1920 The type cell of the so-called dural endothelioma. Journal of Medical Research 41: 349–364

Neapolitano L, Kyle R, Fisher E R 1964 Ultrastructure of meningiomas and the derivation and nature of their cellular components. Cancer 17: 233–241

New G B, Devine K D 1947 Neurogenic tumors of the nose and throat. Archives of Otolaryngology 46: 163–179

Popoff N A, Malinin T I, Rosomoff H L 1974 Fine structure of intracranial haemangiopericytoma and angiomatous meningioma. Cancer 34: 1187–1197

Rosalki S B, McGee L E 1962 Meningioma presenting as nasopharyngeal tumour. Report of two cases. Journal of Laryngology and Otology 76: 133–139

Russell D S, Rubinstein L J 1977 Tumours of the meninges and related tissues. In Pathology of Tumours of the Nervous System, 4th ed. ch 3, p 65–100

Saksela E, Holmström T, Grahne B 1972 Growth pattern of meningiomas penetrating the skull base. Acta Otolaryngologica 74: 363–370

Schmidtmann M 1928 Endotheliome. In Henke F, Lubarsch O (ed.) Handbuch der speziellen pathologischen Anatomie und Histologie, Band III, Teile 1, seite 242–245

Shaheen H B 1931 Psammoma in the maxillary antrum. Journal of Laryngology and Otology 46: 117

17

Lymphoreticular tumours of the nose and sinuses

LYMPHORETICULAR TUMOURS OF THE
NOSE AND SINUSES

Introduction

Freeman, Berg and Cutler (1972) estimated that about one quarter of malignant lymphomas arise in extranodal sites, of which the nasal and paranasal region is one of the less common. Lymphoid tumours in this location began to be reported in the literature in the latter half of the nineteenth century. Heath (1869) described a recurrent round celled tumour in the ethmoid region and this may well have been the first malignant lymphoma in this site to be reported. In 1889, Bosworth included three round celled tumours in his review of 'sarcoma' of the nasal region and, in 1897, Schmidt collected five cases of nasal 'lymphosarcoma'. The relative rarity of the condition was clearly the main reason for the paucity of its documentation and its ultimate definition had to await the broader understanding of lymphoid tumours in general. Geschicter (1935) included seven cases of 'lymphosarcoma' in his review of tumours of the nose and sinuses, thus emphasizing the lymphocytoid form of the tumours originally described but Greifenstein (1937) appears to have been the first to report 'reticulum cell sarcoma' occurring in the ethmoid region.

Terminology

In the context of lymphoma generally, a large number of terms and classifications have been and still are being introduced. Many lymphomas in this region have been reported in terms based on the classification of Gall and Mallory (1942). In terms of non-Hodgkins lymphoma, which is probably exclusively relevant to the present context, the last mentioned authors' subdivision consisted of follicular, lymphocytic, lymphoblastic and 'reticulum cell sarcoma' consisting of clasmatocytic and stem cell types. Of the more recent classifications (Bennett, Farrer-Brown, Henry and Jelliffe, 1974; Gerard-Marchant, Hamlin, Lennert, Rilke, Stansfeld and Van Unnik, 1974; Lukes and Collins, 1975), the one presented by Bennett and his colleagues is most highly favoured at the present time and, being derived from the Gall and Mallory scheme, is more readily adaptable in the present context. The classification offered by Bennett et al. (1974) is briefly summarized as follows:

Follicular Lymphoma	
Diffuse Lymphoma	
Lymphocytic, well differentiated	Grade I malignancy
Lymphocytic, intermediate differentiation	
Lymphocytic, poorly differentiated	
Mixed small and undifferentiated large cell	
Undifferentiated large cell	Grade II malignancy
Histiocytic	
Plasma cell	
Unclassified	

Follicular lymphomas have not been reported as occurring in the nose and sinuses and are presumed not to exist in this location.

Incidence

The nasal region is clearly an unusual site of election for this group of tumours. Gall and Mallory (1942) found only three out of 618 cases of malignant lymphoma (0.48 per cent) primarily involving the nose or sinuses. As is inevitable with rare conditions, reports on relative frequency in the present location show considerable variation. Von Zange and Scholtz (1963) claimed nearly ten per cent of all malignant tumours of the nose and sinuses whilst Sofferman and Cummings (1975) found an incidence of eight per cent of malignant tumours of the sinuses alone. The I.L.O. material (excluding plasma cell tumours) represented less than three per cent of all malignant tumours of the nose and sinuses.

Clinical features

There are no particular signs which would aid in distinction from other malignant tumours in the region. Age distribution is broadly based but the greater proportion of cases occur between the ages of 50 and 70 years and there is no significant sex difference. Nasal obstruction, swelling of the cheek, proptosis and pain are commonly encountered but epistaxis is relatively uncommon. The duration of symptoms is usually measured in months.

Anatomical site of origin

Some of these tumours appear to arise primarily in and even remain confined to the nasal cavity. Fifty per cent of the series presented by von Zange and Scholtz (1963) were apparently of nasal origin. However, paranasal origin would seem to be more common (Wang, 1971) and the 17 cases reported by Ringertz (1938) were of naso-ethmoidal origin. In the ten cases comprising the I.L.O. material, four were of nasal and six of paranasal origin. Within the nasal cavity, such tumours may arise from the septum, floor or lateral wall whilst paranasal tumours are usually of antro-ethmoidal origin. Wang (1971) reported two cases of involvement of the frontal sinus.

Gross appearances

The naked eye features are variable and in no way pathognomonic. In situ, there may be a diffuse mucosal swelling or granulomatous masses associated with radio-opacity. Harrison (1953) reported an unusual case of total excision of a malignant lymphoma in the ethmoidal region and the operation specimen presented a large white circumscribed mass which resembled a carcinoma on gross inspection. More often, however, the pathologist is presented with irregular fragments of tissue whose nature can only be determined by microscopical examination.

Histopathology

One of the major problems of histology in this context is related to the nature and state of the tissue available for examination. The tumour tissue may not only be fragmented but may also be secondarily infected, resulting in necrosis and inflammatory infiltration. Hence, interpretation and classification may prove to be more difficult than in the case of nodal lymphomas. Nevertheless, the microscopical features show variation within the range of recognized types of malignant lymphoma. The largest series of twenty-four nasal lymphomas (Eichel, Harrison, Devine, Scanlon and Brown, 1966) contained representatives of all types within the Gall and Mallory classification with the exception of the follicular lymphoma. Occasionally, nasal or paranasal tumours may show a predominance of mature lymphocytes (Fig. 17.1), representing the lymphocytic, well differentiated type in the Bennett classi-

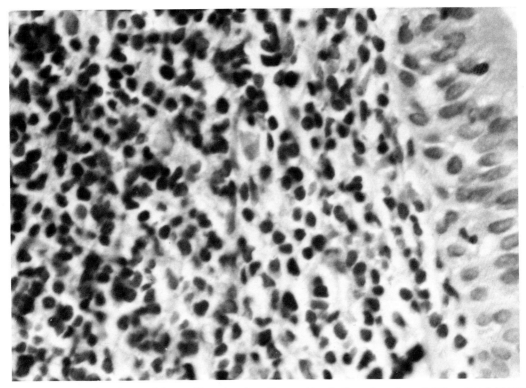

Fig. 17.1 Malignant lymphoma of the maxillary sinus in a 60 year-old male. Lymphocytic, well differentiated. M ×825

fication. More frequently, the cells exhibit a less mature appearance consistent with the intermediate or poorly differentiated lymphocytic type (Figs. 17.2 & 17.3). Occasional mixed small and large cell types may be encountered (Figs. 17.4 & 17.5) but the most commonly reported tumour is the 'reticulum cell' type which would include the large undifferentiated cell or immunoblastic variety (Fig. 17.6), the histiocytic type and possibly even some of the poorly differentiated lymphocytic tumours. As in nodal lymphomas, plasmacytoid differentiation may be observed.

There have been a number of reports of Hodgkin's Disease involving the nose and sinuses (Lautz, 1958; Eichel et al., 1966; Stewart and Stuart, 1971; Tiwari, 1973) but all appear to have had evidence of lymphoid tumour in other sites and in some cases the diagnosis was debatable as far as the nasal lesion was concerned. No convincing example of primary isolated Hodgkin's Disease in the nasal region has been presented.

Necrosis in nasal or paranasal lymphomas may occasionally be found, not infrequently in association with secondary inflammatory infiltration, thus bringing the possibility of midfacial granuloma syndrome into the differential diagnosis. However, the pleomorphic pattern characterizing the infiltrate in the Stewart type granuloma is not usually seen in the malignant lymphoma.

Aetiology and pathogenesis

No specific factors have so far emerged in relation to the causation of this uncommon location of malignant lymphoma. In contrast with Waldeyer's ring, nasal and paranasal mucosa does not normally contain recognizable lymphoid tissue. Nevertheless, in the presence of allergic rhinitis and chronic inflammation, well developed lymphoid follicles may be found and it was suggested by Sofferman and Cummings (1975) that this might be the starting point of neoplasia. However, there is no evidence that malignant lymphoma in this region is necessarily preceded by rhinitis of sinusitis and the observation merely establishes the relative ease with which lymphoid tissue may appear where it is not a normal feature of the part. The abnormal development of lymphoid tissue in the nasal and paranasal region is never as extensive as in the thyroid (Hashimoto's Disease) or in the parotid (Sjögren's Syndrome) nor would it appear to have the same significance but Gall and Mallory (1942) found equal frequency of malignant lymphoma in all three sites.

The diagnosis of primary malignant lymphoma of the

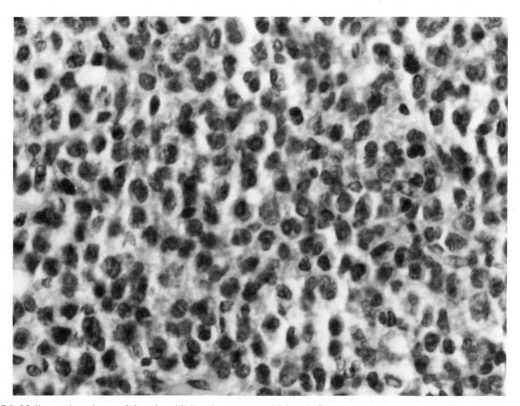

Fig. 17.2 Malignant lymphoma of the ethmoid sinus in a 67 year-old female. Lymphocytic, intermediate differentiation. M × 825

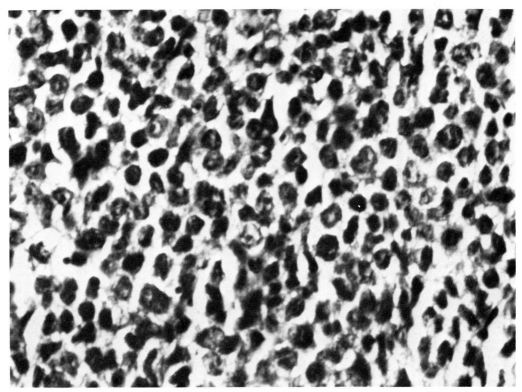

Fig. 17.3 Malignant lymphoma of the nasal cavity in a 54 year-old female. Lymphocytic, poorly differentiated. M ×825

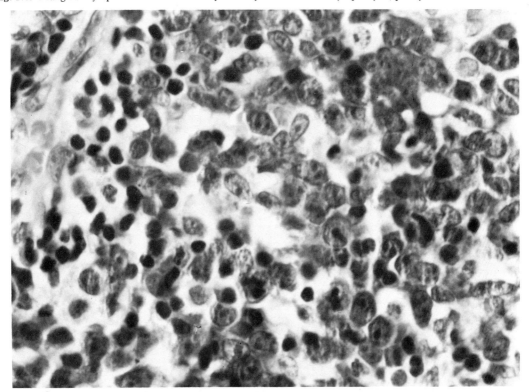

Fig. 17.4 Malignant lymphoma of the nasal cavity in a 72 year-old female. Mixed small and large cell type. M ×825

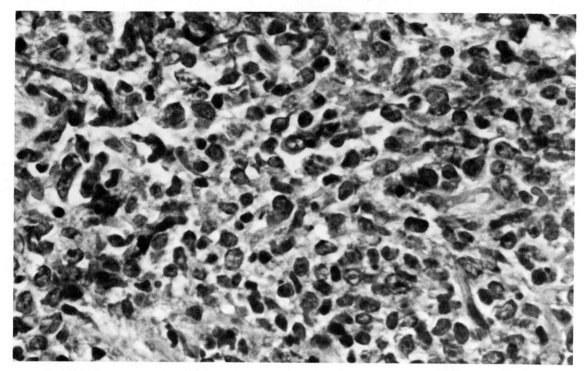

Fig. 17.5 Malignant lymphoma of the nasal cavity in a 75 year-old male. Mixed small and large cell type. M × 595

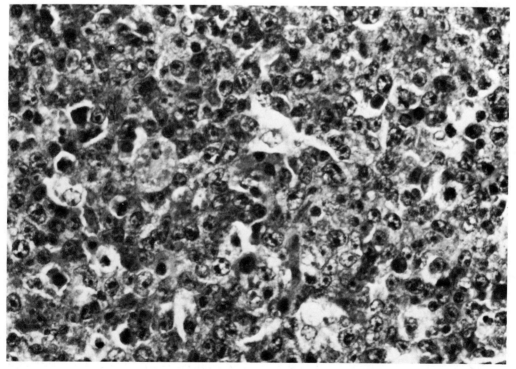

Fig. 17.6 Malignant lymphoma of the nasal cavity in a 71 year-old male. Large, undifferentiated cell type – immunoblasts. M × 520

nasal region depends on the absence of lymphoreticular disease elsewhere and investigations to this end may sometimes have their limitations as might be suggested by the subsequent occurrence of disseminated disease.

Behaviour

Although initially localized, there may be subsequent spread of the tumour to adjacent regions. Unilateral extension from one cavity to another is not uncommon and the orbit may be invaded as a result of involvement of its floor and medial wall. Malignant lymphoma of the maxillary sinus may extend through the anterior wall to involve the cheek and the palate may be invaded through the antral floor.

Regional lymphnode involvement occurs in approximately 20 per cent of cases, usually at a later stage and a generalized lymphadenopathy may sometimes follow. Remote or systemic involvement may occur in any part of the body such as skin, brain, bone and various internal organs. In the I.L.O. material such an event was ultimately observed in nearly 50 per cent of the cases, in one of which leukaemia developed and death occurred after five months. In the last mentioned case, the available evidence pointed to a primary antral involvement but the course of events may well be reversed as in the case reported by Meran, Wey and Speck (1977) and probably also in a case discussed by Sofferman and Cummings (1975).

Crude survival figures show fairly wide variations but a considerable proportion of patients do not die directly of their disease. Eichel et al. (1966) reported a five year survival rate of 41 per cent in nasal lymphomas whilst only two out of eight paranasal 'reticulosarcomas' published by Birt (1970) survived for five years. In the I.L.O. material, four out of ten patients died of their disease in less than one year. Three died of unrelated causes after periods ranging from five to eleven years whilst three patients with paranasal tumours have so far survived for two to twenty-two years. Because of difficulties of classification inherent in the available material, correlation between survival and histological type is not as close as would be expected in nodal lymphomas.

BIBLIOGRAPHY

Bennett M H, Farrer-Brown G, Henry K, Jelliffe A M 1974 Classification of non-Hodgkin's lymphoma. Lancet 2: 405–406

Birt B D 1970 Reticulum cell sarcoma of the nose and paranasal sinuses. Journal of Laryngology and Otology 84: 615–630

Bosworth F H 1889 Sarcoma of the nasal passages in diseases of the nose and throat. W. Wood & Co, ch 36, p 437–452

Eichel B S, Harrison E G, Devine K D, Scanlon P W, Brown H A 1966 Primary lymphoma of the nose, including a relationship to lethal midline granuloma. American Journal of Surgery 112: 597–605

Freeman C, Berg J W, Cutler S J 1972 Occurrence and prognosis of extranodal lymphomas. Cancer 29: 252–260

Gall E A, Mallory T B 1942 Malignant lymphoma. American Journal of Pathology 18: 381–429

Gerard-Marchant R, Hamlin I, Lennert K, Rilke F, Stansfeld A G, Van Unnik J A M 1974 Classification of non-Hodgkin's lymphomas. Lancet 2: 406–408

Geschicter C F 1935 Tumors of the nasal and paranasal cavities. American Journal of Cancer 24: 637–660

Greifenstein A 1937 Die Klinik der Retothelsarkome, dergestellt auf Grund von 31 eigenen Beobachtungen. Archiv für Nasen-, Ohren- und Kehlkopfheilkunde 143: 189–215

Harrison D F N 1953 Two cases of lymphosarcoma of the ethmoid. Journal of Laryngology and Otology 67: 225–228

Heath C 1869 Recurrent sarcomatous tumour involving the orbits, frontal sinuses and cranium. Transactions of the Pathological Society of London 20: 257–259

Lautz H A 1958 Nasal and laryngeal involvement in abdominal Hodgkin's disease. Archives of Otolaryngology 67: 78–80

Lukes R J, Collins R D 1975 New approaches to the classification of lymphomata. British Journal of Cancer 31: Supplement II, 1–28

Meran A, Wey W, Speck B 1977 Zur Manifestation maligner lymphatischer Erkrankungen im Nasennebenhöhlen-Bereich. Hals-, Nasen-, Ohrenheilkunde 25: 206–209

Ringertz N 1938 Tumours arising in lymphatic tissues in pathology of malignant tumours arising in the nasal and paranasal cavities and maxilla. Acta Otolaryngologica Supplement 27: 209–225

Schmidt M 1897 Die Neubildungen in den oberen Luftwegen in Die Krankheiten der oberen Luftwege. Zweite Auflage Kap 18: 620–654

Sofferman R A, Cummings C W 1975 Malignant lymphoma of the paranasal sinuses. Archives of Otolaryngology 101: 287–292

Stewart I A, Stuart A E 1971 Hodgkin's disease in the nose. Journal of Laryngology and Otology 85: 1069–1073

Tiwari R M 1973 Hodgkin's disease of the maxilla. Journal of Laryngology and Otology 87: 85–88

Von Zange J, Scholtz H J 1963 25 Jahre Behandlung bösartiger Geschwülste der Nase und Nebenhöhlen in Jena und ihr Ergebnis. Zeitschrift für Laryngologie, Rhinologie und Otologie 42: 613–626

Wang C C 1971 Primary malignant lymphoma of the oral cavity and paranasal sinuses. Radiology, 100: 151–153

PLASMACYTOMA OF THE NOSE AND SINUSES

Introduction

The existence of neoplasms composed of plasma cells has been known for well over a century, dating back to the description of 'Mollities Ossium' by Dalrymple (1846). For a long time, attention was centred on the bone marrow and the multiplicity of osseous lesions, commonly associated with abnormal protein production and Bence Jones proteinuria. As reported cases began to accumulate, it was gradually realized that solitary tumours of similar structure occurred not only in the skeletal system but also in the soft tissues. With the acceptance of the extramedullary plasmacytoma as an entity, it was soon established that such tumours most commonly occurred in the upper respiratory tract and to a lesser extent in the alimentary system. It is not surprising, therefore, that the first solitary extramedullary plasmacytoma was reported as having arisen in the nasal cavity. Schridde (1905), in the course of a dissertation on plasma cells, used material from a nasal tumour in a 40 year-old man to demonstrate their characteristics. The patient did not have proteinuria and so the author did not relate the tumour to the osseous myeloma. Subsequently, a number of solitary cases were reported and included in the earliest review by Claiborn and Ferris (1931).

Terminology

Although the expressions myeloma and plasma cell myeloma are in common use with both multiple and solitary bone tumours, the extramedullary tumour is, by common consent, referred to as plasmacytoma.

Incidence

This is an uncommon tumour in the nasal region. Estimates of the proportion of extramedullary tumours arising in the upper air passages have ranged from 50 to 75 per cent (Hellwig, 1943; Carr, Hancock, Henry and Ward, 1977). Heatly (1953) claimed that over 50 per cent of extramedullary tumours occurred in the nose and sinuses. On the other hand, Castro, Lewis and Strong (1973) found the nose and sinuses to be involved in only 37.5 per cent of plasmacytomas of the head and neck region. In the I.L.O. material, seven cases represented less than one per cent of all tumours in the nose and sinuses but two per cent of all malignant tumours, as was reported by Ringertz (1938).

Clinical features

Age distribution is broadly based with a peak in the fifth and sixth decades whilst males predominate in the ratio of 2:1. Nasal obstruction, discharge, epistaxis and swelling of the face are common features and, less frequently, pain may occur. The duration of symptoms may range widely from a few days to years.

Anatomical site of origin

These tumours may arise anywhere in the upper respiratory tract but the nasal cavity is the commonest site. In a review of 175 tumours of the upper respiratory tract, Heatly (1953) found 61 per cent in the nasal cavity. Of the paranasal tumours, the greater proportion arise in the maxillary sinus, a smaller number are found in the ethmoid sinuses whilst involvement of the frontal and sphenoid sinuses is very rare.

Gross appearances

In situ, the tumour often appears lobulated but there are no characteristic naked eye features. The tissue is usually firm in consistency and dark in colour.

Histopathology

Closely packed, ovoid or polyhedral cells may form multiple sheets (Fig. 17.7) with a fine connective tissue stroma containing numbers of small blood vessels around which the tumour cells may sometimes form a palisade. The nuclei are often eccentrically placed in a relatively abundant cytoplasm after the manner of normal plasmacytes, although the classical 'cartwheel' arrangement of the heterochromatin is often absent. A well developed Golgi complex often produces an irregular pale area close to the nucleus. This is often referred to as a 'halo' although it rarely completely surrounds the nucleus. An element of pleomorphism is usually present and the nuclei are frequently double or even triple (Fig. 17.8). A gradation may be seen between typical plasmacytes fulfilling the criteria of Marschalko (1895) and lymphoid cells (B-lymphocytes) in the process of transition. Pyronine staining produces a bright red cytoplasm due to the presence of rough endoplasmic reticulum which is a prominent feature in electronmicrographs (Fig. 17.9). In so far as certain cells in the lymphoid series may also be pyroninophilic, the stain is not specific for plasma cells. Similarly, the immunoperoxidase technique for demonstrating immunoglobulins also shows an overlap (Taylor, 1974). Plasmacytoid differentiation in a malignant lymphoma may lead to confusion with plasmacytoma.

Distinction may sometimes have to be made between plasmacytoma and intense plasmacytic inflammatory infiltration. The inflammatory lesion usually shows (a) intermingling with other inflammatory cells, (b) predominance of normal classical plasmacytes with typical nuclear appearance, (c) absence of pleomorphism and multinucleated cells (d) the presence of Russell bodies which are only rarely seen in plasmacytomas. Rawson, Eyler and Horn (1950) emphasized the replacement of tissue by plasmacytoma in contrast with the plasmacytic

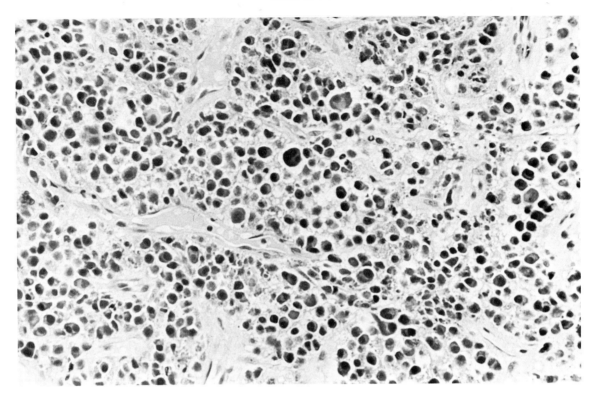

Fig. 17.7 Plasmacytoma of the nasal cavity in an adult male. M ×250

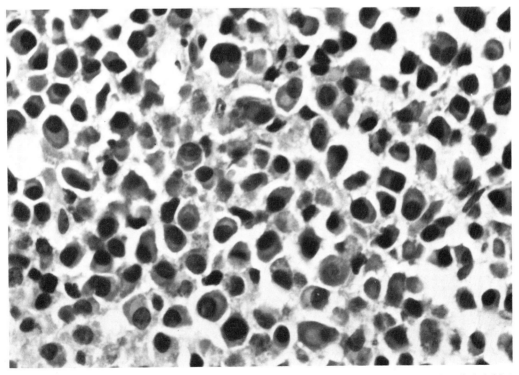

Fig. 17.8 Plasmacytoma of the nasal cavity in a 56 year-old male, showing multiple nuclei and juxtanuclear 'halos'. M ×650

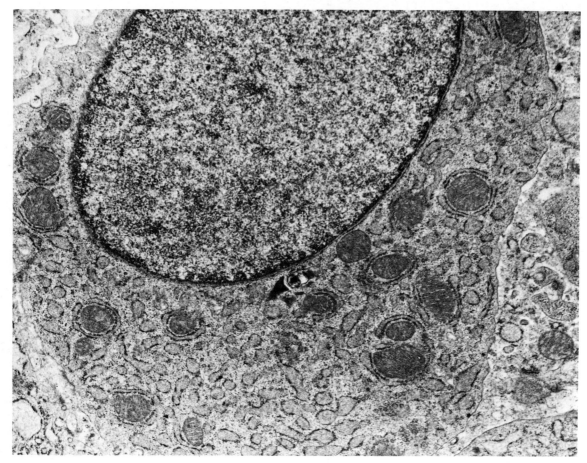

Fig. 17.9 Plasmacytoma of the nasal cavity in a 56 year-old male: numerous profiles of rough endoplasmic reticulum in a plasmacell. M × 17 500

infiltration in inflammatory lesions although plasmacytoma may infiltrate persistent normal tissue.

There are no cytological features in plasmacytomas which correlate with aggressive tendencies and it would seem prudent to regard all tumours of this histological type as being at least potentially malignant.

Aetiology and pathogenesis

No causal agent has been identified. It has been pointed out that inflammatory plasmacytic infiltration is not uncommon in the region but there is no evidence of any relationship of this event to neoplasia. It is of interest to note that plasmacytic infiltration is very common in chronic otitis media but plasmacytoma of the middle ear is extremely rare.

The ill-defined relationship of these extramedullary tumours to plasmacytomas of bone and systematized disease (classical multiple myeloma) have added to the confusion and the problem of prognosis. Occasional cases already have multiple involvement at the time of presentation with a tumour in the nasal region and, in some, remote osseous lesions may well have preceded the nasal or paranasal manifestations, as in one of the cases reported by Dolin and Dewar (1956). Ewing and Foote (1952) suggested that cases of multiple myeloma may well present with tumours in the head and neck region since other lesions are likely to remain silent until revealed by pathological fracture. However, these observations do not invalidate the entity of primary solitary plasmacytoma in the nose and sinuses. There are differences of opinion on the relationship between extramedullary plasmacytoma, solitary plasmacytoma of bone, multiple myelomatosis and plasma cell leukaemia. Some regard all these conditions as variants of the same disease but the enigma concerns the relationship between them, particularly in the individual case. It would appear that extramedullary plasmacytoma is not necessarily the primary manifestation of systematized disease. Carr et al. (1977) believe that extramedullary plasmacytomas are distinct from solitary plasmacytomas of bone and that the frequency of subsequent diffuse involvement with immunoglobulin abnormalities is very low. However, once the histological diagnosis has been made, it is necessary to exclude multiple involvement. Radiographic survey is mandatory and, in the event of even a single remote bone lesion, marrow biopsy is advisable. The electrophoretic composition of the serum proteins must be determined and, where appropriate, the immunoglobulin pattern investigated. Even when an abnormality is found, urinary excretion may be undetectable unless a concentration method is used. Non-secretory myelomatosis is rare.

Behaviour

The course of these tumours is not readily predictable. They may remain localized with or without adjacent bone involvement but there may be spread beyond the confines of the region. One unresolved problem is whether tumour remote from the primary site represents multiple origin or metastasis. Wachter (1914) reported multiple tumours in the nose, larynx and nasopharynx in a 40 year-old woman. Regional lymphnode involvement is usually regarded as being metastatic. Stout and Kenney (1949) found regional lymphnode involvement in 23 per cent of plasmacytomas of the upper respiratory tract and oral cavity whist Dolin and Dewar claimed 29.5 per cent in tumours of the nose and sinuses although only two cases were histologically confirmed. Cervical lymphadenopathy developed in one of the I.L.O. cases.

Remote bone involvement at a later date has been frequently reported, the event taking place at greatly varying time intervals. Stout and Kenney (1949) found 15 examples amongst their 104 cases. Exclusive to the nose and sinuses, Carson, Ackerman and Maltby (1955) reported four out of six cases whilst Castro et al. (1973) found only two out of 14 plasmacytomas in the region. In the I.L.O. material, three out of seven cases showed distant bone lesions, one exhibiting abnormal immunoglobulin in serum and urine (IgG) whilst another showed reversal of the albumin-globulin ratio. Castro et al. (1973) reported two cases of reversed ratio whilst Carson et al. (1955) noted systematized disease in one of their six cases. Immunoglobulin disturbance may well be underestimated and extramedullary plasmacytomas may produce light chain molecules only.

Against this behavioural background, prognosis is clearly difficult to assess. Carson et al. (1955) reported only one of their cases, involving the nasal region, as surviving for more than five years. Batsakis, Fries, Goldman and Karlsberg (1964) reported similar survival in two out of six cases. Castro et al. (1973) gave a five year survival rate of 54 per cent. In the I.L.O. material (four cases of which have been previously reported by Booth, Cheesman and Vincenti, 1973) two patients died at five years and only three out of seven are known to have survived for five years or more. It is interesting to note that the longest survivor (17 years) is the patient who developed systematized disease with abnormal protein pattern. This is in conformity with the observation of Stout and Kenney (1949) that such cases do not necessarily follow the rapidly fatal course of the classical multiple myelomatosis.

BIBLIOGRAPHY

Batsakis J G, Fries G T, Goldman R T, Karlsberg R C 1964 Upper respiratory tract plasmacytoma. Archives of Otolaryngology 79: 613–618

Booth J B, Cheesman A D, Vincenti N H 1973 Extramedullary plasmacytoma of the upper respiratory tract. Annals of Otology, Rhinology and Laryngology 82: 709–715

Carr I, Hancock B W, Henry L, Ward A M 1977 Myelomatosis and other monoclonal gammopathies. Lymphoreticular Disease. Blackwell, ch 8, p 141–152

Carson C P, Ackerman L V, Maltby J D 1955 Plasma cell myeloma. American Journal of Clinical Pathology 25: 849–888

Castro E B, Lewis J S, Strong E W 1973 Plasmacytoma of Paranasal sinuses and nasal cavity. Archives of Otolaryngology 97: 326–329

Claiborn L N, Ferris H W 1931 Plasma cell tumors of the nasal and nasopharyngeal mucosa. Archives of Surgery 23: 477–499

Dalrymple J 1846 On the microscopical character of mollities ossium. Dublin Quarterly Journal of Medical Science 2: 85–95

Dolin S, Dewar J P 1956 Extramedullary plasmacytoma. American Journal of Pathology 32: 83–103

Ewing M R, Foote F W 1952 Plasma cell tumors of the mouth and upper air passages. Cancer 5: 499–513

Fu Y S, Perzin K H 1978 Non epithelial tumours etc. part 9. Plasmacytomas. Cancer 42: 2399–2406

Fu Y S, Perzin K H 1979 Non epithelial tumours etc. part 10. Malignant lymphomas. Cancer 43: 611–621

Heatly C A 1953 Primary plasma cell tumors of the upper air passages with particular reference to involvement of the maxillary sinus. Annals of Otology, Rhinology and Laryngology 62: 289–306

Hellwig G A 1943 Extramedullary plasma cell tumors as observed in various locations. Archives of Pathology 35: 95–111

Marschalko T 1895 Über die sogenannten Plasmazellen, ein Beitrag zur Kenntnis der Herkunft der entzündlichen Infiltrationzellen. Archiv für Dermatologie und Syphilogie 30: 3–52

Rawson A J, Eyler P W, Horn R 1950 Plasma cell tumors of the upper respiratory tract. American Journal of Pathology 26: 445–461

Ringertz N 1938 The pathological anatomy of the mucous membrane plasmacytoma. Pathology of malignant tumours in the nasal and paranasal cavities and maxilla. Acta Otolaryngologica Supplement 27: 234–249

Schridde H 1905 Weitere Untersuchungen über die Körnelungen der Plasmazellen. Zentralblatt für allgemeine Pathologie und pathologische Anatomie 16: 433

Stout A P, Kenney F R 1949 Primary plasma cell tumors of the upper air passages and oral cavity. Cancer 2: 261–278

Taylor C R 1974 The nature of Reed-Sternberg cells and other malignant 'reticulum' cells. Lancet 2: 802–807

Wachter H 1914 Ein Fall von multiplen Plasmazytom der oberen Luftwege. Archiv für Laryngologie und Rhinologie 28: 69–73

18

Vascular tumours of the nose and sinuses

VASCULAR TUMOURS OF THE NOSE AND SINUSES

Under this heading there are a variety of different lesions linked by their close vascular associations. Recognition of the existence of congenital malformations had a profound effect on concepts of vascular tumours many of which have come to be regarded as hamartomas rather than true neoplasms. Such a view, however, is an over-simplification of the situation which obtains in the nasal region where a substantial number of vascular lesions appear to be acquired rather than congenital. In order to establish perspective in this anatomical region, both true tumours and malformations must be considered and in the present context the following classification has been adopted, synonymous terms being included in parenthesis.

1. Haemangioma (Angioma, capillary haemangioma, Haemangio-endothelioma)
2. Angiosarcoma (Haemangio-endothelioma)
3. Haemangiopericytoma
4. Glomus Tumour
5. Chemodectoma (Paraganglioma)
6. Juvenile Angiofibroma (Nasopharyngeal fibroma)
7. Osler's Disease (Hereditary haemorrhagic telangiectasia)

With regard to terminology, the expression 'haeman-gio-endothelioma' merits some comment. Unfortunately, this term has been used in both benign and malignant contexts without, necessarily, being appropriately prefixed. Although for many 'Haemangio-endothelioma' has a malignant connotation, confusion is inevitable. The WHO classification includes the term as a synonym for angiosarcoma and, notwithstanding the logic and desirability of indicating the cell of origin, the present authors have preferred to follow the practice adopted by a number of other writers who have opted for the use of the term 'angiosarcoma'. The WHO alternative is used occasionally in the interests of clarity but never in a benign context.

HAEMANGIOMAS OF THE NOSE AND SINUSES

Introduction

Tumours or tumour-like proliferations of blood vessels are important in Ear, Nose and Throat practice since they are a source of nasal bleeding. Many of these lesions occur on the nasal septum and have long been recognized clinically under the title of 'bleeding polyp of the septum'. Hasslauer (1900) collected 57 vascular lesions of the nasal septum although histological details were not given in the majority. In retrospect, however, there is little doubt that most were probably genuine haemangiomas. Many solitary cases were reported subsequently but Baum (1922) did not accept true haemangioma as a common entity in the nasal cavity. Cases continued to be reported under such titles as haemangioma or capillary haemangio-endothelioma but in 1950 Ash and Old presented 14 cases of haemangioma of the septum which they regarded as true tumours.

Incidence

In a review of over a thousand vascular tumours, Watson and McCarthy (1940) found that there was a disproportionate incidence in the head and neck region which amounted to 56 per cent. Undoubtedly the nasal region occupied a prominent position in that anatomical distribution. In I.L.O. haemangiomas accounted for 14 per cent of all tumours in the nose and sinuses and, in so far as they were almost exclusive to the nasal cavity, they constituted about 20 per cent of all benign neoplasms in that part. In their survey of non-epithelial tumours, Fu and Perzin (1974) found haemangiomas to comprise 32 per cent but the comparable figure in the present authors' material is over 60 per cent.

Clinical features

The age distribution is fairly broadly based but shows a peak in the fifth decade. In fact, the greater proportion of cases present at over the age of 40 years. There is no sex difference. In most cases the complaint is epistaxis with or without attendant nasal obstruction and the duration of symptoms is usually measured in months. The patient commonly presents with a reddish blue polypoid swelling with a smooth surface which may sometimes be ulcerated.

Anatomical site of origin

The tumours are almost invariably confined to the nasal cavity in which the septum is the major site of election. In a series reported by one of us (Osborn 1959), 65 per cent involved the septum whilst the remainder were distributed between the lateral wall and the vestibule. Haemangiomas involving the paranasal sinuses are extremely rare. In the I.L.O. series, one such tumour involved the ethmoid sinus in a 71 year-old male; Afshin and Sharmin (1974) reported a haemangioma of the maxillary sinus in a 15 year-old male whilst Fu and Perzin (1974) recorded a diffuse lesion of the maxilla which involved the antrum as well as the nasal cavity. Primary origin in adjacent bone is occasionally encountered; Azaz and Lustman (1976) reported a case arising in the maxilla but not involving the sinus whilst haemangioma of the nasal bone has also been recorded (Neivert and Bilchick, 1936; Dorfman, Steiner and Jaffe, 1971; Bridger, 1976).

Gross appearances

Almost invariably dark in colour due to its marked vascularity, the surface is usually smooth with occasional granular patches indicating ulceration. Very occasionally, when there is minimal engorgement, the tissue appears pale and the diagnosis is not even suspected prior to microscopy.

Histopathology

Most tumours exhibit the readily recognizable structure of the capillary haemangioma of which the most characteristic feature is the presence of compact cellular masses separated by loose connective tissue giving an impression of lobularity. Each lobule is composed essentially of closely packed capillary type vessels lined by apparently normal endothelial cells. The lumina vary in size, a small number being distended and sinusoidal in appearance whilst the majority are small and amongst the aggregation of endothelial structures may only be identifiable by the presence of occasional red cells (Fig. 18.1). In identifiable lumina, the lining cells usually have a normal flattened appearance but areas may be seen in which no obvious lumen is present. Such apparently solid areas have been interpreted as excessive endothelial proliferation, prompting the use of the term benign haemangioendothelioma (Ash and Old, 1950; Fu and Perzin, 1974). A more probable explanation, however, is that they represent non-patent capillary tissue (Fig. 18.2). The existence of partially canalized haemangiomas

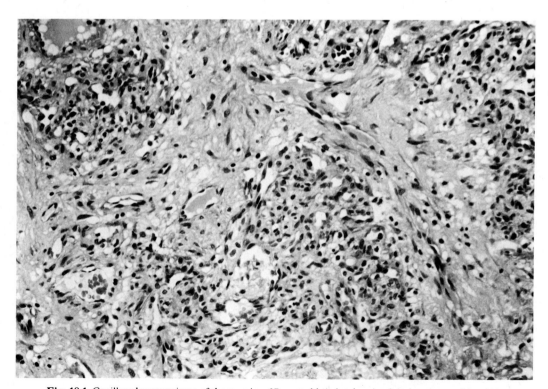

Fig. 18.1 Capillary haemangioma of the nose in a 27 year-old male, showing lobular pattern. M × 200

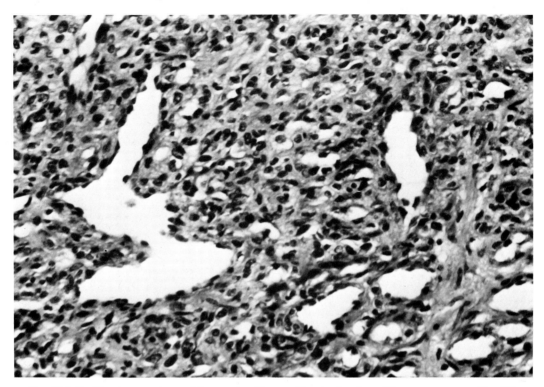

Fig. 18.2 Capillary haemangioma of the nose in a 31 year-old male, showing solid, non-patent area. M × 333

was propounded by Willis to explain the apparent growth in some cases due to subsequent opening up of vascular channels which had not previously contained blood. Extensive areas of non-patent tissue are not very common but in the the authors' view there is nothing to be gained by introducing a confusing subdivision of simple capillary haemangiomas with the term haemangio-endothelioma which for many has malignant connotations.

Apart from a few scattered lymphocytes, there is usually a notable absence of inflammatory cells. In some cases, however, ulceration of the overlying epithelium is followed by the development of inflammatory granulation tissue which mingles with the angiomatous component to give a mixed picture and, occasionally, these secondary inflammatory changes may dominate the scene so that the underlying primary lesion is only identified with difficulty. When ulceration has occurred, pseudo-epitheliomatous hyperplasia of residual epithelium may be a prominent feature. The loose connective tissue stroma may sometimes become more densely fibrous, an event which has sometimes led to an erroneous diagnosis of 'angiofibroma'.

Cavernous haemangiomas, as defined by Crawford (1976), are extremely uncommon in the nasal cavity, if indeed they ever occur. The last mentioned author

pointed out the resemblance to penile erectile tissue and, by the same token, there is likely to be confusion with the nasal erectile tissue when it becomes grossly distended.

Aetiology and pathogenesis
The cause of this benign vascular lesion is at present unknown. Some confusion has been caused due to the use of the term 'pyogenic granuloma', an expression universally adopted by dermatologists in connection with the solitary or multiple, protuberant vascular lesions of the skin. Lever (1949) pointed out that many of these lesions are indistinguishable microscopically from capillary haemangiomas. In his original description, Hartzell (1904), observed infiltration of the vascular element by moderate numbers of polymorphonuclear leucocytes but subsequent writers have noted an absence of inflammatory cells (Rowe, 1958; McGoech, 1968). It is quite clear that whatever dermatological justification there might be for the retention of this term, the vascular lesions in the nasal cavity are neither pyogenic nor primarily granulomatous but are simple capillary haemangiomas.

The question remains as to whether they are to be regarded as of congenital origin (hamartomas) or true acquired neoplasms. Willis (1948) expressed the belief that all the benign vascular tumours were malformations but Ash and Old (1950) did not accept this view in the context of haemangiomas of the nasal septum which they considered to be neoplastic. The peak age distribution in middle life and the relatively short duration of symptoms were factors which led one of the present authors (Osborn 1959) to the same conclusion that these lesions are not congenital but acquired.

Behaviour

The majority of nasal haemangiomas do not recur after removal but an occasional case does present again for a second excision. This is undoubtedly due to incomplete initial removal and is probably comparable with the recurrence of skin lesions (the so-called pyogenic granulomas) with satellite formation (Warner and Wilson Jones, 1968).

BIBLIOGRAPHY

Afshin H, Sharmin R 1974 Haemangioma involving the maxillary sinus. Oral Surgery, Oral Medicine & Oral Pathology 38 : 204–208
Ash J E, Old J W 1950 Haemangiomas of the nasal septum. Transactions of the American Academy of Ophthalmology and Otolaryngology 54 : 350–356
Azaz B, Lustman J 1976 Central haemangioma of the maxilla. International Journal of Oral Surgery 5 : 240–244
Baum H L 1922 The histopathology and histogenesis of benign growths of the nose and accessory sinuses. Annals of Otology, Rhinology and Laryngology 31 : 371–390
Bridger M W 1976 Haemangioma of the nasal bone. Journal of Laryngology and Otology 90 : 191–200
Crawford T 1976 Vascular hamartomas and neoplasms. In : Symmers W St C (ed) Systemic Pathology, 2nd edn. Churchill Livingstone, Edinburgh, ch 3, p 161
Dorfman H D, Steiner G C, Jaffe H L 1971 Vascular tumours of bone. Human Pathology 2 : 349–376
Fu Y, Perzin K H 1974 Non-epithelial tumors of the nasal cavity, paranasal sinuses and nasopharynx. Cancer 33 : I. General Features and Vascular Tumours 1275–1305

Hartzell 1904 Granuloma pyogenicum (botryomycosis of French authors). Journal of Cutaneous Diseases 22 : 520–525
Hasslauer 1900 Die Tumoren der Nasenscheidewand mit Ausschluss der bösartigen Neubildungen. Archiv für Laryngologie und Rhinologie 10 : 60–118
Lever W F 1949 Histopathology of the skin. J B Lippincott
McGeoch A H 1961 Pyogenic granuloma. Australian Journal of Dermatology 6 : 33–40
Neivert H, Bilchick E B 1936 Primary haemangioma of the nasal bone. Archives of Otolaryngology 24 : 495–501
Osborn D A 1959 Haemangiomas of the nose. Journal of Laryngology and Otology 73 : 174–179
Rowe L 1958 Pyogenic granuloma. Archives of Dermatology and Syphilology 78 : 341–347
Warner J, Wilson-Jones E 1968 Pyogenic granuloma recurring with multiple satellites. British Journal of Dermatology 80 : 218–227
Watson W L, McCarthy W D 1940 Blood and lymph vessels tumours. Surgery, Gynecology and Obstetrics 71 : 569–588
Willis R A 1948 The pathology of tumours. Butterworth, London

ANGIOSARCOMA

Introduction

Under the title of 'haemangio-endothelioma', Mallory (1908) described tumours arising from the vascular endothelium, including both benign and malignant varieties. Against the background of multiple angiomatoid syndromes and the concept of hamartomas there has been an obvious reluctance to diagnose malignant tumours of the vascular system and many observers have pointed out the danger of misinterpretation in highly vascular sarcomas. However, notwithstanding their rarity, malignant vascular neoplasms have been recognized in a wide variety of anatomical locations of which the commonest appears to have been the skin. Six out of the eighteen malignant tumours (haemangio-endotheliomas) reported by Stout (1943) were of cutaneous origin but, of the remainder, none involved the nose and sinuses. The earliest reference to angiosarcoma of the nasal cavity appears to have been by MacCoomb and Martin (1942) though no diagnostic details were given in any of the three cases mentioned.

Incidence

This is a very rare tumour in the nasal region and in the English language literature there are less than ten fully reported cases. In their review of 56 malignant vascular tumours, McCarthy and Pack (1950) found 20 angiosarcomas of which 5 had their origin in the nose or sinuses. Fu and Perzin (1974) recorded two cases, comprising 2 per cent of malignant, non-epithelial tumours of the nose and sinuses. In the I.L.O. material, there has been only one case representing less than 0.1 per cent of all tumours of the nose and sinuses and about 2 per cent malignant, non-epithelial tumours. Jackson, Fitz-Hugh and Constable (1977) found one case amongst 115 malignant tumours of the nose and sinuses.

Clinical features

The age distribution is broadly based and there is no sex difference. The published cases have shown an almost even spread between the second and the eighth decades. Nasal bleeding is the common form of presentation with the addition of nasal obstruction when that cavity is involved. Patients with antral tumours may present with swelling of the cheek whilst occasional orbital involvement may result in proptosis. Pain is not a common feature.

Anatomical site of origin

There does not appear to be any particular site of election; in the small number of published cases, distribution is almost equally divided between the nose and sinuses.

Gross appearances

To the naked eye such tumours present as highly vascular or haemorrhagic masses of extremely friable consistency.

Histopathology

The microscopical appearances vary somewhat according to the degree of differentiation (Wilson Jones, 1964). One obvious essential is the presence of vascular channels which vary from the readily identifiable to the poorly formed and ill-defined (Fig. 18.3). Stout (1943) emphasized the existence of irregular anastomotic channels lined by atypical endothelial cells. In the better differentiated examples, such cells may be seen to range from

the normal, flattened type to larger, bulkier cells which show a tendency to pile up and form projections into the lumen (Fig. 18.4). Nuclei may be enlarged with varying irregularity and mitoses may be present. Delineation of vascular spaces may be assisted by reticulin stained preparations in which endothelial proliferation is seen to take place within the basement membrane (Fig. 18.5). In the less well differentiated tumour, vascular channels are less evident amongst sheets of large, irregular, closely packed cells, often with large, palely stained nuclei and prominent nucleoli. Interspersed are irregular slit-like spaces in which the presence of red cells may sometimes indicate the existence of poorly formed vessels, whilst occasional normal-looking capillaries may be seen (Fig. 18.6). The reticulin pattern in such cases tends to reflect the vascular deficiency with fine fibrils often lying between individual cells.

Ultrastructural studies have been reported by Ramsay (1966) in a tumour involving the spinal cord and by Rosai, Sumner, Kostianovsky and Perez-Mesa (1976) on tumours of cutaneous origin. A spectrum of change may be observed ranging from normally appearing, flattened endothelial cells with their pinocytic vesicles, fine filaments and occasional junctional complexes to atypical or bizarre cells which are no longer flattened, have no attachment zones and contain irregular clumps

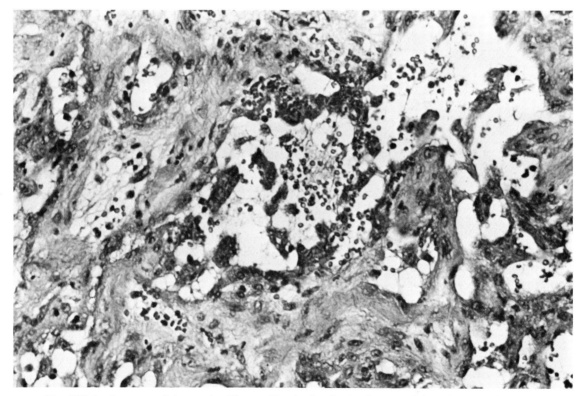

Fig. 18.3 Angiosarcoma of the nose in a 91 year-old male, showing involvement of the endothelium. M × 575

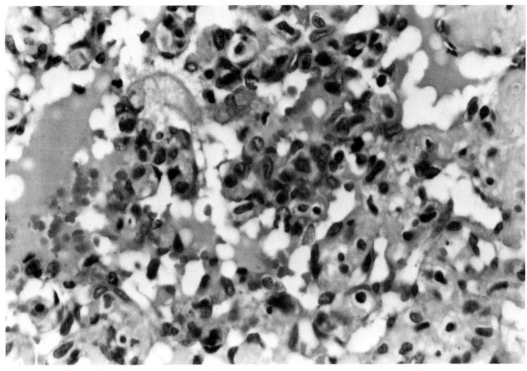

Fig. 18.4 Angiosarcoma of ethmoid region in a 17 year-old female, showing projection of tumour cells into the lumen. M × 537

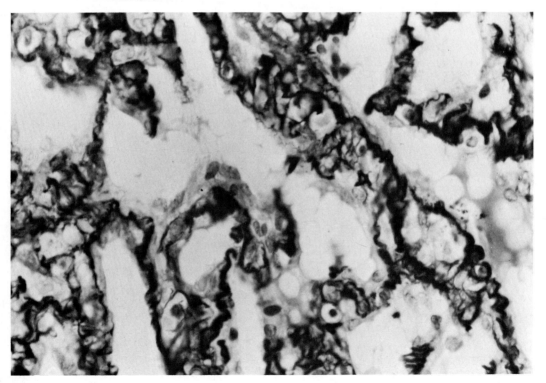

Fig. 18.5 Angiosarcoma of the ethmoid region in a 17 year-old female (see Fig. 18.4). Reticulin stain showing proliferation of tumour within the basement membrane. M × 670

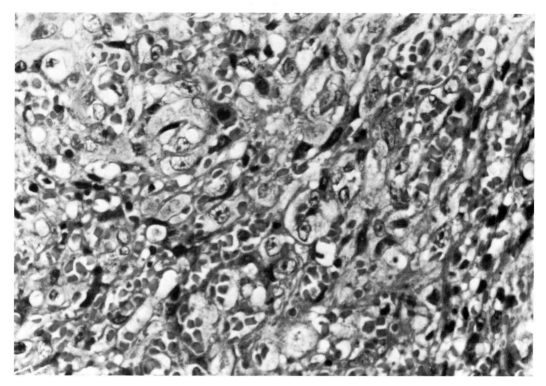

Fig. 18.6 Angiosarcoma of the nose in a 49 year-old female, showing interspersion of relatively normal capillaries. M × 528

of filaments, lysosomes and polyribosomes. The plasma membranes often show numerous intraluminal projections which may form a complex fenestrated pattern.

Aetiology and pathogenesis

Although a number of relevant observations have been made, causal factors in the development of this tumour remain speculative. In two of the five cases recorded by McCarthy and Pack (1950), the appearance of the tumours coincided with pregnancy, thus raising the question of hormonal influence which has been a not infrequent issue in connection with vascular lesions generally. Although workers exposed to vinyl chloride gas in the plastics industry are liable to develop hepatic angiosarcomas (Creech and Johnson, 1974; Lee and Harry, 1974), there have been no reports of nasal or paranasal involvement. This is, perhaps, surprising in view of the portal of entry and the fact that vinyl chloride has been shown experimentally to have a multifarious oncogenic potential (Viola, Bigotti and Caputo, 1971). In the experimental field, the liver has been the main target and the results would not seem to have any particular relevance to the nose and sinuses but, in addition to vinyl chloride induced tumours (Maltoni and Lefemine, 1974), it is interesting to note the development of hepatic angiosarcomas due to dimethyl nitrosamine (Taylor, Lijinsky, Netteschein and Snyder,

1974). This work calls to mind the nitrosamine-induced nasal papillomas in hamsters (see Chapter 12).

It is generally accepted that these tumours are derived from the endothelial cell and Ramsay (1966), in her ultrastructural studies, observed tumour cells appearing to stream from the vascular endothelium. Stout (1943) believed that the growth of malignant vascular tumours took place by sprouting as occurs in granulation tissue rather than in the manner vessels develop in embryonic tissue by formation of cords which subsequently become canalized. On the other hand, he conceded that endothelial cells may proliferate to such an extent that vascular lumina become obscured. Thus we are left with the problem of interpretation of solid cellular areas; do they represent truly solid masses, unexpanded lumina or obliterated channels?

Behaviour

Although these tumours sometimes appear to be localized within the mucous membrane, they are capable of widespread extension, involving more than one cavity in the region as in the case of the 13 year-old boy reported by McCarthy and Pack (1950) in whom the nose, antrum and orbit were involved. As in angiosarcomas generally, bloodborne and lymphatic spread may occur in paranasal tumours (Bomer and Arnold, 1971).

The prognosis in angiosarcoma is generally poor.

McCarthy and Pack (1950) noted that the average survival time was $2\frac{1}{2}$ years. These authors found a five-year cure rate of 9 per cent although they considered that therapeutic results were better in those tumours arising in the nose and sinuses. Two of their five cases survived 3 and 5 years without recurrence. MacCoomb and Martin (1942) also claimed one 5-year survival without recurrence whilst the one case in the I.L.O. series has survived seven years without recurrence. Farr, Carandang and Huvos (1970) compared the behaviour of angiosarcoma and haemangiopericytoma in various

locations within the head and neck region. Both the five and ten year survival rate of angiosarcoma was 50 per cent whereas, in the case of the haemangiopericytoma, the rate fell from 82 per cent at five years to 18 per cent at ten years.

The response of angiosarcomas to irradiation seems to be variable. In three of McCarthy and Pack's cases the tumours appeared to be relatively resistant but, on the otherhand, McClatchy, Batsakis, Rice and Olsen (1976) reported a good response in an angiosarcoma involving the maxillary sinus.

BIBLIOGRAPHY

Bomer D L, Arnold G E 1971 Rare tumours of the ear, nose and throat. Acta Otolaryngologica Supplement 289: 5–25

Creech J L, Johnson M N 1974 Angiosarcoma of the liver in the manufacture of polyvinyl chloride. Journal of Occupational Medicine 16: 150–151

Farr H W, Carandang C M, Huvos A G 1970 Malignant vascular tumors of the head and neck. American Journal of Surgery 120: 501–504

Fu Y, Perzin K H 1974 Non-epithelial tumors of the nasal cavity, paranasal sinuses and nasopharynx 1. general features and vascular tumours. Cancer 33: 1275 1305

Jackson R T, Fitz-Hugh G S, Constable W C 1977 Malignant neoplasms of the nasal cavities and paranasal sinuses. Laryngoscope 87: 726–736

Lee F I, Harry D S 1974 Angiosarcoma of the liver in a vinyl chloride worker. Lancet 1: 1316–1318

McCarthy W D, Pack G T 1950 Malignant blood vessel tumors. Surgery, Gynecology and Obstetrics 91: 465–482

McClatchey K D, Batsakis J G, Rice D H, Olsen N R 1976 Angiosarcoma of the maxillary sinus. Journal of Oral Surgery 34: 1019–1021

MacCoomb W S, Martin H E 1942 Cancer of the nasal cavity. American Journal of Roentgenology 47: 11–23

Mallory F B 1908 The results of the application of special histological methods to the study of tumors. Journal of Experimental Medicine 10: 575–593

Maltoni C, Lefemine G 1975 Carcinogenicity bioassays of vinyl chloride. Annals of the New York Academy of Sciences 246: 195–218

Ramsay H J 1966 Fine structure of haemangiopericytoma and haemangio-endothelioma. Cancer 19: 2005–2018

Rosai J, Sumner H W, Kostianovsky M, Perez-Mesa C 1976 Angiosarcoma of the skin. Human Pathology 7: 83 109

Stout A P 1943 Haemangio-endothelioma: a tumor of blood vessels featuring vascular endothelial cells. Annals of Surgery 118: 445–464

Taylor H W, Lijinsky W, Netteschein P, Snyder C M 1974 Alteration of tumor response in rat liver by carbon tetrachloride. Cancer Research 34: 3391–3395

Viola P L, Bigotti A, Caputo A 1971 Oncogenic response of rat skin, lungs and bones to vinyl chloride. Cancer Research 31: 516–522

Wilson–Jones E 1964 Malignant angio-endothelioma of the skin. British Journal of Dermatology 76: 21–39

HAEMANGIOPERICYTOMA OF THE NOSE AND SINUSES

Introduction

This tumour was first recognized by Stout and Murray (1942) as a result of their investigations into the origin of the glomus tumour by tissue culture technique (Murray and Stout, 1942). At that time they reported nine cases arising in various parts of the integument but, in 1949, Stout published a larger series including one ethmoidal tumour. This was the first report of such a neoplasm in this region.

Incidence

Although more common than the angiosarcoma, less than 40 cases of nasal or paranasal involvement have been recorded in the English language literature. The largest series is that of Compagno and Hyams (1976) who found 23 cases in the files of the Armed Forces Institute of Pathology in Washington. The relative

frequency of involvement of the nose and sinuses is not certain but Backwinkel and Diddams (1970) reviewed 224 published cases and found 21 (nine per cent) in the orbital, oral, nasal and paranasal cavities. Fu and Perzin (1974) recorded an incidence of 0.78 per cent of non-epithelial tumours of the nose, sinuses and nasopharynx. In the I.L.O. material there have been two cases consituting 0.2 per cent of all tumours of the nose and sinuses and 0.9 per cent of non-epithelial tumours.

Clinical features

The age distribution is broadly based with a definite peak in the sixth decade and a marginal predominance of females. The youngest recorded case was in a four year-old Japanese child (Murashima, 1961). The common form of presentation is a painless swelling causing nasal obstruction and recurrent epistaxis may sometimes be severe. The duration of symptoms shows considerable variation but in many cases it is measured in years, suggesting a slowly growing tumour (Rhodes, Brown and Harrison, 1964; Gill and Mehra, 1968; Benvenista and Harris, 1973). On the other hand, some cases have a short history (Eneroth, Fluur, Sodeberg and Anggård, 1970; Hahn, Dawson, Esterly and Joseph, 1973). In situ, the tumour may appear bluish-red to grey whilst its consistency ranges from soft and friable to firm and rubbery.

Anatomical site of origin
The principal site of election is within the nasal cavity. About half the cases reported by Compagno and Hyams (1976) were confined to this region whilst the remainder were mainly naso-ethmoidal with occasional involvement of the maxillary and sphenoid sinuses. The nasal septum is rarely, if ever, a primary site of origin.

Gross appearances
The excised tumour may vary considerably in size, colour and consistency and sometimes a relative pallor may belie its highly vascular nature.

Histopathology
The microscopical picture varies according to the degree of differentiation. Nevertheless, the essential features are

consistently present. Thin-walled vascular channels, lined by normal flattened endothelium, are separated by sheets of tumour cells which appear polyhedral, stellate or even spindle-shaped and show varying degrees of compactness (Figs. 18.7 & 18.8). Nuclei vary in size and shape, tending to reflect the degree of pleomorphism which may be present whilst mitoses may occasionally be seen. Reticulin staining outlines the basement membranes of the vascular channels, thus emphasizing the extravascular location of the tumour cells and thereby helping to distinguish the tumour from angiosarcoma. Stout (1949) emphasized the variability of the histological picture, largely due to the pleomorphism of the intervascular tumour cells. In the more malignant varieties, the tumour may sometimes be interpreted as a fibrosarcoma (Rhodes et al., 1964). Areas of haemorrhage may be present whilst surface ulceration may be associated with necrosis and inflammatory infiltration. The presence of mast cells has been reported by a number of observers.

Ultrastructural studies have been reported by a number of workers (Ramsay, 1966; Von Haam and Narashima Marthy, 1968; Kuhn and Rosai, 1969; Battifora, 1973) but only one group (Hahn et al., 1973) studied a tumour in the nasal region. Taken as a whole, the descriptions of the fine structure are not entirely

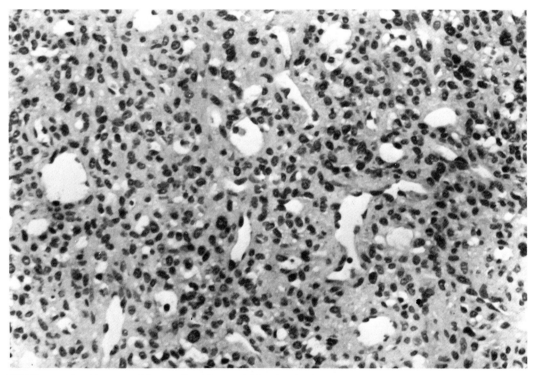

Fig. 18.7 Haemangiopericytoma of the nose in a 33 year-old female, showing numerous vascular spaces separated by tumour cells. M × 333

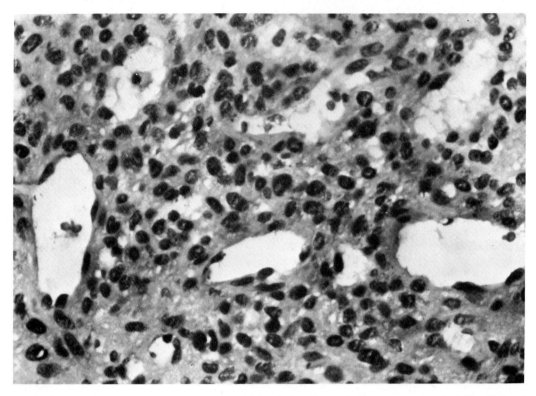

Fig. 18.8 Haemangiopericytoma of the nose in a 33 year-old female (see Fig. 18.7) showing normal endothelium lining the vascular spaces. M × 530

consistent, probably reflecting the variation in differentiation. A consistent feature, however, is the demarcation of relatively normal vascular endothelium from the tumour cells by a basal lamina (Fig. 18.9). The nuclei of·tumour cells may be irregular, often with peripheral aggregation of heterochromatin and well marked nucleoli. Golgi complexes are usually unremarkable whilst profiles of rough endoplasmic reticulum are often collapsed and intermingled with moderate size mitochondria and ribosomes. Intercellular material is invariably present, either as basement membrane-like substance surrounding individual cells or forming more diffuse accumulations of a more flocculent nature (Fig. 18.10) which may be intermingled with collagen fibrils. This lack of uniformity can be related to variability in reticulin staining of light microscopical sections in which widely differing amounts of fibrillar material may be demonstrable amongst the tumour cells.

Opinion is divided on the question of histological distinction between benign and malignant varieties. Enzinger and Smith (1976) claimed the ability to make the distinction on the basis of mitoses, necrosis, haemorrhage and increased cellularity but others (Backwinkel and Diddams, 1970; Walike and Bailey, 1971) have maintained that no valid delineation can be achieved, a view with which the present authors concur.

Aetiology and pathogenesis

The cause of this tumour is not known but there is a definite link with the glomus tumour (q.v.). Murray and Stout (1942) studied the epithelioid cells of glomus tumours in tissue culture and came to the conclusion that the glomus epithelioid cells, the pericytes of Zimmermann (1923) and the 'cellules adventices' of Rouget (1873) are related though separated by degrees of development or differentiation. This led to a consideration of other tumours with a perivascular arrangement which could not be labelled as glomus tumours and to which Stout and Murray gave the name 'haemangiopericytoma'. These authors considered that the glomus tumour and the haemangiopericytoma were simply variants of neoplasms arising from pericytes and, in fact, Stout (1949) noted cells in a haemangiopericytoma which resembled the epithelioid cells of a glomus tumour.

The degree of pleomorphism which may be encountered in the haemangiopericytoma and the varying ultrastructural features have led to much speculation regarding the relationship between pericytes, endothelial cells and smooth muscle cells. The normal pericyte has no intracytoplasmic filaments and is largely invested in a basal lamina (Rhodin, 1968). In the neoplastic pericyte, on the other hand, filaments have sometimes been

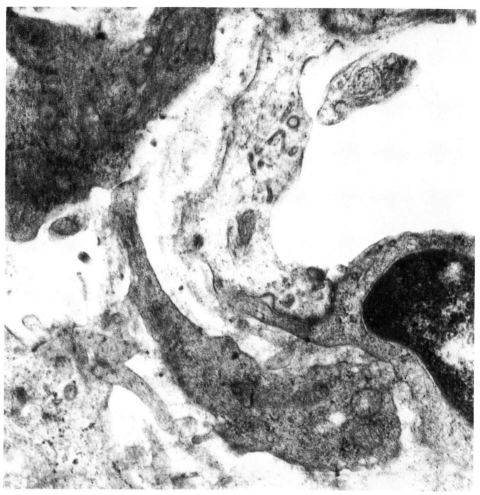

Fig. 18.9 Haemangiopericytoma of the nose in a 33 year-old female (see Fig. 18.7) showing demarcation of normal endothelial cells from tumour cells by the basal lamina (arrow). M ×37 550

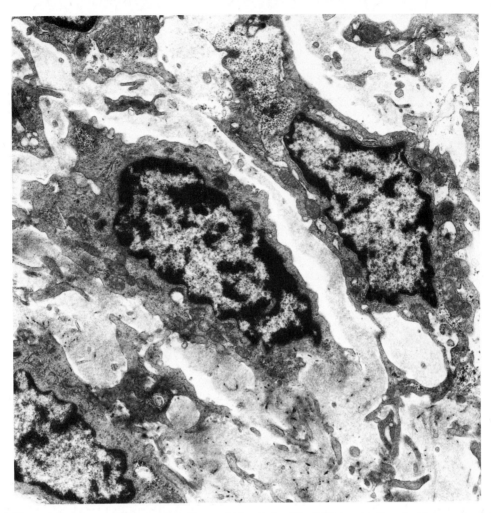

Fig. 18.10 Haemangiopericytoma of the nose in a 33 year-old female (see Fig. 18.7) showing flocculent basement membrane-like material between the tumour cells. M ×9850

reported (Kuhn and Rosai, 1969; Hahn et al., 1973) whilst basal lamina may or may not be found surrounding such cells though basement membrane-like material is invariably present (Fig. 18.10) Kuhn and Rosai also observed that some pericytes may be indistinguishable from fibroblasts, a point which has been noted by the present authors. It would seem that neoplastic pericytes may revert to a more primitive type of cell from which differentiation may procede along different lines.

Behaviour

The course of these tumours is not readily predictable. Some remain localized, with or without strictly local recurrence whilst others involve adjacent parts, as in the original case reported by Stout (1949) in which an ethmoidal tumour invaded the orbit. In general terms, the multiplicity sometimes observed in the glomus

tumour is rarely, if ever, seen in the haemangiopericytoma but metastasis is a well recognized event (O'Brien and Brasfield, 1965; Enzinger and Smith, 1976). So far, there has only been one report of metastasis from a nasal tumour (Eneroth et al., 1970) but there seems to have been some doubt regarding the histological diagnosis. On the other hand, Walike and Bailey (1971) reported a haemangiopericytoma of the frontal sinus which was thought to be a metastasis from a recurrent tumour of the arm.

Recurrence has been reported either as a single or multiple event in about one quarter of the published nasal or paranasal tumours. In the general context, the frequency of recurrence has shown a direct relationship to the duration of follow-up (Backwinkel and Diddams, 1970). This accords with the pattern of survival observed by Farr, Carandang and Huvos (1970) who showed that, compared with the angiosarcoma (q.v.), the haemangiopericytoma is more malignant in the long term. O'Brien and Brasfield (1965) also claimed that the mortality of this tumour had been underestimated. On the other hand, the 18 per cent ten-year survival rate of Farr et al. (1970) contrasts sharply with the corrected survival rate of 70 per cent reported by Enzinger and Smith (1976) on a much larger number of cases of general anatomical distribution. Thus the variability in behaviour is underlined. As far as the nose and sinuses are concerned, survival with or without recurrence has ranged from three weeks (Murashima, 1961) to 19 years (Lenczyk, 1968). Stout's case died at seven years after three recurrences whilst Lenczyk's case had suffered four recurrences but had been free from disease for two years. One of the I.L.O. cases is known to have survived for more than seven years after one early recurrence.

GLOMUS TUMOUR OF THE NOSE AND SINUSES

Introduction

This neoplasm was first described by Masson (1924) under the title of 'Angiomyoneurome artériel' as a tumour originating in the normal glomus, particularly in the extremities. The lesion is characteristically painful.

Incidence

The tumour is extremely rare in the nasal region, only two cases having been reported. Pantazopoulos (1965)

reported an extremely painful tumour in the nose of a fortyfive-year old woman though the histological illustrations were difficult to interpret. In the case described by Fu and Perzin (1974), a mass was present on the septum of a seventy-one year old female. The histology was consistent with the diagnosis but the lesion was painless.

Histopathology

The general structure is not unsimilar to that of the haemangiopericytoma, normal endothelial lined vascular channels being surrounded by tumour cells of a regular polyhedral shape imparting an epithelioid appearance. The more organoid appearance together with the presence of numerous neurofibrils serve to distinguish this neoplasm from the haemangiopericytoma.

Pathogenesis

The tissue culture studies of Murray and Stout (1942) have already been alluded to in connection with the haemangiopericytoma. These authors believed that the epithelioid cell of the glomus and the pericyte represent more highly differentiated forms of Rouget's adventitial cell.

Behaviour

Most glomus tumours are benign in their behaviour (Murray and Stout, 1942). The case of Pantazopoulos had been followed up for less than a year but Fu and Perzin's case had survived for seven years without recurrence following excision.

BIBLIOGRAPHY

Backwinkel K D, Diddams J A 1970 Haemangiopericytoma. Cancer 25 : 896–901
Battifora H 1973 Haemangiopericytoma: ultrastructural study of five cases. Cancer 31 : 1418–1432
Benvinista R J, Harris H E 1973 Nasal haemangiopericytoma. Archives of Otolaryngology 98 : 358–359
Compagno J, Hyams V J 1976 Haemangiopericytoma-like intranasal tumors. American Journal of Clinical Pathology 66 : 672–683
Eneroth C M, Fluur E, Sodeberg G, Anggård A 1970 Nasal haemangiopericytoma. Laryngoscope 80 : 17–24
Enzinger F M, Smith B H 1976 Haemangiopericytoma. Human Pathology 7 : 61–62
Gill B S, Mehra Y N 1968 Haemangiopericytoma in the nasal cavity. Journal of Laryngology and Otology 82 : 839–844
Hahn M J, Dawson R, Esterly J A, Joseph D J 1973 Haemangiopericytoma. Cancer 31 : 255–261
Kuhn C, Rosai J 1969 Tumors arising from pericytes. Archives of Pathology 88 : 653–663
Lenczyk J M 1968 Nasal haemangiopericytoma. Archives of Otolaryngology 87 : 536–539
Masson P 1924 Le glomus neuromyo-artériel des regions tactiles et ses tumeurs. Lyon Chirurgie 21 : 257–280

Murad T M, Von Haam E, Narashima Marthy M S 1968 Ultrastructure of a haemangiopericytoma and a glomus tumor. Cancer 22 : 1239–1249
Murashima J 1961 A case of haemangiopericytoma originating in the nasal cavity and nasal sinus of a small child. Otolaryngology (Tokyo) 33 : 537–539
Murray M R, Stout A P 1942 The glomus tumor – investigation of its distribution and behaviour and the identity of its epithelioid cells. American Journal of Pathology 18 : 183–203
O'Brien P, Brasfield R D 1965 Haemangiopericytoma. Cancer 18 : 249–252
Pantazopoulos P E 1965 Glomus tumor (glomangioma) of the nasal cavity. Archives of Otolaryngology 81 : 83–86
Ramsay H J 1966 Fine structure of haemangiopericytoma and haemangio-endothelioma. Cancer 19 : 2005–2018
Rhodes R E, Brown H A, Harrison E G 1964 Haemangiopericytoma of the nasal cavity. Archives of Otolaryngology 79 : 505–511
Rhodin J A C 1968 Ultrastructure of mammalian venous capillaries, venules and small collecting veins. Journal of Ultrastructure Research 25 : 452–500

Rouget C 1873 Le développement, la structure et les propriétés physiologiques des capillaires sanguins et lymphatiques. Archives de physiologie normale et pathologique 5: 603–663

Stout A P 1949 Haemangiopericytoma. Cancer 2: 1027–1054

Stout A P, Murray M R 1942 Haemangiopericytoma. Annals of Surgery 116: 26–33

Walike J W, Bailey B J 1971 Head and neck haemangiopericytoma. Archives of Otolaryngology 93: 345–353

Zimmermann K W 1923 Der feinere Bau der Blutkapillaren. Zeitschrift für Anatomie und Entwicklungsgeschichte 68: 29–109

CHEMODECTOMA OF THE NOSE AND SINUSES

Introduction

Although comparatively rare, the chemodectoma or 'non-chromaffin' paraganglioma is well recognized especially in the head and neck region. The more common sites of such tumours are the carotid body, the vagal body and the jugulo-tympanic region (glomus jugulare) but other locations include the larynx and the orbit whilst the first report of a genuine chemodectoma of the nasal cavity appears to have been presented by Moran (1962). Since then a small number of cases have been recorded in the world literature.

Incidence

Such tumours arising in the nasal cavity are extremely rare. Volkov and Schechkin (1976) reported three cases but the solitary illustration of the histopathology was difficult to interpret. Lack, Cubilla, Woodruff and Farr (1977) reviewed 69 cases occurring in the head and neck region, collected over nearly forty years. Amongst these authors' material were three tumours involving the nasal cavity.

Clinical features

The age distribution of the cases has been largely in middle life though Moran's patient was a woman of 89 years whilst one of the cases reported by Lack et al. (1977) was only eight years old. Recurrent epistaxis is likely to be the presenting symptom and a firm rubbery tumour may attain a size of several centimetres in diameter. The tumour is usually characterized by a slow rate of growth so that duration of symptoms is likely to be prolonged.

Anatomical site of origin

Most of the tumours so far reported appear to have arisen in the lateral wall but one of the tumours described by Volkov and Schechkin arose in the ethmoid sinus with secondary involvement of the nasal cavity.

Histopathology

The microscopial picture displays the features of a chemodectoma arising in any location. Compact groups of polyhedral cells, of epithelial appearance, are often delineated by a well defined reticulin network and lie in intimate relationship to capillary vessels. The cells usually have a moderately abundant, finely granular cytoplasm. The nuclei are generally rounded but may sometimes exhibit irregularity though conclusion regarding behaviour cannot be drawn from the histological pattern alone. A common feature of all these tumours is their ability to produce catecholamines, a property which they share with the adrenal medulla and tumours derived therefrom though the concentration in the cells of chemodectomas is rarely sufficient to exhibit the chromaffin reaction. Nevertheless, the characteristic secretory granules can be visualized under the electron microscope and can also be demonstrated by the formaldehyde induced fluorescence technique of Falck (1962).

Aetiology and pathogenesis

In the present context, there are no indications as to the cause of this tumour, although there have been reports of enlarged carotid bodies in relation to chronic hypoxaemia (Arias-Stella, 1969) and an increase in the incidence of carotid body tumours at high altitudes (Saldana, Salem and Travezan, 1973).

Chemoreceptor tissue is known to be widely distributed in the body, subserving the same function as the carotid body by responding to chemical changes in the blood. It was on this basis that Mulligan (1950) introduced the term 'chemodectoma'. Chemoreceptor tissue is presumed to be normally present in the nasal cavity though the amount must be too small to be readily identifiable. Unfortunately, there has been some confusion caused by reference to such tissue in certain locations as 'glomus bodies'. The concensus of opinion is that, unlike the glomus tumour and the haemangiopericytoma which derive from the pericyte of mesenchymal origin, the chemodectoma arises from cells which have migrated from the neural crest and is, therefore, neuroectodermal.

Behaviour

Most of the reported cases have remained localized and were presumed to be benign. On the other hand, the ethmoidal tumour of Volkov and Schechkin (1976) not only involved the nasal cavity but spread into the maxillary sinus and the orbit, the patient finally dying with metastases in the brain. Frankly malignant behaviour with lymphatic and systemic metastases is not unknown in such tumours in other primary locations and prognosis must clearly be viewed with caution.

BIBLIOGRAPHY

Arias-Stella J 1969 Human Carotid body at high altitudes. American Journal of Pathology 55: 150

Falck B 1962 Observations on the possibilities of the cellular localization of monoamines by a flourescence method. Acta Physiologica Scandinavica Supplement 197: 1–25

Lack E E, Cubilla A L, Woodruff J M, Farr H W 1977 Paragangliomas of the head and neck region. Cancer 39: 397–409

Moran T E 1962 Non-chromaffin paraganglioma of the nasal cavity. Laryngoscope 72: 201–206

Mulligan R M 1950 Chemodectoma in the dog. American Journal of Pathology 26: 680–681

Scaldana M J, Salem L E, Travezan R 1973 High altitude hypoxia and chemodectomas. Human Pathology 4: 251–263

Volkov Y N, Schechkin V N 1976 Chemodectoma of the nose and of the accessory sinuses. Vestnik Otorinolaringologii 4: 56–59

JUVENILE ANGIOFIBROMA

Introduction

The first recorded description of this fibro-vascular, tumour-like lesion, involving predominantly the post-nasal region, was by Chelius (1847) but, according to Chauveau (1906), surgeons were endeavouring to deal with growths of this nature prior to the nineteenth century whilst Acuna (1956) asserted that removal was practised by Hippocrates. Chelius noted the fibrous nature of the lesion and its common occurrence about the time of puberty. Gosselin (1873) emphasized the occurrence of nasopharyngeal fibrous polyps almost exclusively in young males and noted that whilst some lesions appeared to regress with attainment of adult status, others required surgical intervention. The volume of literature that has accumulated on this relatively rare condition is a measure of the speculation and concern regarding its nature and management.

Terminology

The earlier writers usually referred to 'fibrous polyps' but Chauveau (1906) described such lesions as 'fibromes nasopharyngiens'. The epithet 'juvenile', erroneously attributed to Chauveau, appeared later. A greater appreciation of the vascular component led to the use of the term 'angiofibroma' by Friedberg (1940). For reasons which will become apparent, the present authors use the expression 'juvenile angiofibroma' without specification of the nasopharynx.

Incidence

It has generally been accepted that the condition is relatively rare in the Western World but impressions of a higher incidence in the Middle and Far East have not always been borne out by the published facts. Handousa, Farid and Elwi (1954) estimated an incidence in Egypt of approximately 1:50 000 patients seen for ear, nose and throat conditions. On the other hand, Harma (1959) considered that the incidence in Finland was probably of the order of 1:6000 patients. In the I.L.O. material the frequency was about 1:40 000 patients though this could well be exaggerated due to selection in a specialized institution. In fact, 14 cases were referred for treatment over a period of 27 years (just over one per cent of all tumours of the nose and sinuses). In India, Bhatia, Mishra and Prakash (1967) collected 92 cases at Lucknow over a similar period of time whilst Acuna (1973) has claimed 279 cases over a period of 22 years in Mexico.

Clinical features

The low age distribution is undoubtedly a hall mark of this condition and reports of cases in older subjects are highly questionable. There is general agreement that in most cases the age of onset is in the second decade of life and that there is an overwhelming predominance of males. Many of the cases reported by Pluyette (1887) as examples occurring in females are unacceptable on the grounds of age alone. Larger series usually do not contain cases in females and this has led to the categorical statement that the condition occurs exclusively in pubescent males. Nevertheless, there have been a number of authentic reports of juvenile angiofibroma in females (Finerman, 1951; Parchet, 1951; Osborn and Sokolovsky, 1965; Maniglia, Mazzarella, Minkowitz and Moskowitz, 1969). In the I.L.O. material there were 13 males and one female with ages ranging from 10 to 20 years.

Nasal obstruction is the common presenting symptom, being frequently unilateral. Spontaneous epistaxis is not uncommon but is not necessarily so frequent or severe as to attract particular attention. Severe bleeding, however, may accompany attempted biopsy and, for this reason, some clinicians strongly advocate dispensing with this procedure in favour of less hazardous clinical examination, radiography and angiography. Expansion and extension of the lesion may lead to facial deformity with lateral swelling of the cheek and proptosis producing the so-called 'frog face' appearance, though this is relatively uncommon in the cases encountered in the Western Hemisphere. The gross appearance, when observed clinically, is that of a smooth, dark red swelling commonly occupying part or the whole of the postnasal space from which it may appear as an extension from behind the soft palate. Extensive involvement of the nasal cavity is not uncommon and a mass may even project from the anterior nares. Clinical evidence of sexual underdevelopment was reported in one series (Martin, Ehrlich and Abels, 1948) but many other authors have been unable to confirm this feature.

Anatomical site of origin

The location of the attachment or origin is important both to the surgeon and the pathologist. It has already been noted that the lesion tends to fill the nasopharynx and, in so far as a proportion of cases exhibit unequivocal adherence to the roof of that cavity, it is understandable that the condition has come to be regarded as a nasopharyngeal tumour, Careful assessment, however, reveals that in many cases the principal attachment is around the margins of the choanae, i.e. the medial pterygoid plate, the posterior border of the hard palate, the posterior margin of the vomer and the adjoining part of the roof of the nasopharynx. In the lesions which extend forwards to the front of the nose, more anterior attachments are to be found, particularly on the lateral wall (inferior and middle turbinates) and occasionally on the septum. These have been described by some authors as secondary attachments though such an interpretation is without adequate foundation. In addition to these more common locations, paranasal involvement has been reported on many occasions. Thus, origin in the maxillary sinus has been reported by Munson (1941), Maniglia et al. (1969). Ethmoidal and sphenoid sinuses may also be involved (Gill, Rice, Ritter, Kindt and Russo, 1976; Boles and Dedo, 1976). Extension through the base of the skull into the middle cranial fossa was reported by Hunter, Smyth and Macafee (1963) and there are a number of accounts of apparent extension into the pterygomaxillary fissure and infratemporal fossa, the lesional tissue finding its way round the posterior aspect of the maxilla to produce a swelling in the lateral aspect of the cheek (Handousa et al., 1954; Hora and Weller, 1961; Sardana, 1965; Bhatia et al., 1967; Moktar, Badrawy and Osman, 1972).

Gross appearance

After removal, which may sometimes be necessarily in multiple fragments, the lesion is seen to consist of firm tissue of a tough and obviously fibrous nature in which areas of haemorrhage may be noted (Figs. 18.11 & 18.12). The surface is usually smooth and reddish in colour whilst darker, raw areas may indicate its relatively broad attachment.

Histopathology

The dominating feature is great vascularity in a fibrous background. A common and characteristic finding is the presence of numerous vessels of varying shapes and sizes embedded in the collagenous tissue and being for the

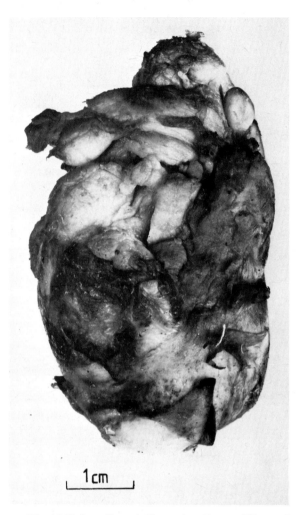

1 cm

Fig. 18.11 Juvenile angiofibroma in a 10 year-old boy.

most part thin-walled, often of no more than endothelial thickness (Fig. 18.13). Endothelial cells may be flattened or swollen and the walls of the vessels may contain small amounts of smooth muscle. The lumina of such vessels are usually empty apart from a few residual red cells but some may contain fibrinous masses indicative of thrombosis whilst, occasionally, a wall appears to have ruptured with resulting haemorrhage. Zones of apparently normal capillary tissue may be seen, not infrequently in relation to areas of haemorrhage and presumably representing reparative granulations. Small numbers of normal vessels of venous or arterial status may be seen but of particular interest is the presence of occasional bizarre-looking vessels in which the distribution of the muscle coat is so irregular that abrupt changes from substantial muscular to mere endothelial thickness are encountered (Fig. 18.14). Such anomalous vessels can usually be found after a careful search. The connective tissue stroma

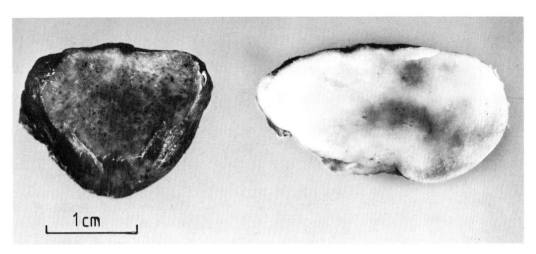

Fig. 18.12 Juvenile angiofibroma in a 14 year-old boy, showing haemorrhage on the cut surface.

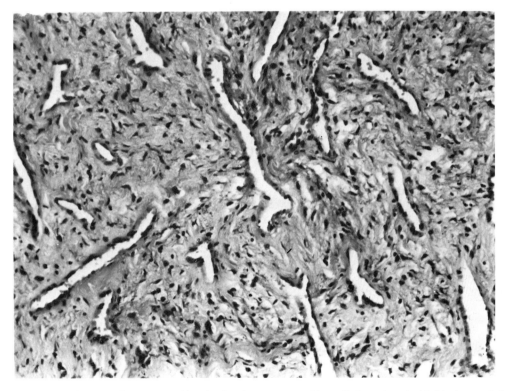

Fig. 18.13 Juvenile angiofibroma in a 15 year-old male, showing numerous thin-walled vessels embedded in dense cellular fibrous tissue. M × 208

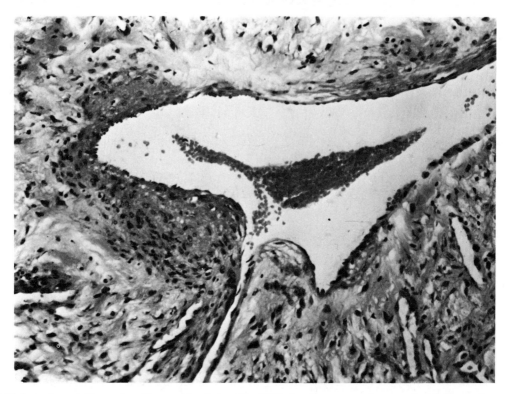

Fig. 18.14 Juvenile angiofibroma in a 15 year-old male (see Fig. 18.13) showing an anomalous vessel with abrupt change in the wall from muscular to mere endothelial thickness. M × 208

which forms the background to the vascular component consists of a collagenous element showing varying degrees of density and cellularity. It is to be noted that the collagen fibres are never whorled as in a fibroma but often tend to form a laminated pattern more consistent with a reparative fibrosis. Sometimes the stromal component appears more loosely arranged and has been described by some writers as myxomatous though the appearance is usually more the result of oedema than the accumulation of mucin. Nevertheless, acid mucopolysaccharides have been demonstrated by Schiff (1959). Some such areas tend to be not only more cellular but noteworthy for the size and shape of the cells. The presence of stellate cells and giant cells, which may be multinucleated, have been noted particularly by several authors (Sternberg, 1954; Hubbard, 1958; Harma, 1959). Their occurrence in appreciable numbers is infrequent but on occasions their appearance may be quite bizarre, arousing anxiety as to possible malignancy (Fig. 18.15). Occasional straplike cells may simulate the elements of a rhabdomyosarcoma but cross striation is absent. Mast cells are sometimes present in considerable numbers.

Aetiology and pathogenesis
Pre-occupation with the fibrous tissue component dominated the earlier theories. Bensch (1878) believed in origin from the embryonic fibrocartilage between the body of the sphenoid and the basi-occiput. The normal ossification in this region around the age of 25 years seemed to fit the pattern of age incidence. Ringertz (1938) suggested origin from the ventral periosteum in the posterior wall of the nasopharynx. Brunner (1942) believed that the lesion originated in the fascia basalis formed by the fusion of the pharyngeal aponeurosis and the buccopharyngeal fascia near the base of the skull. All these theories, however, not only implied an exclusively collagenous nature but assumed a limited origin within the nasopharynx which has not been borne out by subsequent observations. Verneuil (1861) commented on the often poorly defined site of attachment and suggested that the lesion might not arise exclusively from the embryonic fibrocartilage.

The occasional finding of unusual stromal cells has inevitably led to speculation, such as origin from paraganglionic tissue (Girgis and Famy, 1973) but wide experience with simple nasal polyps indicates that bizarre cells may be encountered without special significance, especially in the young. Although many writers have clearly regarded these lesions as true tumours, doubts have been expressed from an early stage (Verneuil, 1861; Sébileau, 1923; Willis, 1948).

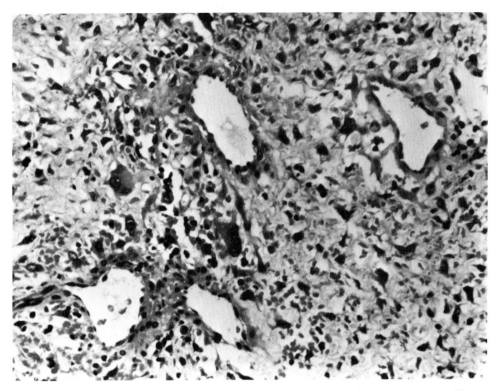

Fig. 18.15 Juvenile angiofibroma in a 16 year-old male, showing bizarre cells in the fibrous stroma. M × 325

Martin et al. (1948) emphasized their clinical impression of sexual underdevelopment and regarded the lesion as angiomatous rather than fibromatous, being the result of oestrogenic stimulation. The hormonal theory was pursued by other writers and Dane (1954) suggested that the abnormal growth was the result of androgenic stimulation consequent upon a disturbed oestrogen-androgen balance. In most subsequent series, including the present authors' cases, no convincing evidence of disturbed sexual development has been observed. Furthermore, no support for the theory of hormonal upset has been found in endocrinological studies (Hunter et al., 1963; Patterson, 1965).

One of the present authors (Osborn, 1959) drew attention to the similarity between the anomalous vessels in these lesions and elements of nasal erectile tissue, suggesting that the condition is a vascular hamartoma. Coincidentally, Schiff (1959) studied the stromal component and came to the conclusion that the lesion was a desmoplastic response to malformed erectile tissue, probably mediated by hormonal activity. Harma (1959) also noted the presence of abnormal vessels but considered the lesion to be a hyperplastic tissue reaction under hormonal influence.

The normal distribution of nasal erectile tissue is indicated in Chapter 1 but it may also be found in paranasal locations and routine biopsies have revealed its presence in maxillary and frontal sinuses. Studies of this tissue in animals (Swindle, 1935 and 1937) have shown that its development is extremely complex with the formation of anastomotic shunts and, at or shortly after birth, a substantial portion of the vasculature undergoes atrophy. Such a tissue could well provide a fertile field for the development of a hamartoma. Anomalous vessels of the type shown in Fig. 18.14 may be regarded as caricatures of Swindle's 'arterio-capillary anastomoses' which may occasionally be seen in normal erectile tissue (Osborn, 1959). Such structures permit the transmission of arterial pressures into capillary type vessels which, under normal conditions, received some support from surrounding elastic tissue. The malformed vessels are not so protected with the inevitable result of leakage or rupture with oedema and haemorrhage. Reparative processes follow with the ultimate formation of scar tissue and a recurring cycle of events leads to a proliferative lesion limited finally by the extent and distribution of the malformed tissue. Ectopic location could well account for paranasal involvement whilst expansile growth results in pressure erosion of bone and disturbance of the normal alignment of the craniofacial structure as in the 'frog face' deformity. Exuberant fibroblasts in the reparative process may account for many of the bizarre stromal cells which are not unknown in lesions of lesser pathological significance. The ob-

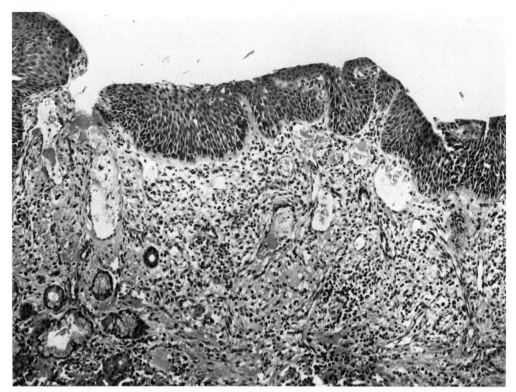

Fig. 18.16 Hereditary haemorrhagic telangiectasia in an 18 year-old male, showing rupture of a distended vessel with haemorrhage onto the surface. M × 130

served regression is explicable on the basis of progressive fibrosis.

The hamartomatous theory is consistent with the age pattern, the distribution of nasal erectile tissue and the self limiting feature of the lesion. The possibility of greater participation of the nasal erectile tissue in sexual orgasm (Osborn, 1959) is speculative but nevertheless represents the only attempt to explain the sex incidence.

Behaviour

Extension of the lesion is largely predetermined by the distribution of malformed tissue. 'Recurrence' is not uncommon and is clearly related to the difficulties of complete surgical removal. Harma (1959) noted that such an event was less likely in those cases exhibiting limited attachment with the postnasal space. Angiographic studies may help to minimize unawareness of the full extent of the lesion (Ward, Thompson, Calcaterra and Kadin, 1974) but the lesional potential of malformed though still intact vascular tissue cannot be recognized in advance. In the I.L.O. material, six out of fourteen cases exhibited a single recurrence.

BIBLIOGRAPHY

Acuna R T 1956 The nasopharyngeal fibroma and its treatment. Archives of Otolaryngology 64: 451–455
Acuna R T 1973 Nasopharyngeal fibroma. Acta Otolaryngologica 75: 119–1123
Bensch H 1878 Beiträge zur Beurtheilung der chirurgischen Behandlung der Nasenrachenpolypen. Breslau
Bhatia M L, Mishra S C, Prakash J 1967 Lateral extensions of nasopharyngeal fibroma. Journal of Laryngology and Otology 81: 99–106
Boles R, Dedo H 1976 Nasopharyngeal angiofibroma. Laryngoscope 86: 364–370

Brunner H 1942 Nasopharyngeal fibroma. Annals of Otology Rhinology and Laryngology 51: 29–63
Chauveau C 1906 Histoire des maladies du pharynx, J. B. Bailliere et fils, Paris, Tome 5, p 562
Chelius M J 1847 A system of surgery, vol 2, p 726. London
Dane W H 1954 Juvenile nasopharyngeal fibroma in state of regression. Annals of Otology, Rhinology and Laryngology 63: 997–1014
Figi F A 1940 Fibromas of nasopharynx. Journal of the American Medical Association 115: 665–671

Finerman W B 1951 Juvenile nasopharyngeal angiofibroma in the female. Archives of Otolaryngology 54: 620–623

Friedberg S A 1940 Nasopharyngeal fibroma. Archives of Otolaryngology 31: 313–326

Gill G, Rice D H, Ritter F N, Kindt G, Russo H R 1976 Intracranial and extracranial nasopharyngeal angiofibroma. Archives of Otolaryngology 102: 371–373

Girgis I H, Famy S A 1973 Nasopharyngeal fibroma: its histopathological nature. Journal of Laryngology and Otology 87: 1107–1123

Gosselin L 1873 Fibrome ou polype fibreux nasopharyngien suffocant et rebelle. Clinique chirurgicale de l'hopital de la charite (Paris), Bailliere et Fils, Tome 1, 92–116

Handousa A, Farid H, Elwi A M 1954 Nasopharyngeal fibroma. Journal of Laryngology and Otology 68: 647–666

Harma R A 1959 Nasopharyngeal angiofibroma. Acta Otolaryngologica, Supplement 146: 7–74

Hora J F, Weller W A 1961 Extranasopharyngeal juvenile angiofibroma. Annals of Otology, Rhinology and Laryngology 70: 164–170

Hubbard E M 1958 Nasopharyngeal angiofibroma. Archives of Pathology 65: 192–204

Hunter K, Smyth G D C, Macafee C A S 1963 Nasopharyngeal fibroma. Journal of Laryngology and Otology 77: 138–145

Maniglia A J, Mazzurella L A, Minkowitz S, Moskowitz H 1969 Maxillary sinus angiofibroma treated with cryosurgery. Archives of Otolaryngology 89: 527–532

Martin H, Ehrlich H E, Abels J C 1948 Juvenile nasopharyngeal fibroma. Annals of Surgery 127: 513–536

Moktar M, Badrawy R, Osman M 1972 The juvenile angiofibroma of the nasopharynx. Journal of the Egyptian Medical Association 55: 692–703

Munson F T 1941 Angiofibroma of the left maxillary sinus. Annals of Otology, Rhinology and Laryngology 50: 561–569

Osborn D A 1959 The so-called juvenile angiofibroma of the nasopharynx. Journal of Laryngology and Otology 73: 295–315

Osborn D A, Sokolovski A Juvenile nasopharyngeal angiofibroma in a female. Archives of Otolaryngology 82: 629–632

Parchet V 1951 L'Angiofibrome nasopharyngien chez la femme. Annales d'Otolaryngologie 68: 60–69

Patterson C N 1965 Juvenile nasopharyngeal angiofibroma. Archives of Otolaryngology 81: 270–277

Pluyette 1887 Des fibromes nasopharyngiens chez la femme. Revue de Chirurgie (Paris) 7: 202–223

Ringertz N 1938 Juvenile nasal fibroma In Pathology of malignant tumours arising in the nasal and paranasal cavities and maxilla. Acta Otolaryngologica, Supplement 27: 158–161

Sardana D S 1965 Nasopharyngeal fibroma. Archives of Otolaryngology 81: 584–588

Schiff M 1959 Juvenile nasopharyngeal angiofibroma. Laryngoscope 69: 981–1016

Sébileau P 1923 Considerations sur les fibromes nasopharyngiens. Annales des Maladies du Oreille et Larynx 42: 553–615

Shaheen H B Nasopharyngeal fibroma. Journal of Laryngology and Otology 45: 259–264

Sternberg S S 1954 Pathology of juvenile nasopharyngeal angiofibroma. Cancer 7: 15–28

Swindle P F 1935 The architecture of the blood vascular networks in the erectile and secretory lining of the nasal passages. Annals of Otology, Rhinology and Laryngology 44: 913–932

Swindle P F 1937 Nasal blood vessels which serve as arteries in some mammals and as veins in others. Annals of Otology, Rhinology and Laryngology 46: 600–628

Verneuil 1861 Les polypes nasopharyngiens. Bulletin de la Societé de Chirurgie de Paris 1: 258–272

Ward P H, Thompson R, Calcaterra T, Kadin M R 1974 Juvenile angiofibroma: a more rational therapeutic approach based on clinical and experimental evidence. Laryngoscope 84: 2182 ff

Willis R A 1948 Pathology of tumours, 1st edn. Butterworth, London, ch 41, p 651–652

Additional references

Albrecht R, Küttner K 1970 Zur Ultrastruktur der juvenilen Nasenrachenfibrome. Zeitschrift für Laryngologie etc. (Stuttgart), 49: 653–661

Küttner K 1973 Ultrahistochemical studies of the nuclear inclusion bodies in juvenile nasopharyngeal fibromas (2nd report). Zeitschrift für Laryngologie etc. (Stuttgart), 52: 748–752

HEREDITARY HAEMORRHAGIC TELANGIECTASIA

This familial disease, which is transmitted to both sexes through an autosomal dominant gene, is not a neoplasm but is of particular interest to those engaged in Ear, Nose and Throat practice because it almost invariably presents with epistaxis, notwithstanding the concurrence of cutaneous and internal haemorrhage. The first description of the disease was by Sutton (1864) who noted the association of epistaxis and haemoptysis and also recorded familial incidence. Subsequently, there were reports by Rendu (1896), Osler (1901) and Weber (1907) which resulted in the eponymous title of 'Rendu-Osler-Weber disease'. The early history of this condition was well reviewed by Harrison (1964).

Although uncommon, the disease is not excessively rare. In 1932, Goldstein estimated that at least 600 cases constituting about 100 families had been reported in the literature. Harrison (1964) reported 20 cases. Although many of the published cases have been of European descent, reports are now world-wide and Asiatic incidence has been established (Sharma, Mahambre, Audi and Borker, 1975).

Multiple haemorrhagic lesions due to malformed capillary vessels are found in the skin and mucous membranes. The nasal fossa is commonly involved but mucosal lesions are found in the oral cavity and gastro-intestinal haemorrhage may occur (Griggs, 1941). Involvement of the lower respiratory, urinary and genital tracts may also be encountered.

Epistaxis is the common presenting symptom, usually dating from childhood though many patients do not seek advice until middle life. Haemorrhage from skin lesions, haemoptysis, haematemesis, haematuria are well recognized manifestations and in females excessive menstruation is not uncommon, as was noted by Sutton (1864).

Histology reveals irregularly distended capillary vessels with areas of haemorrhage (Fig. 18.16) though the microscopic picture is not sufficiently specific to permit diagnosis on histological grounds alone.

Repeated haemorrhage is liable to lead to the development of iron deficiency anaemia and, inasmuch as the nose is the major source of bleeding, alleviation of epistaxis is clearly of material benefit to the patient. The administration of ethanyl oestradiol to sufferers from this disease has been found to be effective in stopping nasal haemorrhage (Harrison, 1964). Based on animal experiments (Harrison, 1959), the rationale is believed to be the induction of squamous metaplasia of the nasal epithelium, forming a protective layer.

BIBLIOGRAPHY

Goldstein H I 1932 Hereditary multiple telangiectasia. Archives of Dermatology and Syphilology 26: 282–308

Griggs D E 1941 Hereditary haemorrhagic telangiectasia with gastro-intestinal bleeding. American Journal of Digestive Disease 8: 344–346

Harrison D F N 1959 The effect of systemic oestrogen upon the nasal mucous membrane and its application to the treatment of familial haemorrhagic telangiectasia. M D Thesis, University of London

Harrison D F N 1964 Familial haemorrhagic telangiectasia. Quarterly Journal of Medicine 33: 25–38

Osler W 1901 On a family form of recurring epistaxis associated with multiple telangiectases of the skin and mucous membranes. Johns Hopkins Hospital Bulletin 12: 333–337

Rendu M 1896 Epistaxis répétées chez un sujet porteur de petits angiomes cutanés et muqueux. Bulletin et Memoires de la Société médicale des Hôpitaux de Paris, 3e Série 13: 731–733

Sharma N G K, Mahambre L, Audi P S, Borker M P 1975 Hereditary haemorrhagic telangiectasia. Journal of the Indian Medical Association 65: 110–112

Sutton H G 1864 Epistaxis as an indication of impaired nutrition and of degeneration of the vascular system. Medical Mirror 1: 769–781

Weber F P 1907 Multiple hereditary development angiomata (Telangiectases) of the skin and mucous membranes associated with recurring haemorrhage. Lancet 2: 160–162

19

Mesenchymal soft tissue tumours of the nose and sinuses

FIBROSARCOMA OF THE NOSE AND SINUSES

Introduction

Sarcomas of this region have been recognized and described in their various forms since the early days of histological studies. One of the earliest accounts was that of Billroth (1869) who reported a spindle celled sarcoma of the nasal septum. Johnston (1904) reviewed 71 cases of 'sarcoma' of the nasal septum, amongst which many were not specified or, as in the case of malignant melanomas, would no longer be acceptable under this heading. On the other hand, this author included some cases which were labelled as either 'fibrosarcoma' or 'spindle cell sarcoma'. In 1927, Portela published a fatal case of nasal and paranasal fibrosarcoma with bilateral involvement and terminal meningitis.

Terminology

Although spindle cells are a characteristic feature of this type of tumour, the use of the term 'spindle cell sarcoma' was strongly criticized by Stout (1948) and has now been largely abandoned. The expression 'fibromatosis' is used by some (Conley, Stout and Healey, 1967; Fu and Perzin, 1976) to indicate a well differentiated, less aggressive type of neoplasm but the term has also been used to denote an occasional post-irradiation effect though the histological appearance is not easily distinguished from fibrosarcoma (Pettit, Chamness and Ackerman, 1954). In the present context, reference is confined to the term 'fibrosarcoma', appropriately qualified according to the degree of differentiation.

Incidence

Fibrosarcoma is not a very common tumour in this region. Stout (1948) found seven out of 218 fibrosarcomas arising in the upper respiratory tract. Swain, Sessions and Ogura (1974) in a retrospective study of 40 patients with fibrosarcoma of the head and neck, seen between 1940 and 1972, found four cases involving the maxillary sinus and one in the nasal cavity, the remainder originating in the mandible, oral cavity, nasopharynx, neck and scalp. Fu and Perzin (1974 and 1976), in their comprehensive study of 256 non-epithelial tumours of the nose, sinuses and naso-pharynx, found 19 cases of which six were classified as fibromatosis and thirteen as fibrosarcoma. Jackson, Fitz-Hugh and Constable (1977) reported three fibrosarcomas amongst 115 malignant tumours of the nose and sinuses. In the I.L.O. material there were five cases, representing approximately 0.5 per cent of all tumours of the nose and sinuses, less than 1.5 per cent of all malignant tumours and 2 per cent of non-epithelial tumours.

Clinical features

There is no significant sex difference and the age distribution tends to be broadly based, matching the pattern which has been observed in respect of all sites (Mackenzie, 1964). The I.L.O. experience was confined to the upper age groups, Fu and Perzin found two cases of 'fibromatosis' occurring in the first two decades and Portela's fatal case involved a 16 year-old male.

The most common presenting sign is a mass either superficially palpable or deeply located and often associated with pain. Being usually of slow growth, the neoplasm is likely to have been present for some time when the patient first seeks advice.

Anatomical site of origin

Paranasal involvement, either primary or secondary, tends to predominate. Of the five cases reported by Swain et al. (1974) only one was of nasal origin whilst the five cases in the I.L.O. material were all paranasal (two in the maxillary sinus and three in the ethmoid region). At the time of presentation, many of these tumours are found to involve more than one cavity (Fu and Perzin, 1976).

Gross appearances

To the naked eye these tumours usually present as firm white fibrous growths but not infrequent haemorrhage may result in discolouration.

Histopathology

Stout's (1948) classification of well differentiated, low grade and poorly differentiated high grade malignant fibrosarcomas may be helpful in the more general context but, in paranasal tumours, correlation with behaviour is much less certain. Furthermore, Fu and Perzin (1976) have admitted that distinction between fibromatosis and fibrosarcoma is probably less valid in respect of tumours of the head region.

The usual microscopical picture consists of slender spindle cells with fine tapering nuclei, running in leashes and intertwining bands (Fig. 19.1) whilst an occasional herringbone pattern may be seen (Fig. 19.2) and even perivascular palisading. Small areas of angiomatoid vascular formations are occasionally observed and variable numbers of thin walled vessels amongst the tumour cells may present a picture requiring distinction from haemangiopericytoma. Haemorrhage is commonly present and areas of necrosis may be found. A suggestion of nuclear palisading is sometimes present, recalling the view of Warren and Sommer (1936) that some fibrosarcomas are of neurogenic origin – a concept which is not generally accepted. In some areas the spindle cells tend to become fusiform with more abundant cytoplasm (Fig. 19.3). Some degree of nuclear irregularity may be present but mitoses are usually scanty. Occasional giant cells may be seen but the presence of many bizarre cells with grotesque nuclei should raise suspicion of an alternative diagnosis such as malignant fibrous histiocytoma (q.v.) or anaplastic carcinoma. The fact that many fibrosarcomas appear to be fairly well differentiated should not mislead since fibroma is 'a dangerous diagnosis' (Mackenzie, 1964).

Intercellular material is variable in amount and often stains feebly with Van Gieson though more positively with Masson Trichrome whilst reticulin preparations usually show a fine intercellular fibrillary pattern (Fig. 19.4). Osteoid and new bone formation may be found at the edge of the lesion due to reactive change in the adjacent bone which may be invaded by the tumour. This is not an integral part of the neoplasm which produces neither bone nor cartilage and is recognized by its more organized appearance as compared with the irregular osteoid production in osteogenic sarcoma (Fig. 21.8). Myxoid areas are very uncommon in fibrosarcoma. Other tumours which may cause confusion include leiomyosarcoma, rhabdomyosarcoma and even neurilemmoma.

Aetiology and pathogenesis

Little is known regarding the causation of nasal and paranasal fibrosarcomas. In the more general context, there is no convincing evidence that trauma plays any part but claims to have produced fibrosarcoma in

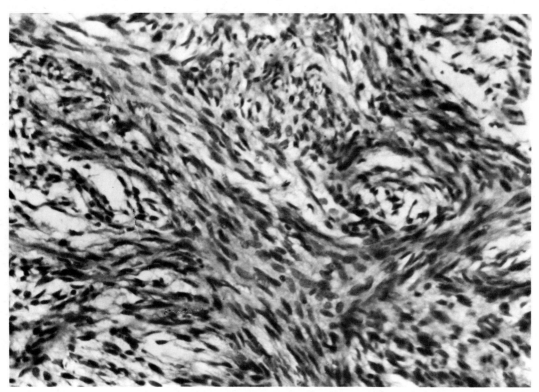

Fig. 19.1 Fibrosarcoma of the ethmoid region in a 44 year-old female. M × 325

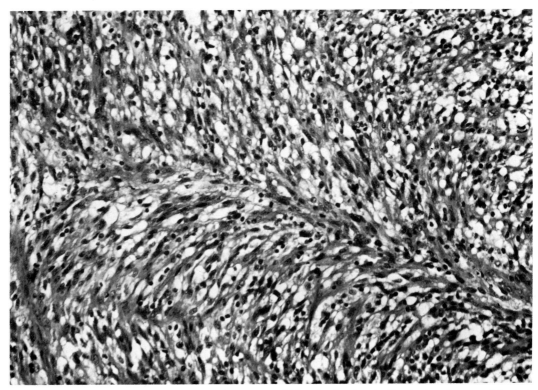

Fig. 19.2 Fibrosarcoma of the maxillary sinus in a 73 year-old female, showing the 'herring bone' pattern. M × 208

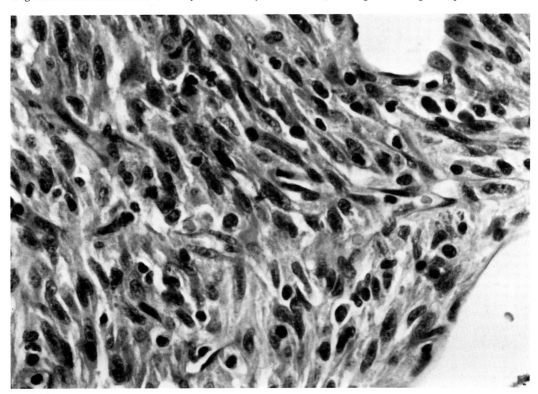

Fig. 19.3 Fibrosarcoma of the maxillary sinus in a 73 year-old female (see Fig. 19.2) showing plump single cells. M × 520

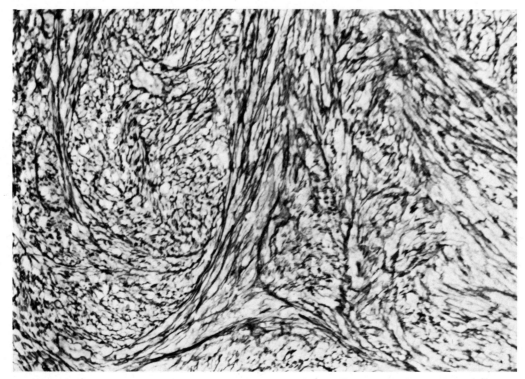

Fig. 19.4 Fibrosarcoma of the maxillary sinus in a 73 year-old female (see Fig. 19.2) showing fine reticulin pattern. M × 208

experimental animals by irradiation have been made by Lacassagne and Vinzent (1929) and later by Burrows, Mayneord and Roberts (1937). No subsequent work along these lines has been published but there have been a number of reports of the development of fibrosarcoma following radiotherapy (Pettit, Chamness and Acker-man, 1954; Cade 1957; Schwartz and Rothstein, 1968). Pettit et al. (1954) reported a tumour involving the ethmoid region of a six year-old child following irradiation for bilateral retinoblastoma and they pointed out that, as in many other cases, the radiotherapy was excessive and poorly managed. On the other hand, although fibrosarcoma is traditionally regarded as being radio-resistant, Windeyer, Dische and Mansfield (1966) reported a favourable response to irradiation.

The precise tissue of origin is a matter for speculation. The tumours are believed to be derived largely from bone, arising either centrally or peripherally from the periosteum with subsequent involvement of nasal or paranasal cavities (Hoggins and Brady, 1962). Origin from mucosal connective tissue has been mooted but is no more than an unconfirmed possibility.

Behaviour

Many of these tumours are slowly growing but their activity is not entirely predictable and confusion with other spindle celled tumours has obviously obscured the picture. Local spread from one cavity to another is a common event. Ethmoidal tumours usually involve the nasal cavity but may also extend into the maxillary and frontal sinuses and the postnasal space.

There is a marked tendency for fibrosarcomas to recur. Mackenzie (1964) found a recurrence rate of 49 per cent in 205 fibrosarcomas of soft tissues in various locations. Two of the five I.L.O. cases exhibited multiple recurrences. Lymphnode metastasis is uncommon. Con-ley et al. (1967) found none in their series of head and neck tumours and none were observed in the I.L.O. material though, in a more general context, Bizer (1971) claimed 11 per cent. Bloodstream spread may involve the lungs, abdominal viscera, brain, other bones and skin. Conley et al. (1967) found systemic metastasis in 18 per cent, Swain et al. (1974) recorded 20 per cent but in the I.L.O. cases none were found.

Survival rates are certainly better than those of paranasal carcinomas. Swain et al. (1974) found a much higher six-year rate (55 per cent) in the better differentiated as compared with the more poorly differentiated fibrosarcomas (11 per cent). In the I.L.O. cases, four out of five survived for more than five years. One patient died of his disease after seven years and another died from an unrelated cause after ten years. The remaining two have survived for 5 and 12 years without recurrence.

BIBLIOGRAPHY

Billroth T 1872 Spindelzellensarkom in der Nase. Chirurgische Klinik (Wien 1869–1870) A Hirschwald, Berlin Band 3, p 73

Bizer L S 1971 Fibrosarcoma. American Journal of Surgery 121: 586–587

Burrows H, Mayneord W V, Roberts J E 1937 Neoplasia following the application of X-rays to inflammatory lesions. Proceedings of the Royal Society, London, Series B 123: 213–217

Cade S 1957 Radiation – induced cancer in man. British Journal of Radiology 30: 393–402

Conley J, Stout A P, Healey W V 1967 Clinicopathologic analysis of eighty-four patients with an original diagnosis of fibrosarcoma of the head and neck. American Journal of Surgery 114: 564–569

Fu Y, Perzin K H 1976 Non-epithelial tumours of the nasal cavity, paranasal sinuses and nasopharynx. Cancer VI. Fibrous tissue tumours 37: 2912–2928

Hoggins G S, Brady C L 1962 Fibrosarcoma of the maxilla. Oral Surgery, Oral Medicine and Oral Pathology 15: 34–38

Jackson R T, Fitz-Hugh G S, Constable W C 1977 Malignant neoplasms of the nasal cavities and paranasal sinuses. Laryngoscope 87: 726–736

Johnston R H 1904 Sarcomata of the nasal septum. Laryngoscope 14: 454–473

Lacassagne A, Vinzent R 1929 Sarcomes provoqués chez des lapins par l'irradiation d'abces a streptobacillus caviae. Comptes Rendus de Societe de Biologie 100: 249–251

Mackenzie D H 1964 Fibroma: A dangerous diagnosis. British Journal of Surgery 51: 607–612

Pettit V D, Chamness J T, Ackerman L V 1954 Fibromatosis and fibrosarcoma following irradiation therapy. Cancer 7: 149–158

Portela J 1927 Fibrosarcome envahissant des fosses nasales, des deux sinus maxillaires, de l'ethmoide et des deux sinus sphenoidaux. Revue de Laryngologie 48: 530–531

Stout A P 1948 Fibrosarcoma. Cancer 1: 30–63

Swain R E, Sessions D G, Ogura J H 1974 Fibrosarcoma of the head and neck. Annals of Otology, Rhinology and Laryngology 83: 439–444

Schwartz E E, Rothstein J D 1968 Fibrosarcomas following radiation therapy. Journal of the American Medical Association 203: 296–298

Warren S, Sommer G N J 1936 Fibrosarcoma of the soft parts. Archives of Surgery 33: 425–450

Windeyer B, Dische S, Mansfield C M 1966 The place of radiotherapy in the management of fibrosarcoma of the soft tissues. Clinical Radiology 17: 32–40

Additional references

Gane N F C, Lindup R, Strickland P, Bennett M H 1970 Radiation-induced fibrosarcoma. British Journal of Cancer 24: 705–711

Prasad U, Kanjilal J K 1969 Fibrosarcoma of the ethmoid. Journal of Laryngology and Otology 83: 627–631

Richardson D, Maguda T A 1970 Fibrosarcoma of the nose and paranasal sinuses. Journal of the Tennessee Medical Association 63: 829–831

MALIGNANT FIBROUS HISTIOCYTOMA OF NOSE AND SINUSES

Introduction

A variety of non-epithelial lesions involving particularly the skin and subcutaneous tissues have been recognized for many years under such names as histiocytoma, sclerosing haemangioma, fibrous xanthoma, dermatofibroma, dermatofibrosarcoma protuberans, fibroxanthosarcoma and xanthogranuloma. Not unsimilar histological patterns have been encountered in deeper soft tissues. Microscopically, the common theme is the presence of histiocyte-like cells and collagen producing cells and a unifying principle has emerged based on the derivation of fibroblastic elements from histiocytes. The first reported case in the nasal region was by Townsend, Neel, Weiland, Devine and McBean (1973) under the title of 'fibrous histiocytoma'.

Incidence

Fu and Perzin (1976) considered that fibrous histiocytoma of the nose and sinuses was extremely uncommon but since 1973 there have been a number of reports of such tumours (Spector and Ogura, 1974; Rice, Batsakis, Headlington and Boles, 1974; Wilmes and Meister, 1978; Crissman and Henson, 1978). Furthermore, review of fibrosarcomas in the I.L.O. material revealed

two cases which were undoubtedly malignant fibrous histiocytomas.

Clinical features

The age distribution is very broadly based, ranging from three to eighty-two years in the published cases whilst the sexes appear to be equally affected. The clinical picture has no specific features, nasal obstruction, epistaxis, local swelling and proptosis being common forms of presentation.

Anatomical site of origin

The maxillary sinus is most commonly involved but the nasal cavity and ethmoid region may also be affected.

Gross appearances

To the naked eye, the tumour appears as a soft tissue mass, usually of fibrous consistency, which could represent a variety of lesions.

Histopathology

A case of M.F.H. in the frontal sinus has been described by Schaefer et al (1980).

The microscopical picture is variegated but a common feature is the presence of spindle cells which may not only resemble fibroblasts but tend to be associated with collagen and reticulin. The cells and their accompanying fibres often run in parallel bundles, lying in various directions and sometimes intertwined but a particular feature is the tendency for the bundles to be arranged at right angles to each other and often seeming to approach a central point (Figs. 19.5 & 19.6). This arrangement has been given various names such as 'cartwheel', 'flower' or 'fan' pattern but Bednář (1957) used the expression 'storiform' (from the Latin *storea* meaning a rush mat) and this has been generally accepted. Occasionally, the bundles approach each other in a spiral pattern prompting the use of such terms as 'pinwheel' or 'spiral nebula'. The storiform pattern is not always immediately obvious not is it entirely exclusive to this particular tumour.

In addition to the complex spindle cell pattern, there are areas of palely eosinophilic, irregularly polyhedral cells of histiocytic type (Fig. 19.7) which may or may not contain lipid material. Foam cells are usually present, either in groups or interspersed amongst spindle cells (Fig. 19.8). Bizarre cells with grotesque nuclei are often present and also multinucleated giant cells of varying appearance (Figs. 19.9 & 19.10) and sometimes of Touton type. Occasional myxoid areas may be encountered (Fig. 19.10b). Mitoses, both normal and atypical

may be present in considerable numbers but there are differences of opinion regarding the significance of this feature in relation to aggressive behaviour.

The spindle cell element has frequently resulted in an initial diagnosis of fibrosarcoma but the presence of histiocyte-like cells which may be seen to blend with the spindle cells, foam cells and a variety of multinucleated giant cells should suggest a reconsideration of the diagnosis. The storiform pattern is an interesting feature but is not a reliable criterion *per se*.

Aetiology and pathogenesis

The wide age distribution offers no clue to the causation of this tumour. The concept of derivation of fibroblasts from histiocytes in this context was put forward by Stout and his colleagues (Kauffman and Stout, 1961; Ozzello, Stout and Murray, 1963; O'Brien and Stout, 1964) and has resulted in a clarification of a hitherto confused picture. The principal variations in the histological pattern are thus explicable on this basis. In such tumours where differentiation has been predominantly fibroblastic, the lesion may be indistinguishable from a fibrosarcoma and it is noteworthy that an occasional storiform pattern is observable in spindle celled tumours which do not exhibit any of the other features of the fibrous histiocytoma. In circumstances where histiocytes have become facultative fibroblasts, it is hardly surpris-

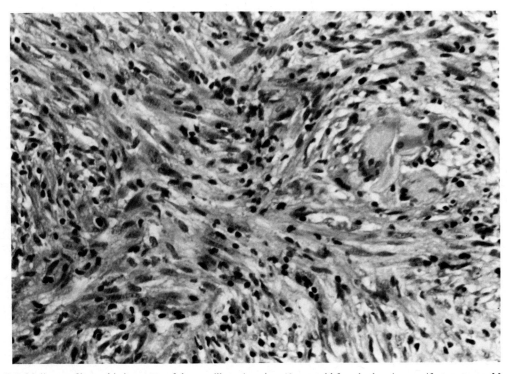

Fig. 19.5 Malignant fibrous histiocytoma of the maxillary sinus in a 49 year-old female showing storiform pattern. M × 320

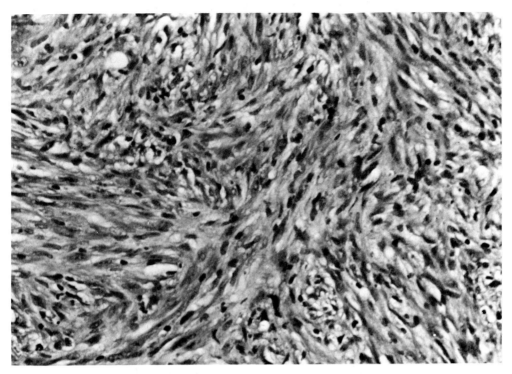

Fig. 19.6 Malignant fibrous histiocytoma of the maxillary sinus in a 49 year-old female (see Fig. 19.5) showing storiform pattern. M × 320

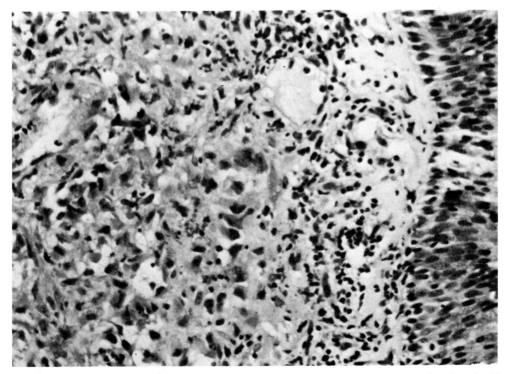

Fig. 19.7 Malignant fibrous histiocytoma of the maxillary sinus in a 49 year-old female (see Fig. 19.5) showing subepithelial accumulation of histiocytic cells. M × 320

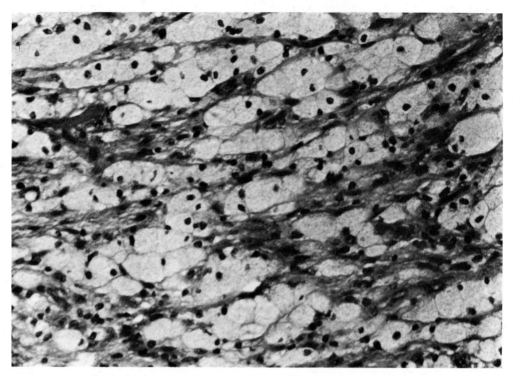

Fig. 19.8 Malignant fibrous histiocytoma of the maxillary sinus in a 41 year-old male, showing aggregation of foam cells. M × 320

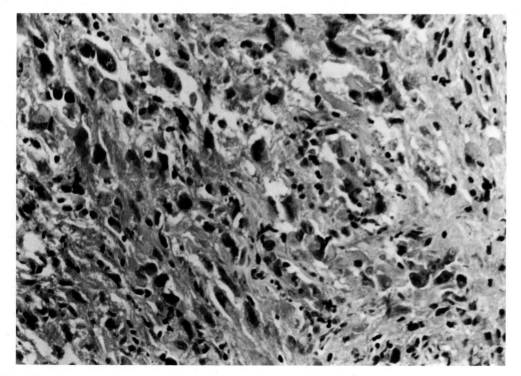

Fig. 19.9 Malignant fibrous histiocytoma of the maxillary sinus in a 49 year-old female (see Fig. 19.5) showing bizarre cells histiocytes and atypical mitoses. M × 320

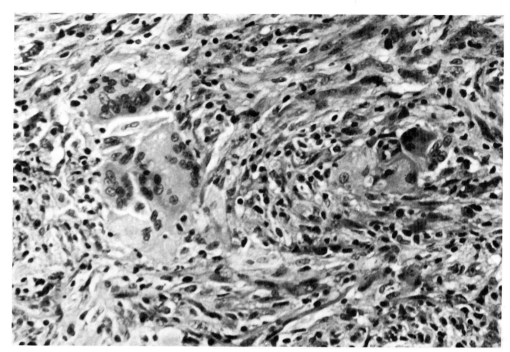

Fig. 19.10a Malignant fibrous histiocytoma of the maxillary sinus in a 49 year-old female (see Fig. 19.5) showing multinucleated giant cells. M × 320

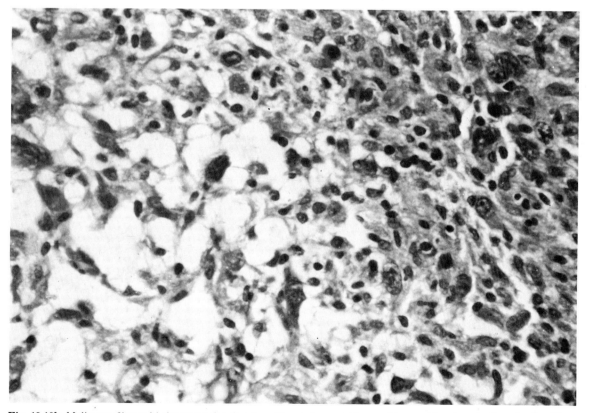

Fig. 19.10b Malignant fibrous histiocytoma showing myxoid and pleomorphic area. Note multinucleated cells and cells with atypical nuclei also in the myxoid field. M × 400

ing if the end products behave exactly as though they had always been fibroblastic elements.

Behaviour

In the present anatomical context, most of these tumours tend to behave like more aggressive fibrosarcomas, spreading from one cavity to another. Multiple lesions are occasionally found involving other parts of the body (Rice et al., 1974). Regional lymphnode metastasis has been reported (Rice et al., 1974; Crissman and Henson, 1978). The last mentioned authors also reported massive deposits of tumour in the pleura, presumably of systemic origin. Of the cases reported so far, none have been recorded as surviving for more than two years and the I.L.O. cases did not survive beyond this period.

In the more general context, recurrence rate is high, metastasis occurs in over a quarter of the cases but survival, with or without persistent disease would appear to be somewhat better (Soule and Enriquez, 1972).

BIBLIOGRAPHY

Bednář B 1957 Storiform neurofibroma of the skin, pigmented and non-pigmented. Cancer 10: 368–376

Crissman J D, Henson S L 1978 Malignant fibrous histiocytoma of the maxillary sinus. Archives of Otolaryngology 104: 228–230

Fu Y, Perzin K II 1976 Non-epithelial tumors of the nasal cavity, paranasal sinuses and nasopharynx. Cancer 37: 1912–2928

Kauffman S L, Stout A P 1961 Histiocytic tumors (Fibrous xanthoma and histiocytoma) in children. Cancer 14: 469–482

O'Brien J E, Stout A P 1964 Malignant fibrous xanthomas. Cancer 17: 1445–1455

Ozzello L, Stout A P, Murray M R 1963 Cultural characteristics of malignant histiocytomas and fibrous xanthomas. Cancer 16: 331–344

Rice D H, Batsakis J G, Headlington J T, Boles R 1974 Fibrous histiocytoma of the nose and paranasal sinuses. Archives of Otolaryngology 100: 398–401

Schaefer S D, Denton R A, Blend B L, Carder H M 1980 Laryngoscope 90: 2021–2026

Soule E H, Enriquez P 1972 Atypical fibrous histiocytoma, malignant fibrous histiocytoma, malignant histiocytoma and epithelial sarcoma. Cancer 30: 128–143

Spector G J, Ogura J H 1974 Malignant fibrous histiocytoma of the maxilla. Archives of Otolaryngology 99: 385–387

Townsend G L, Neel H B, Weiland L H, Devine K D, McBean J B 1973 Fibrous histiocytoma of the paranasal sinuses. Archives of Otolaryngology 98: 51–52

Wilmes E, Meister P 1978 Fibröse Histiozytome der Nase und Nasennebenhöhlen. Laryngologie, Rhinologie und Otologie (Stuttgart) 57: 69–72

MYXOMA OF THE NOSE AND SINUSES

Myxomatous tissue may occur in a variety of neoplasms, usually as one component in the tumour structure but occasionally it is present as an exclusive feature justifying the term myxoma. According to Stout (1948) myxoma ranks third in malignant tumours of soft tissues after fibrosarcoma and liposarcoma. Myxomas are more commonly encountered in cardiac muscle but are also found in other locations such as subcutaneous tissues, aponeuroses and bone, to mention some of the more usual sites of origin. Those of osseous origin are more likely to be found in the bones of the facial skeleton and consequently the nose and sinuses may become involved. The earliest report of a myxoma in the nasal region was that of Hajek and Polyak (1910) who carried out a postmortem study in a patient dying of generalized tuberculosis. Harbert, Gerry and Dimmette (1949) recorded a myxoma of the maxilla which filled the maxillary sinus and found five previously published cases involving the paranasal sinuses.

Incidence

Notwithstanding its relative position amongst the connective tissue tumours generally, myxoma is not a common tumour in the nose and sinuses. Fu and Perzin (1977) collected six myxomas amongst their 256 cases of non-epithelial tumours of the nose, sinuses and nasopharynx. The jaws are not infrequently affected; three out of the 49 cases reported by Stout (1948) involved the maxilla whilst Zimmerman and Dahlin (1958) presented 26 myxomas of the jaws of which 15 were located in the maxilla and several involved the maxillary sinus.

Clinical features

The age distribution is largely confined to the lower age groups. Four of Fu and Perzin's cases were under the age of 25 years, the youngest being 15 months old. The ages of Zimmerman and Dahlin's series were almost entirely within the second to the fourth decades. No sex difference has been observed. Presentation is often with facial, intranasal or intra-oral swelling which may or may not be painful.

Anatomical site of origin

For reasons which will be apparent from the views on pathogenesis, the maxillary sinus is the most frequently reported site in the present context although the other cavities may also be involved as in the case of Hajek and Polyak (1910) in which the tumour involved the nasal septum, the ethmoid region and the body of the sphenoid.

Gross appearance
To the naked eye these tumours appear as greyish masses of consistency ranging from gelatinous to firm and fibrous. They are not encapsulated and, although some have been described as being 'enucleated' their borders may be difficult to define.

Histopathology
Microscopically, stellate and spindle cells are randomly distributed in a loose mucoid stroma (Figs. 19.11 & 19.12). Varying amounts of fibrous tissue may be present whilst reticulin staining reveals a delicate fibrillar network. Distinction from myxoid areas in other types of tumour depends on the absence of any other recognizable, differentiated cellular elements. In the case of fibrosarcoma, the myxoid component is never dominant, if present at all, whilst the presence of mature or immature fat cells will assist in the identification of a liposarcoma. Very occasionally, pleomorphic salivary or mucosal gland tumours may exhibit a prominent myxoid picture but the epithelial component can usually be found if searched for with diligence. The mucoid ground substance is composed of acid mucopolysaccharides (hyaluronic acid and chondroitin sulphate A and C) which exhibit hyaluronidase-labile metachromasia with Toluidine Blue. Ultrastructural studies (Harrison, 1973; White, Chan, Mohnac and Miller, 1975) have shown that many of the stellate or spindle cells contain prominent rough endoplasmic reticulum.

Aetiology and pathogenesis
No direct causal factors have been identified but, in the region under discussion, myxomas are presumed to have originated in the adjacent bone. Thoma and Goldman (1947) considered that myxomas in the head region were largely odontogenic in origin whilst a small number were osteogenic. According to these authors, the embryonic mesenchyme from which the dental papilla and the periodontal membrane are derived may give rise to an odontogenic fibroma. The latter may differentiate into either a dentinoma or a cementoma or it may dedifferentiate into a myxoma. In the more general context, Stout (1948) regarded myxomas as arising from primitive mesenchyme in whatever location. On the other hand, Fu and Perzin (1977) regarded their pathogenesis as uncertain.

Behaviour
Many myxomas are regarded as being benign in so far as they do not metastasize. For this reason, Stout (1948)

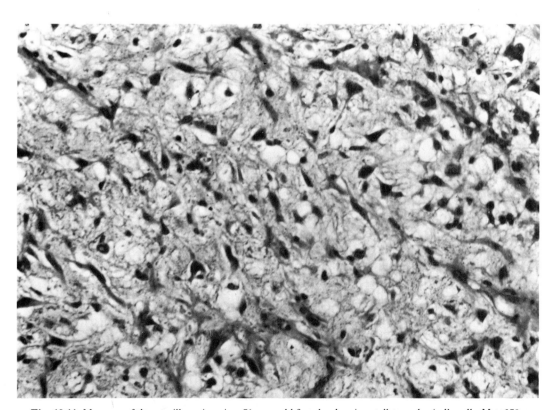

Fig. 19.11 Myxoma of the maxillary sinus in a 51 year-old female, showing stellate and spindle cells. M × 350

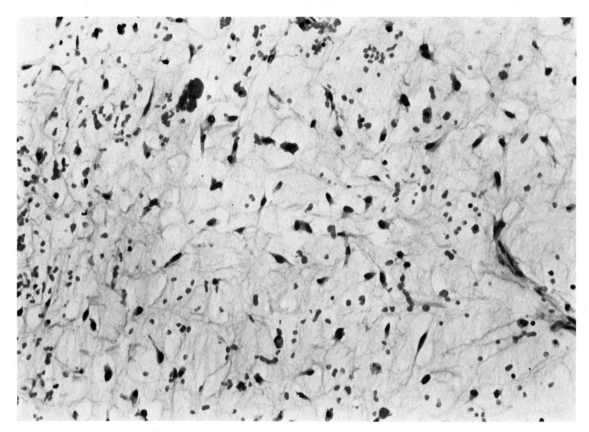

Fig. 19.12 Myxoma of the maxilla in a 40 year-old male. M × 225

maintained that myxoma was not synonymous with myxosarcoma, the existence of which as an entity is debatable. Of their 26 myxomas of the jaws, Zimmerman and Dahlin (1958) found 20 to be benign whilst six were classified as initially malignant though of low grade. Even though they do not metastasize, many myxomas are locally invasive and are likely to recur if not completely removed and it would seem that, in the present context, the term benign is purely relative. In Stout's series, only one patient died as the direct result of this tumour although 20 per cent had persistent disease. In Fu and Perzin's cases, survival without recurrence was recorded in five out of six for periods ranging from four to nine years. These authors advised wide resection of such tumours which are not radio-sensitive.

BIBLIOGRAPHY

Fu Y, Perzin K H 1977 Non-epithelial tumours of the nasal cavity paranasal sinuses and nasopharynx. VII Myxomas. Cancer 39: 195–203

Hajek M, Polyak L 1910 Myxoma lymphangiectaticum des Nasengerüstes. Archive fur Laryngologie und Rhinologie 23: 43–56

Harbert F, Gerry R G, Dimmette R M 1949 Myxoma of the maxilla. Oral Surgery, Oral Medicine and Oral Pathology 2: 1414–1421

Harrison J D 1973 Odontogenic myxoma: ultrastructural and histochemical studies. Journal of Clinical Pathology 26: 570–582

Stout A P 1948 Myxoma, the tumour of primitive mesenchyme. Annals of Surgery 127: 706–719

Thoma K H, Goldman H M 1947 Central myxoma of the jaw. American Journal of Orthodontics (Oral Surgery Section) 33: 532–540

White D K, Chan S, Mohnac A M, Miller A S 1975 Odontogenic myxoma. Oral Surgery, Oral Medicine and Oral Pathology 39: 901–917

Zimmerman D C, Dahlin D C 1958 Myxomatous tumours of the jaws. Oral Surgery, Oral Medicine and Oral Pathology 11: 1069–1080

TUMOURS OF ADIPOSE TISSUE

Whether benign or malignant such tumours are extremely uncommon in the nose and sinuses and only a very few cases have been reported, the majority being benign.

Although a common tumour elsewhere in the body, lipomas have only rarely been reported in the paranasal sinuses and only solitary cases have been published by Goldstein (1915), Silbernagel (1938), Fu and Perzin (1977). The case recorded by the last mentioned authors was one out of 256 non-epithelial neoplasms of the nose, sinuses and nasopharynx. All three cases occurred in the maxillary sinus but, in Silbernagel's case, the patient had had a lipoma removed from the neck many years previously. Histologically, such tumours resemble mature adipose tissue, hence interpretation at microscopical level could be debatable.

Liposarcomas of the nose and sinuses are very rare. They are more common in soft tissues particularly in the gluteal region, thigh and retroperitoneum. In the more general context, these tumours represent one of the commonest malignant neoplasms of soft tissues (Spittle, Newton and Mackenzie, 1970). The report on 53 cases by Enterline, Culberson, Rochlin and Brady (1960) contained five cases arising in the head region but none involved the nose and sinuses. In a recent review of liposarcoma, Baden, Newman and Hackensack (1977) found that the head and neck region accounted for less than four per cent of all sites of origin. Giardino and Manfredi (1967) reported a liposarcoma arising in the cheek and subsequently invading the maxillary sinus. Fu and Persin (1977) have recorded the only liposarcoma primarily involving the maxillary sinus.

The liposarcoma is essentially a tumour of adult life, being rare in children. In the largest series of tumours affecting the lower limb and retroperitoneal region, Enzinger and Winslow (1962) found a peak age incidence in the sixth decade with no cases under the age of twenty.

The microscopical features of liposarcoma were first described by Virchow (1857 and 1865) who noted the mucoid element which is frequently present. The variegated histological picture has long been recognized and has led to the introduction of several classifications (Stout, 1944; Enterline et al., 1960; Enzinger and Winslow, 1962; Spittle et al., 1970). Many liposarcomas have two main components: fat cells of varying maturity, ranging from recognizable adipose tissue of adult type to rounded lipoblasts of assorted sizes and myxoid tissue composed of stellate and spindle cells in a mucoid background containing acid mucopolysaccaride. The combination of these two components in varying proportions and degrees of maturity constitutes the myxoid variant which is the most common type. Stout (1944) introduced four histological subdivisions: Well and poorly differentiated myxoid types, a round cell type composed of rounded lipoblasts of varying sizes but no myxoid tissue and a mixed type containing the features of the first three groups and exhibiting pleomorphism. Enterline et al. (1960) distinguished a fifth type which they called 'lipoma-like' although it seems to resemble a highly differentiated myxoid type. In the less well differentiated variants are to be found many bizarre nuclei and multinucleated giant cells. Intracellular fat can be demonstrated in frozen sections and its accumulation leads to rounding of the cells and peripheral displacement of the nucleus, producing the characteristic signet ring form.

Overlap in these classifications undoubtedly occurs and this might imply that such subdivisions were arbitrary and academic but the exercise nevertheless has a practical justification. Stout (1944) maintained that the well differentiated myxoid type rarely metastasized. Enterline et al. (1960) also found a much lower frequency of metastasis in the myxoid variety and a degree of correlation has been found between survival and the histological pattern. Spittle et al. (1970), in a review of 60 cases of general distribution, showed that the five-year survival rate in the myxoid group was over 80 per cent but in the pleomorphic group it was under 50 per cent, the average for all types being 64 per cent.

Local spread by direct extension may occur as in any malignant neoplasm and was well illustrated in the case described by Fu and Perzin (1977) in which the tumour ultimately involved the ethmoid region, sphenoid sinus, temporal bone and cranial cavity. Although there appeared to be some regression following irradiation, the patient died within six months of presentation.

BIBLIOGRAPHY

Baden E, Newman R, Hackensack N J 1977 Liposarcoma of the oropharyngeal region. Oral Surgery, Oral Medicine and Oral Pathology 44: 889–902
Enterline H T, Culberson J D, Rochlin D B, Brady L W 1960 Liposarcoma. Cancer 13: 932–950

Enzinger F M, Winslow D J 1962 Liposarcoma. Archive für pathologische Anatomie 335: 367–388
Fu Y, Perzin K H 1977 Non-epithelial tumours of the nasal cavity, paranasal sinuses and nasopharynx; VIII Adipose tissue tumours. Cancer 40: 1314–1317

Giardino C, Manfredi C 1967 Liposarcoma della guancia con invasione secondaria del seno mascellare. Giornale Italiano Chirurgia 23: 743–758

Goldstein M A 1915 Lipoma of the maxillary antrum. Laryngoscope 25: 142–144

Silbernagel C E 1938 Lipoma of the maxillary antrum. Laryngoscope 48: 427–428

Spittle M F, Newton K A, Mackenzie D H 1970 Liposarcoma. British Journal of Cancer 24: 696–704

Stout A P 1944 Liposarcoma – the malignant tumour of lipoblasts. Annals of Surgery 119: 86–107

Virchow R 1857 Ein Fall von bösartigen zum Teile in der Form des Neurons auftretenden Fettgeschwülsten. Archiv für pathologische Anatomie 11: 281–288

Virchow R 1865 Myxoma lipomatodes malignum. Archiv für pathologische Anatomie 32: 545–546

20

Cartilaginous tumours of the nose and sinuses

CARTILAGINOUS TUMOURS OF THE NOSE
AND SINUSES

Introduction

Although benign and malignant varieties are now well
recognized in the general context, the distinction was
not made or appreciated for a very long time. Their
cartilaginous nature was readily apparent in many cases
but none were regarded as inherently malignant and,
regardless of behaviour, many tumours were reported
under the name of enchondroma. Nevertheless, Volkmann (1855) reported a fatal case of enchondroma of the
metacarpal; the patient died of post-operative pyaemia
and, at autopsy, was found to have multiple tumour
deposits in the lungs of almost identical appearance.
Paget (1870) included in his account of cartilaginous
tumours an enormous tumour of the innominate bone,
weighing about 20 kilograms. From his illustration of
the microscopy there is little doubt that it was a
chondrosarcoma. Although malignant cartilaginous tumours subsequently achieved recognition, it was not
until 1930 that Phemister established chondrosarcoma
as an entity separate from osteogenic sarcoma.

The rarity of cartilaginous tumours in the upper jaw
was noted by Paget (1870) but the earliest account was
probably that of Morgan (1836 and 1842) in which a
tumour began as a slowly growing swelling in the nostril
of a 15 year-old boy. The lesion produced a hideous
distortion of the face and local excision was followed by
massive recurrence from which the patient died 15 years
later. The hard lobulated character of the tumour
depicted in a postmortem cast was certainly suggestive
of a chondrosarcoma. Under the title of enchondroma,
Heath (1887) described four cartilaginous tumours of
the nasal and paransal region but at least three of these
were probably chondrosarcomas. The first paransal
chondrosarcoma reported as such was by Mollison
(1916), an antroethmoidal tumour having invaded the
orbit of a 19 year-old girl who died shortly after
operation.

Terminology

The early comprehensive use of the term enchondroma
or chondroma has, unfortunately, been perpetuated by
some writers. Where adequate investigation is possible,
benign tumours composed of mature cartilage are
chondromas whilst malignant varieties should be designated chondrosarcomas. Mesenchymal chondrosarcoma (Dahlin and Henderson, 1962) is a variant of the
malignant group with a distinctive histological picture.
Chondromyxoid fibroma and benign chondroblastoma
to which the former is apparently related (Dahlin, 1956)
are quite distinct, both clinically and pathologically,
from the common chondroma; they are usually benign
in character and have not been reported in the nasal or
paranasal region (Schutt and Frost, 1971) although one
of the present authors had an opportunity of studying
such a tumour in the antro-ethmoidal region of a 13
year-old boy (Figs. 20.8 and 20.9).

Incidence

Although chondromas are relatively common in other
locations, doubt has been cast on their existence in the
nasal region, notwithstanding the fact that a number of
reports have appeared in the literature. Fu and Perzin
(1974) found seven cases amongst their 256 non-
epithelial tumours, four of which were located in the
nasopharynx whilst the remaining three arose in the
nasal septum. The question as to whether they should be
regarded as true neoplasms was, in fact, raised by the
last mentioned author. In the I.L.O. material, one
tumour of the nasal septum was found, to which the
label chondroma could be conceivably applied.

As regards chondrosarcoma, this is also an uncommon
tumour in the nose and sinuses. In a review of 288 cases
of chondrosarcoma, Henderson and Dahlin (1963)
found only four tumours in the head region. Evans,
Ayala and Romsdahl (1977) included six cranial tumours
in their series of 81 cases in various sites. Fu and Perzin
(1974) found ten cases involving the nose and sinuses
whilst the I.L.O. material contained only three chondrosarcomas of the paranasal sinuses.

Clinical

Chondromas in the nasal region tend to occur at a
somewhat earlier age than their malignant counterparts.

In Fu and Perzin's cases the ages ranged from 10 to 46 years, all except one being female. In the general context, the chondrosarcomas reported by Henderson and Dahlin (1963) showed a broadly based age distribution covering the first to the ninth decade with a peak in the sixth. The ten malignant tumours of Fu and Perzin (1974) ranged in age from 20 months to 69 years. Males tend to be affected more commonly than females though the difference is of doubtful significance.

The common form of presentation is a slowly increasing mass leading to nasal obstruction, swelling of the cheek or proptosis with visual disturbance in advanced cases. The lesion may or may not be associated with pain.

Anatomical site of origin

Chondromas are most frequently located in the nasal cavity usually arising from the septum. Reports of paranasal chondromas are often difficult to assess because although bone destruction may result purely from pressure erosion, the suspicion remains that some at least were low grade chondrosarcomas. The latter may arise in the nasal cavity (septum, floor, lateral wall or cribriform plate), the ethmoid sinuses, maxilla and antrum or sphenoid region. Nevertheless, at the time of presentation there is frequently multiple involvement of cavities. In Fu and Perzin's series, the nasal cavity was involved in six cases, the ethmoid in one, the maxillary sinus in two and the sphenoid in one. In the I.L.O. cases the ethmoid sinuses were involved in two and the maxillary sinus in one. Antral tumours are often secondary to primary maxillary origin.

Gross appearances

Cartilaginous tumours, especially chondromas, may show a resemblance to normal cartilage. Malignant varieties often show a coarsely lobulated pattern composed of bluish-white masses of tissue and presenting a coarsely globular surface (Fig. 20.1). This lobular

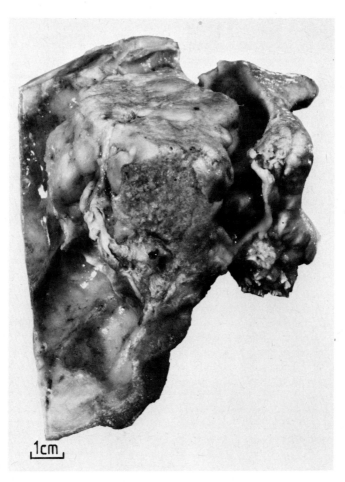

1cm

Fig. 20.1 Chondrosarcoma of the ethmoid sinus in a 47 year-old male.

tendency has been emphasized by many observers including Barnes and Catto (1966). The consistency may be hard with varying degrees of calcification and ossification or it may be soft and gelantinous, particularly in the centres of lobules.

Histopathology

The identification of a chondroma depends partly on its gross appearance and partly on the lack of orderly arrangement of otherwise normal appearing cartilage cells in their lacunae. The important problem is the distinction between benign and malignant tumours and attention should be concentrated on the cells rather than the intercellular substance, a point which was emphasized by Lichtenstein and Jaffe (1943) who stressed the fact that cartilaginous tumours were frequently underdiagnosed. In the well differentiated examples, malignancy is to be suspected in the presence of many cells with plump nuclei; more than occasional cells with two such nuclei; giant cartilage cells with large single or multiple nuclei or with irregular clumps of chromatin (Fig. 20.2). Nuclear irregularity and prominence of nucleoli (Fig. 20.3 & 20.4) are additional suggestive features of malignancy. Myxoid changes and high cellularity are not significant per se, nuclear atypia being more important. Mitoses are usually scanty. Lobularity

is often a feature at microscopical level (Fig. 20.5), the periphery of lobules often showing high cellularity and cytological irregularities. Invasion of adjacent bone is a common feature (Fig. 20.6 & 20.7) whilst calcification and ossification may be present in varying degree, ranging from a powdery deposit of calcareous particles to mature bone. The formation of the latter follows the normal course of development in preformed cartilage and osteoid production is only encountered at the periphery of the tumour where it represents reactive change in adjacent tissue.

In the more anaplastic tumours, the cells tend to become more spindle-shaped, the lacunae less obvious whilst the lobular pattern may disappear. In the highly malignant type, marked cellular pleomorphism, nuclear atypia and tumour giant cells may be present whilst mitoses may also be found.

Attempts at histological grading have been made by Fu and Perzin (1974) and by Evans et al. (1977). The last mentioned authors introduced three categories. Grade I is characterized by a marked preponderance of cells with small densely staining nuclei and occasional multiple nuclei within one lacuna. There is increased cellularity towards the periphery of the tumour lobules whilst calcification and bone formation are common. Grade II shows higher cullularity with increased cell

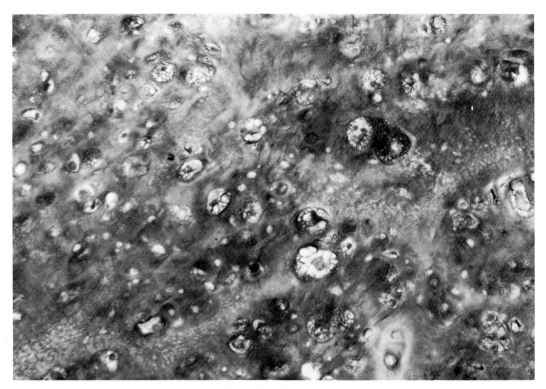

Fig. 20.2 Chondrosarcoma of the ethmoid sinus in a 39 year-old male. M × 325

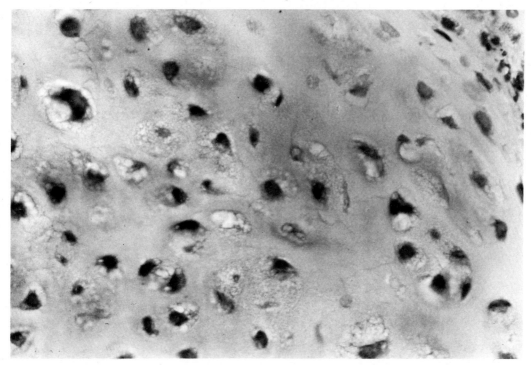

Fig. 20.3 Chondrosarcoma of the ethmoid sinus in a 39 year-old male (see Fig. 20.2). Lacunae contain plump irregular cells which are occasionally binucleate. M × 520

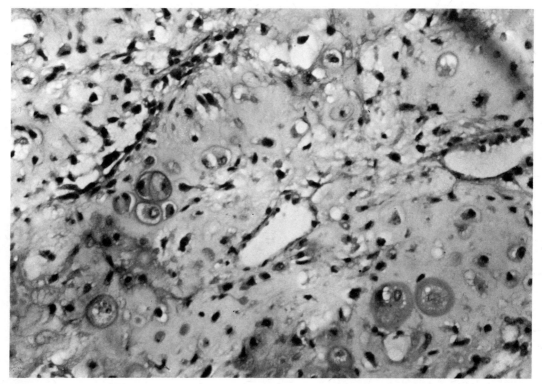

Fig. 20.4 Chondrosarcoma of the ethmoid sinus in a 47 year-old male (see Fig. 20.1) showing a less well differentiated tumour. M × 260

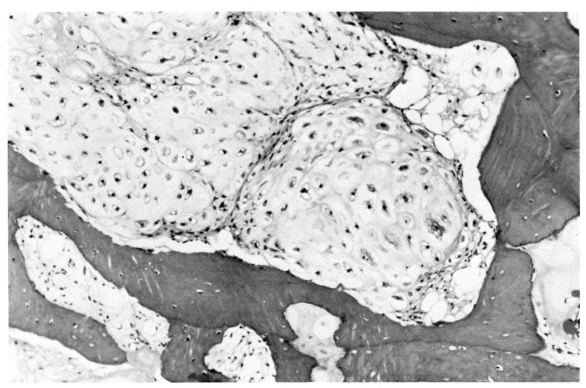

Fig. 20.5 Chondrosarcoma of the nose in a midele-aged male, showing lobulated cartilaginous tissue M ×135

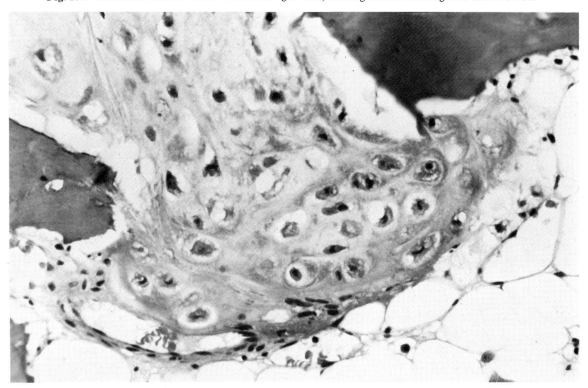

Fig. 20.6 Chondrosarcoma of the nose in a midele-aged male (see Fig. 20.5) showing the cartilaginous tumour breaking through the bone. M ×360

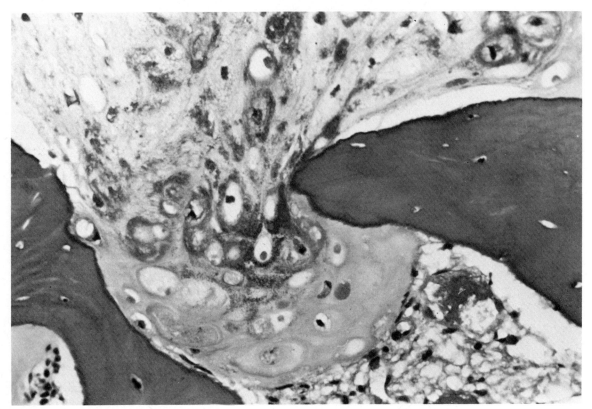

Fig. 20.7 Chondrosarcoma of the nose in a middle-aged male, showing invasion of bone and commencing calcification. M ×
360

size and moderate sized nuclei but mitoses are infrequent. In Grade III, the principal feature is the presence of two or more mitoses per ten high power fields (× 40 objective) with greater cellularity and greater nuclear size together with features resembling fibrosarcoma. It would appear that this system of grading has some prognostic significance.

It can be difficult to distinguish between chondroma and chondrosarcoma of low grade malignancy. Large biopsies may be required, preferably from the growing margin of the lobules (O'Neal and Ackerman, 1951). Biopsies are misleading when a small fragment of tissue is taken from a cartilaginous area of an osteogenic sarcoma, thus leading to the erroneous diagnosis of chondrosarcoma (Barnes and Catto, 1966). In the general context, areas of nuclear irregularity which are sometimes encountered in the chondromyxoid fibroma (Jaffe and Lichtenstein, 1948) have occasionally been mistakenly diagnosed as chondrosarcoma but the former tumour is not common in the nasal region. The microscopical features of the chondromyxoid fibroma consist of lobules of myxoid tissue containing spindle or stellate cells, occasionally lying in lacunae. The intercellular mucoid becomes collagenized and hyalinized (Figs.

20.8 & 20.9), giving the impression of cartilage. The precise origin of this benign tumour is not certain.

A variant on the theme of malignancy in these tumours is the mesenchymal chondrosarcoma, first reported by Lichtenstein and Bernstein in 1959. The tumour is characterized by the presence of sharply defined areas of relatively mature cartilage in a highly cellular background composed of small rounded, oval or spindle cells with occasional areas of transition between the two types of tissue. Such tumours are unquestionably malignant, tending to occur at an earlier age than the common chondrosarcoma. Primary involvement of the maxilla has been reported by Dahlin and Henderson (1962) and by Salvador, Beabout and Dahlin (1971). Olszewski (1969) recorded one such tumour arising in the maxillary sinus and the antroethmoidal neoplasm reported by Wirth and Shimkin (1943) was clearly of the same histological type.

Aetiology and pathogenesis
A factor in the causation of some of these tumours would appear to be irradiation. Hatcher (1945) reported three cases of chondrosarcoma following irradiation and, in a review of 24 or other cases of post-irradiational sarcoma

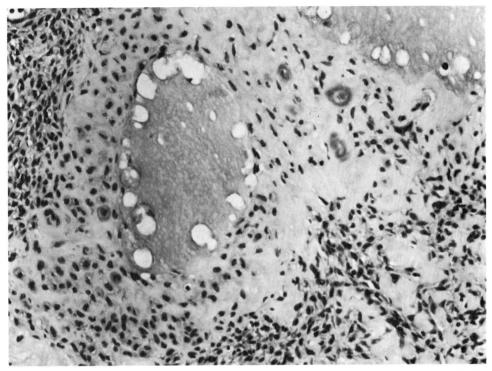

Fig. 20.8 Chondromyxoid fibroma in the antro-ethmoid region of a 13 year-old boy, showing myxoid areas with advancing collagenization. M × 260

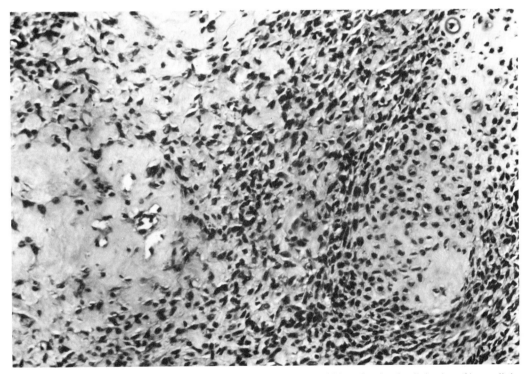

Fig. 20.9 Chondromyxoid fibroma in the antro-ethmoid region of a 13 year-old boy showing hyalinization of intercellular collagen. M × 260

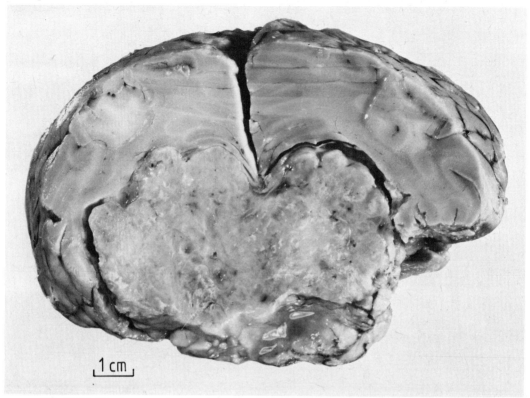

Fig. 20.10 Chondrosarcoma of the ethmoid sinus in a 47 year-old male showing invasion of the brain.

of bone, he commented on the fact that nine were chondrosarcomas. Cohen and d'Angio (1961) described an atypical chondrosarcoma in a 13 year-old boy who had received irradiation following nephrectomy for a Wilm's tumour during the first year of his life.

According to Lichtenstein and Jaffe (1943) chondrosarcomas arise from mature cartilage. It is to be expected, therefore, that such tumours might be found in locations where cartilage is normally present, e.g. the nasal cavity. On the other hand, the occurrence of chondrosarcomas in the maxilla which is not preformed in cartilage cells requires further explanation and Miles (1950) considered in detail the various mechanisms by which cartilage could appear in this location. He suggested that cartilaginous remnants might be carried into the maxilla in the fourth month of development by the outgrowth from the nasal capsule which ultimately develops into the maxillary sinus.

Behaviour

The rate of growth of chondrosarcoma can be extremely variable. In the nasal region it is commonly a slowly growing tumour, the time interval being measured in years but, occasionally, rapid growth may occur leading to the patient's demise in a matter of months. Local invasion leads to multiple involvement of bones and

cavities which is often apparent at presentation. Local recurrence is frequent, sometimes after many years so that five-year cure rates are of limited value. Evans et al. (1977) found no correlation between recurrence and histological grading. Systemic metastasis may occur particularly to the lungs (Batsakis and Dito, 1962; Henderson and Dahlin, 1963; Evans et al., 1977). The last mentioned authors found a significant correlation between metastasis and histological grading; their grade I showing no metastases whilst grade III produced 71 per cent.

In the general context, Evans et al. (1977) also found a significant correlation between survival and histological pattern. Their overall survival rates, tumours of all sites, were 77 per cent at five years and 67 per cent at ten years but ten year survival rates were 83 per cent for grade I, 64 per cent for grade II and 29 per cent for grade III. In the nose and sinuses, survival is not greatly different from that of other locations. Fu and Perzin (1974) found a five year survival rate of 57 per cent whilst an analysis by these authors of 16 reported cases have a five year survival rate of 62 per cent. The I.L.O. cases illustrate the extreme variability; one ethmoidal and one antral tumour have survived without recurrence for 19 and 10 years respectively; the other ethmoidal tumour grew rapidly, invading the undersurface of the brain (Fig.

20.10) and leading to the death of the patient in four months from the time of presentation.

As regards treatment, the main reliance is on surgery since chondrosarcomas are generally regarded as being radio-resistant although there have been occasional claims to the contrary (Harmer, 1935; Paddison, 1971).

BIBLIOGRAPHY

Barnes R, Catto M 1966 Chondrosarcoma of bone. Journal of Bone and Joint Surgery 48B: 729–764

Batsakis J G, Dito W R 1962 Chondrosarcoma of the maxilla. Archives of Otolaryngology 75: 55–61

Cohen J, d'Angio G J 1961 Unusual bone tumours after roentgen therapy of children. American Journal of Roentgenology 86: 502–512

Dahlin D C 1956 Chondromyxoid fibroma of bone with emphasis on the morphological relationship to benign chondroblastoma. Cancer 9: 195–203

Dahlin D C, Henderson E D 1962 Mesenchymal chondrosarcoma. Cancer 15: 410–417

Evans H L, Ayala A G, Romsdahl M M 1977 Prognostic factors in chondrosarcoma of bone. Cancer 40: 818–831

Fu Y, Perzin K H 1974 Non-epithelial tumours of the nasal cavity, paranasal sinuses and nasopharynx. III Cartilaginous tumours. Cancer 34: 453–463

Harmer W D 1935 Treatment of malignant disease of the upper jaw. Lancet 1: 129–133

Hatcher C H 1945 Development of sarcoma in bone subjected to roentgen or radium irradiation. Journal of Bone and Joint Surgery 27: 179–195

Heath C 1887 Lectures on diseases of the jaws. British Journal of Dental Science 30: 756–761

Henderson E D, Dahlin D C 1963 Chondrosarcoma of bone – a study of 288 cases. Journal of Bone and Joint Surgery 45A: 1450–1458

Jaffe H L, Lichtenstein L 1948 Chondromyxoid fibroma of bone. Archives of Pathology 45: 541–551

Lichtenstein L, Bernstein D 1959 unusual benign and malignant chondroid tumours of bone. Cancer 12: 1142–1157

Lichtenstein L, Jaffe H L 1943 Chondrosarcoma of bone. American Journal of Pathology 19: 553–574

Miles A E W 1950 Chondrosarcoma of the maxilla. British Dental Journal 88: 257–269

Mollison W M 1916 Some cases of growth of the upper jaw and ethmoid region. Dental Record 36: 44–47

Morgan 1836 Exostosis of the bones of the face. Guy's Hospital Reports 1: 403–406

Morgan 1842 Case follow-up. Guy's Hospital Reports 7: 491

Olszewski W 1969 Chondrosarcoma mesenchymale Patologia Polska 20: 23–27

O'Neal L W, Ackerman L V 1952 Chondrosarcoma of bone. Cancer 5: 551–557

Paddison G M, Hanks G E 1971 Chondrosarcoma of the maxilla. Cancer 28: 616–619

Paget J 1870 Cartilaginous tumours. Lectures on surgical pathology, 3rd edn. Longmans Green & Co pp 498–528

Phemister D B 1930 Chondrosarcoma of bone. Surgery, Gynecology and Obstetrics 50: 216–233

Salvador A H, Beabout J W, Dahlin D C 1971 Mesenchymal chondrosarcoma. Cancer 28: 605–615

Schutt P G, Frost H M 1971 Chrondromyxoid fibroma. Clinical Orthopaedics 78: 323–329

Volkmann R 1855 Akutes schmerzhaftes Enchondrom des Metacarpus; Enchondrom der Lunge. Deutsche Klinik 7: 577–578

Wirth J E, Shimkin M B 1943 Chondrosarcoma of nasopharynx simulating juvenile angiofibroma. Archives of Pathology 36: 83–88

Additional references

Aretsky P J, Kantu K, freund R H, Polisar I A 1970 Chondrosarcoma of the nasal septum. Annals of Otology, Rhinology and Laryngology 79: 382–388

Coates H L, Pearson B W, Devine K D, Unni K K 1977 Chondrosarcoma of the nasal cavity, paranasal sinuses and nasopharynx. Transactions of the American Academy of Ophthalmology and Otology 84: 919–926

Coyas A J 1965 Chondrosarcoma of the nose. Journal of Laryngology and Otology 79: 69–72

Faccini J M, Williams J L 1973 Nasal chondroma. Journal of Laryngology and Otology 87: 811–815

Gray R, Leonard G 1977 Chondrosarcoma of the nasal septum. Journal of Laryngology and Otology 91: 427–431

Hickey H L 1940 Chondroma of ethmoid. Archives of Otolaryngology 31: 645–652

Hopmann E 1931 Enchondrom des Keilbeins, der Siebbeine und der Nasenscheidewand. Zeitschrift fur Laryngologie, Rhinologie und Otologie 21: 454–458

Howarth W 1930 Chondroma of the nasal septum. Journal of Laryngology and Otology 45: 191–192

Jaffe H L, Lichtenstein L 1943 Solitary enchondroma of bone. Archives of Surgery 46: 480ff

Jones H M 1973 Cartilaginous tumours of the head and neck. Journal of Laryngology and Otology 87: 135–151

Keiller V H 1925 Cartilaginous tumours of bone. Surgery, Gynecology and Obstetrics 40: 510–521

Klaue H 1924 Ein Chondrom des rechten Siebbeins. Zeitschrift fur Laryngologie, Rhinologie, Otologie und ihre Grenzgebiete 13: 121–127

Kragh L V, Dahlin D C, Erich J B 1960 cartilaginous tumours of the jaws and facial regions. American Journal of Surgery 99: 852–856

Lapidot A, Ramm C, Fani K 1966 Chondrosarcoma of maxilla. Journal of Laryngology and Otology 80: 743–747

Lott S, Bordley J E 1972 A radiosensitive chondrosarcoma of the sphenoid sinus and base of skull. laryngoscope 82: 57–60

Menne F R, Frank W W 1937 So-called primary chondroma of ethmoid. Archives of Otolaryngology 26: 170–178

Paradzik 1929 Uber ein Chondrom des Siebbeins. Zeitschrift fur Hals-, Nasen- und Ohrenheilkunde 22: 505–506

Podesta E 1927 Sopra un caso di encondroma delle fossa nasali. Archivio Italiano di Otologia, Rinologia e Laringologia 38: 548–582

Sandler H C 1957 Chondrosarcoma of maxilla. Oral Surgery, Oral Medicine and Oral Pathology 10: 97–103

Sicard J 1897 Des tumeurs cartilagineuses (enchondromes) des fosses nasales. Thèse, Paris, No. 235, Bailière et filsUffenorde W 1908 Die Chondrome der Nasenhöhle und Mitteilung eines Falles von Enchondrom des Siebbeins mit allgemeiner Besprechung der Operationsmethoden für die Nasennebenhöhle. Archive für Laryngologie und Rhinologie 20: 255–274

Wolfowitz B L 1973 Osteosarcoma and chondrosarsoma of the maxilla. Journal of Laryngology and Otology 87: 409–416

21

Osteogenic tumours of the nose and sinuses

OSTEOMAS OF THE NOSE AND SINUSES

Introduction

Benign osseous tumours of the cranio-facial bones have been recognized for a very long time. Baillie (1799) illustrated a massive ivory tumour of the fronto-ethmoid region which had grown into the orbits and the cranial cavity. One of the earliest detailed descriptions was that of Hilton (1836) who reported an enormous tumour in the naso-antroethmoidal region which had been growing slowly for over 20 years in a young male adult. The tumour finally fell out of his face and was found to have a circumference of more than 28 centimetres. It was described as having an ivory consistency and weighed 418 grams. Reported involvement of the paranasal cavities soon began to indicate the frontal sinus as the principal location and Harris (1928) reviewed osteomata in this site collected over a period of about 50 years. Malan (1938) published an even larger review covering all the paranasal sinuses.

Incidence

Osteomata occur predominantly in skull bones and large scale surveys of radiographs of paranasal sinuses (Childrey, 1939; Eckel and Palm, 1959) revealed the presence of such tumours in about 0.4 per cent of the cases examined. Fu and Perzin (1974) found 31 osteomata amongst their 256 non-epithelial tumours (12 per cent). In the I.L.O. material there were 23 osteomata constituting about two per cent of all tumours of the nose and sinuses and about nine per cent of all non-epithelial tumours.

Clinical

These tumours tend to be encountered largely in middle age. Samy and Mostafa (1971), in a review of 128 osteomata of the sinuses, noted a high incidence in the second and fourth decades, rising to a maximum in the fourth with a predominance of males (1.7:1). In the I.L.O. cases the peak occurrence was also in the fourth decade with a male to female ratio of 2:1. The cases

reported by Fu and Perzin (1974) ranged in age from 32 to 64 years with a predominance of females.

The tumours are often asymptomatic in the early stages but slow expansile growth may lead to local pain or headache and encroachment on adjacent areas may result in disturbance of anatomical structures such as displacement of the eye. External swelling may be present and X-rays commonly show sharply defined opacities. In the I.L.O. material, local swelling was present in 45 per cent, pain or headache in 41 per cent and nasal obstruction in 23 per cent; one case had proptosis.

Anatomical site of origin

The commonst site of origin is undoubtedly the frontal sinus. In a review of 653 published cases, Eckel and Palm (1959) found osteomata in the frontal sinus in 51.9 per cent, the ethmoid sinuses in 22 per cent, the maxillary sinus in 5.1 per cent, the sphenoid sinus in 1.7 per cent and the nasal cavity in 0.6 per cent, the remainder being of external or indeterminate origin. In more recent times, however, the relative positions of the antrum and ethmoids have been reversed (Samy and Mostafa, 1971; Fu and Perzin, 1974). The nasal cavity and the sphenoid sinus have clearly emerged as rare sites of origin. Guthrie (1930) reported an osteoma of the posterior part of the nasal septum whilst Mikaelian, Lewis and Behringer (1976) presented the postmortem findings in a case of osteoma of the sphenoid sinus.

A proportion of tumours in the frontal sinus arise in the region of the junction with the ethmoid bone but a considerable number arise from the roof, the floor and the interfrontal septum (Eckel and Palm, 1959). Of the 23 cases in the I.L.O. material, 22 tumours originated in the frontal sinus (in various positions) and one in the ethmoid region. At the time of presentation, some tumours have already involved more than one cavity. Thus Leroux (1956) reported an osteoma arising in the anterior wall of the sphenoid sinus and growing into the upper part of the nasal cavity whilst, in a more common situation, Olumida, Fajemisin and Adeloye (1975) described a fronto-ethmoidal tumour. A number of reports of such tumours have appeared in the literature and presumably reflect origin at the junction of the frontal and ethmoid bones.

Multiple osteomata in the paranasal sinuses are uncommon but, when present, may be associated with polyposis of the large intestine, subcutaneous desmoid tumours and epidermoid cysts (Fitzgerald, 1943; Gardner and Plenk, 1952). The inheritance is through a simple dominant gene and, in so far as the polyposis is linked to colonic carcinoma, cases of multiple osteomata should be fully investigated.

Gross appearances

Considerable variation in size has been reported (Malan, 1938), the tumours commonly ranging from about 0.5 to several centimetres in maximum diameter. The massive tumours seen in former times are no longer encountered and were obviously related to late presentation and diagnosis. Where the tumour presents a free unrestrained surface, it is often lobulated (Fig. 21.1) the consistency is hard and the cut surface shows either a solid ivory-like appearance or a coarse granularity due to trabeculated structure (Fig. 21.2).

Histopathology

The microscopical picture shows an element of variability, not only from one tumour to another but often within the same lesion, especially in those arising in the frontal sinus. Various histological classifications have been suggested; Malan (1938) offered four subdivisions comprising eburnated, compact, spongy and mixed whilst Fu and Perzin (1974) divided their cases into ivory, mature (cancellous) and fibrous. The concensus of opinion is that there are two main structural types, the solid, ivory or eburnated and the coarsely trabeculated or cancellous.

The ivory type shows solid bone with irregularly disposed small vascular spaces (Fig. 21.3). The bone is usually mature with lamellar structure but areas of woven bone may be present. There is usually little or no osteoblastic activity and numbers of irregular cement lines may be present. The cancellous type shows usually coarse trabeculae with predominantly lamellar structure and irregular cement lines (Fig. 21.4). Definitive osteoblasts may be seen lining the bone fragments with marginal osteoid production, indicating active apposition (Fig. 21.5). Interosseous spaces of varying size may often contain distended thin-walled vessels in a stroma ranging from loose connective tissue to cellular, dense fibrous tissue (Fig. 21.6). The latter may sometimes be a dominant feature resulting in the use of the label 'fibrous osteoma' though it is not generally recognized as a separate entity (Jaffe, 1958). The presence of bone marrow in the interosseous spaces is not an integral

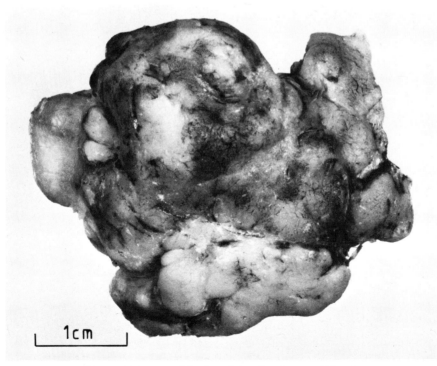

1cm

Fig. 21.1 Osteoma of the frontal sinus in a 56 year-old female.

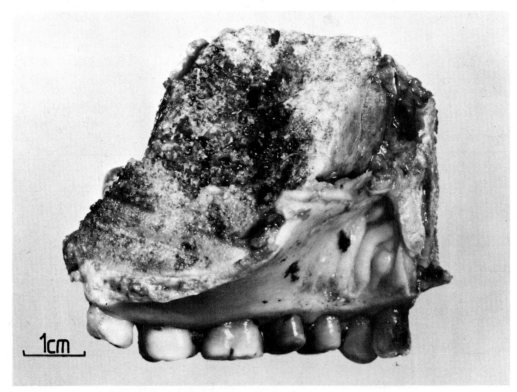

Fig. 21.2 Osteoma of the maxillary sinus in a 43 year-old female.

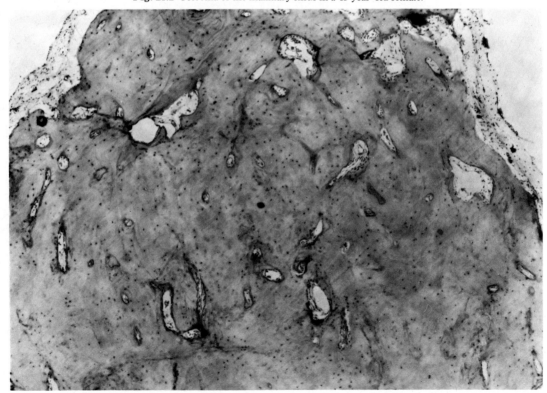

Fig. 21.3 Compact (ivory) osteoma of the frontal sinus in a 52 year-old male. M ×55

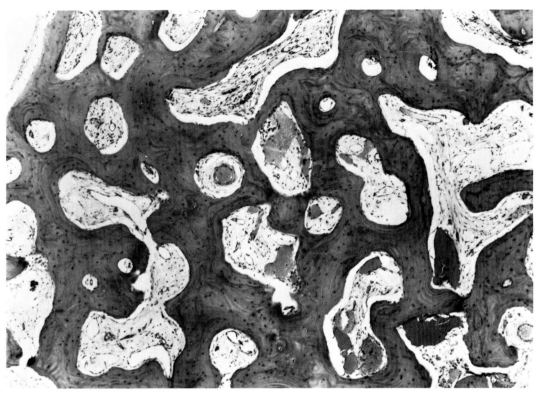

Fig. 21.4 Cancellous osteoma of the maxillary sinus in a 43 year-old female (see Fig. 21.2) showing lamellar bone with loose connective tissue spaces. M ×55

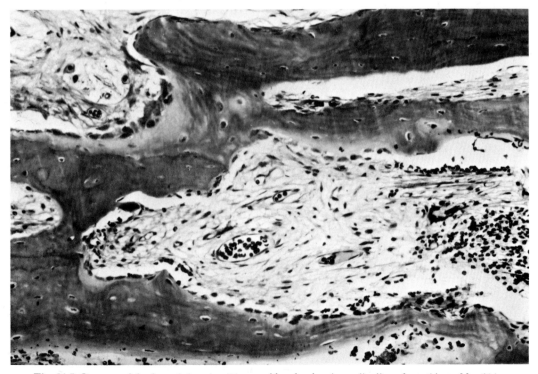

Fig. 21.5 Osteoma of the frontal sinus in a 54 year-old male, showing palisading of osteoblasts. M ×214

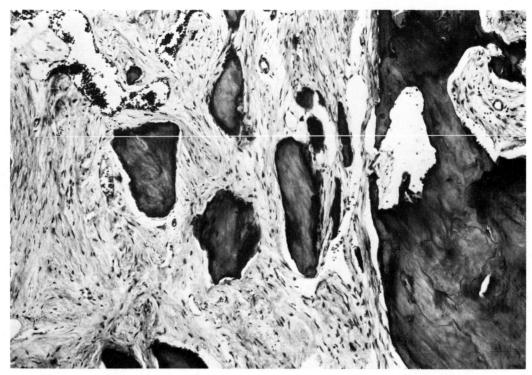

Fig. 21.6 Fibrous osteoma of the frontal sinus in a 30 year-old male, showing a densely fibrous stroma. M × 134

feature and probably represents a junctional zone with normal bone.

There is frequently a mixed picture giving an impression of a continuous spectrum from ivory to cancellous types. In the I.L.O. material, over 50 per cent of cases showed such a pattern.

Aetiology and pathogenesis

Osteomata are largely confined to the bones of the skull which have a somewhat complex system of development. The widely held view is that these tumours are developed from cartilage and the direct apposition of cartilaginous and membranous bones may result in the enclavement of cartilaginous fragments in the membranous portion. The other two theories of origin are trauma and infection. The evidence for injury being a significant factor is inadequate and unconvincing. The infective theory is based on the belief that local inflammation may provoke abnormal activity in the periosteum with resulting osteogenesis. However, the protagonists may well have confused cause with effect. There is an association between osteomata and infection in a small number of cases; Mehta and Grewal (1963) found 50

osteomata amongst 5086 patients with symptoms of sinusitis. The infection may nevertheless be secondary, having been predisposed to by inadequate drainage.

Behaviour

Osteomata are slowly growing tumours which in the early stages may give no indication of their presence. Later, the expanding lesion may give rise to pressure effects leading to bone erosion or displacement of anatomical structures, e.g. proptosis. Obstruction of ostia may lead to the development of a mucocele (Poole, Potanos and Kreuger, 1962) and subsequent infection may result in a pyocele. Occasionally, upward extension into the cranial cavity may lead to erosion of the dura mater, fistulous communication between the sinus and the brain producing a pneumocele, brain abscess or meningitis with concomitant neurological disturbance (Bartlett, 1971).

Inasmuch as the treatment of these tumours is limited to local excision which may or may not be technically simple, total extirpation cannot always be guaranteed. Nevertheless, recurrence is rarely seen, thus reflecting the essentially benign nature of the lesion.

BIBLIOGRAPHY

Baillie M 1799 Series of engravings accompanied with explanations intended to illustrate the morbid anatomy of some of the most important parts of the human body. Fasciculus 10, Fig. 2. W Bulmer & Co

Bartlett J R 1971 Intracranial neurological complications of frontal and ethmoidal osteomas. British Journal of Surgery 58: 607–613

Childrey J H 1939 Osteoma of the sinuses, the frontal and sphenoid bone. Archives of Otolaryngology 30: 63–72

Eckel W, Palm D 1959 Statistische und röntgenologische Untersuchungen zu einigen Fragen des Nebenhöhlenosteoms. Archiv für Ohren-, Nasen-, Kehlkopfheilkunde 174: 440–457

Fitzgerald G M 1943 Multiple composite odontomes coincident with other tumorous conditions. Journal of the American Dental Association 30: 1408–1417

Fu Y, Perzin K H 1974 non-epithelial tumours of the nasal cavity, paranasal sinuses and nasopharynx; II osseous and fibro-osseous lesions. Cancer 33: 1289–1305

Gardner E J, Plenk H P 1952 Hereditary pattern for multiple osteomas in a family group. American Journal of Human Genetics 4: 31–36

Guthrie T 1930 A case of osteoma of the nasal septum. Journal of Laryngology and Otology 45: 189–190

Harris R 1928 Osteoma of the frontal sinus. Laryngoscope 38: 331–346

Hilton J 1836 A large bony tumour of the face. Guy's Hospital Reports 1: 493–506

Jaffe H L 1958 Tumours and tumourous conditions of the bones and joints. Lea and Febiger, Philadelphia

Leroux L 1956 Ostéome naso-sphenoïdal. Annales d'Otolaryngologie 73: 310–311

Malan E 1938 Chirurgia degli osteomi delle cavite pneumatiche perifacciali. Archivio Italiano di Chirurgia 48: 1–124

Mehta B S, Grewal G S 1963 Osteoma of the paranasal sinuses along with a case report of an orbito-ethmoidal osteoma. Journal of Laryngology and Otology 77: 601–610

Olumida A A, Fajemisin A A, Adeloye A 1975 Osteoma of the ethmofrontal sinus. Journal of Neurosurgery 42: 343–345

Pool J L, Potanos J N, Kreuger E G 1962 Osteomas and mucoceles of the frontal paranasal sinuses. Journal of Neurosurgery 19: 130–135

Samy L L, Mostafa H 1971 Osteomata of the nose and paranasal sinuses with a report on twenty-one cases. Journal of Laryngology and Otology 85: 449–469

Additional references

Arnold J 1873 Zwei Osteome der Stirnhöhlen. Archiv für Pathologische Anatomie 57: 145–163

Bickett J 1871 Exostosis of the frontal bone growing into the cranial cavity. Guy's Hospital Gazette 16: 503–520

Karmody C S 1969 Osteoma of the maxillary sinus. Laryngoscope 79: 427–434

Seward M H 1965 An osteoma of maxilla. British Dental Journal 118: 27–30

Souček C D 1974 Pneumocephalus with osteomas. Journal Kansas Medical Society 75: 123–124

OSTEOID OSTEOMA AND BENIGN OSTEO-BLASTOMA

Introduction

The term osteoid osteoma was first introduced by Jaffe in 1935 although Bergstrand described two cases in 1930. In the course of subsequent studies, there came to light another bone lesion which was very similar histologically but differed in its clinical and radiological presentation. Initially, the latter lesion was designated osteogenic fibroma by Lichtenstein (1951) and giant osteoid osteoma by Dahlin and Johnson (1954) but was subsequently named benign osteoblastoma by Jaffe (1956) and Lichtenstein (1956).

Incidence

Neither of these bone lesions is very common and occurrence in the nasal or paranasal region would appear to be a rare event. Byers (1968) noted that the occurrence of osteoid osteoma was nearly three times as frequent as that of benign osteoblastoma.

Clinical features

The age distribution of osteoid osteoma shows a maximum occurrence in the second decade with very few cases over the age of 40 years and a male predominance of about two to one (Jaffe, 1945; Sherman, 1947; Flaherty, Pugh and Dockerty, 1956). Benign osteoblastoma shows a similar age distribution but without the predominance of males (Jaffe, 1956; Lichtenstein, 1956).

The common form of presentation is pain which is often more severe in the osteoid osteoma, causing the patient to wake up during the night. The benign osteoblastoma reported by Fu and Perzin (1974) presented with painless displacement of the eye.

Radiological appearances have presented a variable pattern but the common finding in both conditions is a localized lesion. Osteoid osteoma often shows a radiolucent area surrounded by a zone of increased density, with or without some central opacity but the extent of the surrounding bone reaction may depend on the site of the lesion (Flaherty at el., 1956). The radiographic features of the benign osteoblastoma have been discussed by Lichtenstein (1956) and by Pochaczevsky, Yen and Sherman (1960) and there are clearly differing views on the specificity of the pattern observed. This lesion is less often demarcated by surrounding sclerosis though it may exhibit central opacity.

Anatomical site of origin

About two-thirds of all osteoid osteomas occur in the lower limbs but, although Flaherty et al. (1956) recorded one such lesion in the mandible, there have been no reports of occurrence in the nasal or paranasal region. Benign osteoblastoma shows a predilection for the vertebral column though other sites are also affected including the head region, especially the calvarium (Pochaczevsky et al., 1960; Lichtenstein and Sawyer, 1964). Involvement of the maxilla has been reported by Borello and Sedano (1967) and by Kent, Castro and Girotti (1969) whilst Fu and Perzin (1974) found one such tumour in the ethmoid region. In the I.L.O. material, there was one case involving the frontal sinus.

Gross appearances

Byers (1968) emphasized the distinction between osteoid osteoma and benign osteoblastoma on the basis of size. Those lesions of one centimetre or less in diameter more or less fit the clinical and radiological pattern of osteoid osteoma whilst those of more than one centimetre in diameter appear to fall into the group of benign osteoblastomas. The tissue as removed appears granular and gritty and its marked vascularity imparts a red or brown colour.

Histopathology

Microscopically, there are no reliable distinguishing features. Numerous trabeculae of osteoid or immature bone form a relatively regular pattern and are surrounded by osteoblasts. The intervening spaces are occupied by a highly vascular stroma containing numbers of multinucleated giant cells resembling osteoclasts (Fig. 21.7). The vessels are usually thin walled and engorged whilst stromal cells may resemble osteoblasts and may form compact groups with or without deposition of osteoid. Irregular calcification of osteoid trabeculae is often seen.

The picture may be confused, particularly on the basis of small biopsies, with giant cell tumours or osteogenic sarcoma. Apart from clinical or radiological features, the presence of osteoid or bony trabeculae would be inconsistent with giant cell tumour whilst the absence of nuclear irregularity and paucity of mitoses amongst the stromal cells, together with the fairly regular trabecular arrangement, would make osteogenic sarcoma less likely. The aetiology of these two lesions is completely unknown and although early minority views suggested an inflammatory process it is now generally accepted that both are neoplastic.

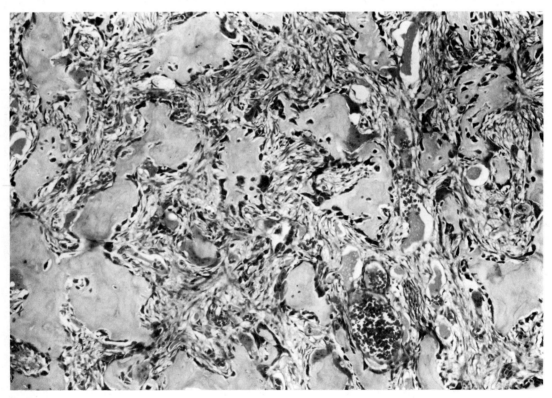

Fig. 21.7 Benign osteoblastoma of the frontal sinus in a 44 year-old male showing palisading of osteoblasts around masses of osteoid in a fibrous stroma. M × 130

Behaviour

Sherman (1947) suggested that the low age distribution might imply that the lesions tended to regress though there is no clear evidence of such an event since most cases are subjected to local surgery, following which the lesion does not recur (Lichtenstein, 1956).

BIBLIOGRAPHY

Bergstrand H 1930 Über eine eigenartige wahrscheinlich bisher nicht beschriebene osteoblastische Krankheit in den langen Knochen der Hand und des Fusses. Acta Radiologica 11: 596–613

Borello E D, Sedano H O 1967 Giant osteoid osteoma of the maxilla. Oral Surgery, Oral Medicine and Oral Pathology 23: 563–566

Byers P D 1968 Solitary benign osteoblastic lesions of bone: Osteoid osteoma and benign osteoblastoma. Cancer 22: 43–57

Dahlin D C, Johnson E W 1954 Giant osteoid osteoma. Journal of Bone and Joint Surgery 36A: 559–572

Flaherty R A, Pugh D G, Dockerty M B 1956 Osteoid osteoma. American Journal of Roentgenology 76: 1041–1051

Fu Y, Perzin K H 1974 Non-epithelial tumors of the nasal cavity, paranasal sinuses and nasopharynx. II. Osseous and fibroosseous lesions. Cancer 33: 1289–1305

Jaffe H L 1935 Osteoid osteoma. A benign osteoblastic tumor composed of osteoid and atypical bone. Archives of Surgery 31: 709–728

Jaffe H L 1945 Osteoid osteoma of bone. Radiology 45: 319–334

Jaffe H L 1956 Benign osteoblastoma. Bulletin of the Hospital for Joint Diseases 17: 141–151

Kent J N, Castro H F, Girotti W R 1969 Benign osteoblastoma of the maxilla. Oral Surgery, Oral Medicine and Oral Pathology 27: 209–219

Lichtenstein L 1951 Classification of primary tumors of bone. Cancer 4: 335–341

Lichtenstein L 1956 Benign osteoblastoma. Cancer 9: 1044–1052

Lichtenstein L, Swayer W R 1964 Benign osteoblastoma. Journal of Bone and Joint Surgery 46A: 755–765

Pochaczevsky R, Yen Y M, Sherman R S 1960 The roentgen appearance of benign osteoblastoma. Radiology 75: 429–437

Sherman M S 1947 Osteoid osteoma. Journal of Bone and Joint Surgery 29: 918–930

OSTEOGENIC SARCOMA OF THE NOSE AND SINUSES

The early history of osteogenic sarcoma is necessarily obscure because although sarcomatous tumours have been recognized for over a hundred years no precise distinction was made between osteoblastic, fibroblastic or chondroblastic varieties. It is only in relatively recent times that osteogenic sarcoma has been defined in terms of osteoid or bone production (Lichtenstein, 1965).

Terminology

The terms osteosarcoma and osteogenic sarcoma are used synonymously but the latter is preferable in so far as it emphasizes the basic characteristic of these tumours. Although they may be divided histologically according to the predominant form of differentiation, expressions such as 'osteo-chondro-fibrosarcoma' are no longer acceptable.

Incidence

Although the commonest primary tumour of the bony skeleton, it is much less common in the nose and sinuses. Hatfield and Schulz (1970) estimated the incidence of osteogenic sarcoma, irrespective of location, as about 0.5 per 100 000 of the population. In a review of 1000 bone tumours, Christiansen (1925) found 441 osteogenic sarcomas and of these ten had their origin in the maxilla whilst a further eight involved other bones of the skull. More than 50 per cent of osteogenic sarcomas involve the long bones but between six and seven per cent have their origin in the jaws (Garrington, Scofield, Cornyn and Hooker, 1967; Curtis, Elmore and Sotereanos, 1974). The upper jaw is affected less frequently than the lower. Richards and Coleman (1957) reported 17 cases of osteogenic sarcoma of the jaws, of which only four involved the maxilla. Reported examples of osteogenic sarcoma of the maxilla do not necessarily involve the maxillary sinus, thereby reducing still further the number of cases which may come within the purview of the Ear, Nose and Throat Surgeon. Fu and Perzin (1974) found 11 cases amongst their 256 non-epithelial tumours (about 4 per cent). In the present authors' material, osteogenic sarcoma of the nose and sinuses accounted for 2.5 per cent of non-epithelial tumours and about 0.5 per cent of all tumours in the region.

Clinical features

Osteogenic sarcoma, in the general context, shows a peak age distribution in the second decade (Christiansen, 1925; Dahlin and Coventry, 1967) but in those cases involving the nasal and paranasal region the mode has shifted to the third decade. There is, nevertheless, a wide scatter as indicated in the six cases reported by LiVolsi (1977) where the ages ranged from 10 to 75 years. Caron, Hajdu and Strong (1971) found no significant difference in age incidence in relation to sites of origin within the head region. Most series show a male predominance but Dehner (1973) reported an osteogenic sarcoma in the maxilla of a girl of 15 years.

The common presenting feature is a local swelling. Caron et al. (1971) noted swelling with or without pain in 13 out of 15 maxillary tumours. Early symptoms may include pain and loosening of teeth or dentures. Epistaxis or bloody nasal discharge may be the presenting signs before external swelling is apparent but involvement of the nasal cavity will sooner or later lead to obstruction. Diplopia and proptosis result from orbital extension.

Serum calcium and alkaline phosphatase levels are sometimes raised (McKenna, Schwinn, Soong and Higinbotham, 1966; Caron et al., 1971).

Anatomical site of origin

Published accounts reveal the maxilla to be the principal location within the nasal and paranasal region and nearly 100 osteogenic sarcomas of this bone have been reported. The series presented by Kragh, Dahlin and Erich (1958) contained 23 maxillary tumours (nine involving the antrum) and two ethmoidal neoplasms. Garrington et al. (1967) included 18 maxillary tumours in their series of osteosarcomas of the jaws but only four of these appear to have involved the maxillary sinus. On the other hand, seven out of nine maxillary tumours reported by Roca, Smith and Jing (1970) had involved the antrum. Wolfe and Platt (1949) reported two osteogenic sarcomas of the nasal bones. In the series published by Fu and Perzin (1974), seven involved the antrum, two the nasal cavity, one the ethmoid region whilst one showed multiple siting. In the present authors' material, five had their origin in the antrum and one in the nasal cavity. The frontal sinus appears to be a rare site of election. Caron et al. (1971) reported frontal bone involvement in their series whilst Bone, Biller and Harris (1973) described a tumour involving the frontal sinus in a 58 year-old woman.

Gross appearance

The naked eye features vary according to the composition of the tumour. Commonly, the tissue presents a firm grey gritty mass which may be mottled by vascularity and haemorrhage. Predominance of fibroblastic or chondroblastic elements may produce resemblance to tumours of those types.

Histopathology

Microscopically, the tumour is composed of frankly malignant, usually spindle-shaped or pleomorphic mesenchymal cells associated with osteoid and immature neoplastic bone formation (Fig. 21.8). The pleomorphic tumour cells contain large, angular, hyperchromatic nuclei and mitoses may be numerous. Although malignant osteoplastic elements usually predominate, fibro-

blastic or chondroblastic differentiation is frequently observed and may give rise to errors in diagnosis on biopsy material (Fig. 21.9). The essential feature is the production of osteoid by the neoplastic cells and, once this has been established, the tumour is designated osteogenic sarcoma irrespective of the presence of other features consistent with fibro- or chondrosarcoma. The reported proportions of these differential elements has shown considerable variation. Thus Kragh et al. (1958) found chondroblastic differentiation in 50 per cent but osteoblastic differentiation was found in over 50 per cent by subsequent writers (Garrington et al., 1967; Dahlin and Coventry, 1967). Clearly, osteoid or bone formation by the tumour cells may be slight or intensive (Fig. 21.10). The primary maxillary lesion in one of the cases described by Fu and Perzin (1974) only showed fibrosarcoma in the biopsy specimen and osteogenic areas were identified only at autopsy in the pulmonary metastases. In another two of their cases only chondroblastic tissue was found in the biopsy material as was also found in one of the present authors' cases (Fig. 21.9).

The stroma is usually vascular in varying degree and areas of angiosarcomatous pattern may occur. Giant cells, which may be multi-nucleated, are not infrequently present and could occasionally cause confusion in diagnosis. Garrington et al. (1967) found such cells to be present in 42 per cent of cases. Electron microscopical studies by Ghadially and Mehta (1970) showed that the tumour cells resembled normal osteoblasts in so far as they were multi-processed and contained well marked Golgi complexes and abundant rough endoplastic reticulum. They deviated, however, due to de-differentiation with pleomorphic mitochondria, numerous free ribosomes, cytolysosomes and nuclear variations.

Aetiology and pathogenesis

Many osteogenic sarcomas appear to arise without any particular cause but a wide variety of aetiological factors have been put forward, including trauma, genetic factors, previously existing benign lesions and irradiation. Especially in the present context, the last mentioned factor is undoubtedly the most important.

The role of irradiation in the development of osteogenic sarcoma has been clearly established (Cahan, Woodward, Higinbotham, Stewart and Coley, 1948; Cruz, Coley and Stewart, 1957; Arlen, Higinbotham, Huvos, Marcove, Miller and Shah (1971). Radiotherapy had been given for either benign lesions or malignant, non-osteogenic tumours. A not inconsiderable proportion of extracranial sarcomas have resulted from irradiation of giant cell tumours of long bones whilst cranial osteogenic sarcomas have quite often developed after irradiation of retinoblastomas in childhood (Soloway, 1966). Cahan et al. (1948) included one case of ethmoidal sarcoma following irradiation of a retinoblastoma and

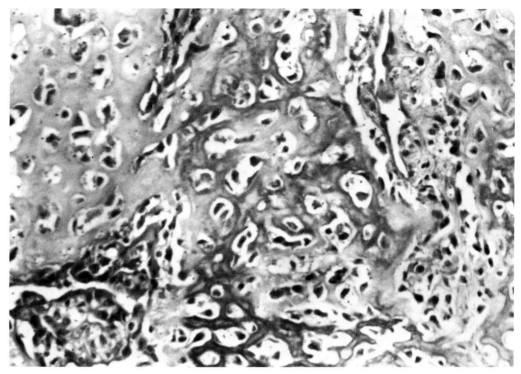

Fig. 21.8 Osteogenic sarcoma of the maxillary sinus in a 29 year-old male, showing osteoid production by tumour cells. M × 330

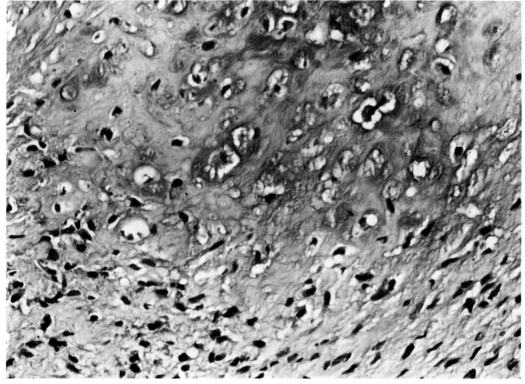

Fig. 21.9 Osteogenic sarcoma of the maxillary sinus in a 29 year-old male (see Fig. 21.8) showing a 'chondrosarcomatous' area. M × 425

other cases, arising in similar circumstances, have been reported (Skolnik, Fornatto and Heydemann, 1956; Hatfield and Schulz, 1970; LiVolsi, 1977). LiVolsi pointed out that 14 of the published cases of osteogenic sarcoma of the maxilla (including her own) had received irradiation, in five instances for retinoblastoma and in four for fibrous dysplasia. In their series of postradiation sarcomas, Sabanas, Dahlin, Childs and Ivins (1956) included two maxillary tumours whose primary diagnoses were fibrous dysplasia and giant cell reparative granuloma. The two cases of sarcoma of the nasal bones reported by Wolfe and Platt (1949) had been irradiated many years previously for intractable skin lesions. In the present authors' material, one case had been irradiated eleven years previously for a non-osteogenic tumour of the antrum which was thought to belong to the lymphoma group (Fig. 21.11). In the published cases, the interval between irradiation and the development of sarcoma has ranged widely from about five to forty years.

Schwartz and Alpert (1964) reviewed 26 sarcomas preceded by fibrous dysplasia of bone, adding two cases of their own. Some, including maxillary lesions, had progressed naturally to malignancy but nearly 40 per cent had been irradiated for their primary condition, as illustrated by the case reported by Yannopoulos, Bom, Griffiths and Crikelair (1964).

The propensity for Paget's Disease of bone to develop sarcoma has long been established. Jaffe and Selin (1951) considered that the incidence was between five and ten per cent in cases of polyostotic disease. Osteogenic sarcoma arising in Paget's Disease of the maxilla has been reported by Karpawich (1958) and LiVolsi (1977). One of the cases in the present authors' series was also associated with polyostotic Paget's Disease (Fig. 21.12).

As with many types of neoplasm, trauma has been invoked as a possible cause though the evidence is usually far from convincing. Badgley and Batts (1941) found a history of injury in 36 per cent of their cases but they pointed out that it was usually of a minor nature and often antedated the onset of symptoms by a matter of weeks. Although there have been several reports of familial occurrence of osteogenic sarcoma (Robbins, 1967), the tumours have all been extracranial.

Behaviour

The tumour may occupy the whole of the maxilla and may extend into the ethmoid sinuses, the orbit and the nasopharynx. Spread to the opposite side is not uncom-

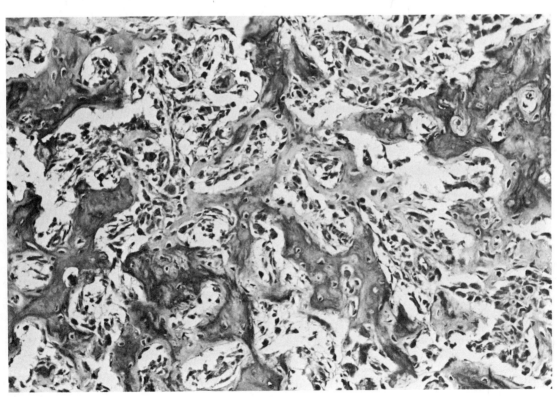

Fig. 21.10 Osteogenic sarcoma of the maxillary sinus in a 22 year-old female, showing irregular osteoid and bone production. M ×180

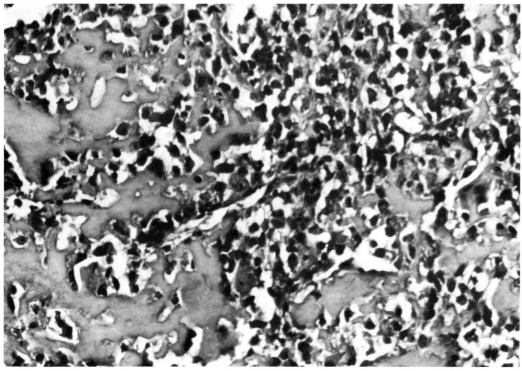

Fig. 21.11 Osteogenic sarcoma of the maxillary sinus in a 59 year-old female, 10 years after irradiation for a non-osteogenic tumour, showing marked osteoid production. M × 330

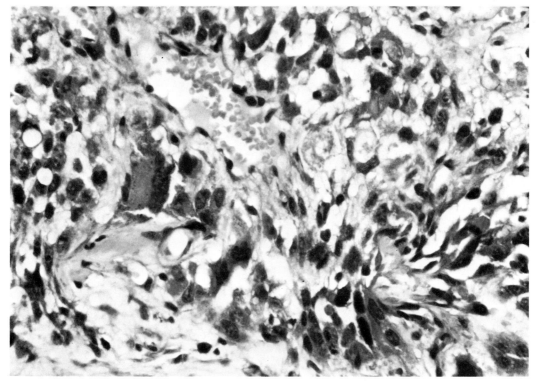

Fig. 21.12 Osteogenic sarcoma of the maxillary sinus in a 58 year-old female following Paget's Disease. Note intercellular hyaline material suggestive of osteoid. M × 325

mon and extension into adjacent soft tissues such as the cheek may also occur. One of Fu and Perzin's cases exhibited multiple involvement at presentation.

Metastasis to regional lymphnodes has been reported by several authors (Garrington et al., 1967; Caron et al., 1971; Fu and Perzin, 1974) but dissemination via the bloodstream is much more common, especially to the lungs, brain and other bones. Patients dying of osteogenic sarcoma very often have pulmonary metastases.

Recurrence is frequent and Caron et al. (1971) noted this event in 80 per cent of maxillary tumours. A number of workers have attempted histological grading (Meyerding, 1938; Kragh et al., 1958; Garrington et al., 1967; Dahlin and Coventry, 1967). Although it is admittedly

difficult to apply the method of Broders (1925) to non-epithelial tumours, the results of some of these workers showed some correlation with survival. Kragh et al. (1958) found an overall five year survival rate of about 31 per cent in sarcomas of the jaws and facial bones. Garrington et al. (1967) reported a five year survival rate in maxillary tumours of 25 per cent whilst Caron et al. (1971) found a rate of 33 per cent for sarcomas in the same site. Of the eleven cases reported by Fu and Perzin (1974) only one was known to be living after ten years. These authors emphasized the poorer prognosis when the nose and sinuses are involved. Only one of the present authors' cases has survived five years, three dying in less than twelve months.

BIBLIOGRAPHY

Arlen M, Higinbotham N L, Huvos A C, Marcove R C, Miller T, Shah I C 1971 Radiation-induced sarcoma of bone. Cancer 28: 1087–1099

Badgley C E, Batts M 1941 Osteogenic sarcoma. Archives of Surgery 43: 545–550

Bone R C, Biller H F, Harris B L 1973 Sarcoma of the frontal sinus. Annals of Otology, Rhinology and Laryngology 82: 162–165

Broders A C 1925 The grading of carcinoma. Minnesota Medicine 8: 726–730

Cahan W G, Woodward H Q, Higinbotham N L, Stewart F W, Coley B L 1948 Sarcoma arising in irradiated bone. Cancer 1: 3–29

Caron A S, Hajdu S I, Strong E W 1971 Osteogenic sarcoma of the facial and cranial bones. American Journal of Surgery 122: 719–725

Christiansen C F 1925 Bone tumours. Analysis of one thousand cases with special reference to location, age and sex. Annals of Surgery 81: 1074–1092

Cruz M, Coley B L, Stewart F W 1957 Postradiation bone sarcoma. Cancer 10: 72–88

Curtis M L, Elmore J S, Sotereanos G C 1974 Osteosarcoma of the jaws. Journal of Oral Surgery 32: 125–130

Dahlin D C, Coventry M B 1967 Osteogenic sarcoma. Journal of Bone and Joint Surgery 49A: 101–110

Dehner L P 1973 Tumours of the mandible and maxilla in children. II a study of 14 primary and secondary malignant tumors. Cancer 32: 112–120

Fu Y, Perzin K H 1974 non-epithelial tumors of the nasal cavity, paranasal sinuses and nasopharynx. Cancer 33: II. Osseous and Fibroosseous Lesions 1289–1305

Garrington G E, Scofield H H, Cornyn J, Hooker S P 1967 Osteosarcoma of the jaws. Cancer 20: 377–391

Ghadially F N, Mehta P N 1970 Ultrastructure of osteogenic sarcoma. Cancer 25: 1457–1467

Hatfield P M, Schulz M D 1970 Postirradiation sarcoma. Radiology 96: 593–602

Jaffe H L, Selin G 1951 Tumours of bones and joints. Bulletin of New York Academy of Medicine 27: 165–174

Karpawich A J 1958 Paget's disease with osteogenic sarcoma of maxilla. Oral Surgery, Oral Medicine and Oral Pathology 11: 827–834

Kragh L V, Dahlin D C, Erich J B 1958 Osteogenic sarcoma of the jaws and facial bones. American Journal of Surgery 96: 496–505

Lichtenstein L 1965 Bone tumours. 3rd C V Mosby

LiVolsi V A 1977 Osteogenic sarcoma of the maxilla. Archives of Otolaryngology 103: 485–488

McKenna R J, Schwinn C P, Soong K Y, Higinbotham N L 1966 Sarcomata of the osteogenic series. Journal of Bone and Joint Surgery 48A: 1–26

Meyerding H W 1938 The results of treatment of osteogenic sarcoma. Journal of Bone and Joint Surgery 20: 933–948

Richards W G, Coleman F L 1957 Osteogenic sarcoma of the jaw. Oral Surgery, Oral Medicine and Oral Pathology 10: 1156–1165

Robbins R 1967 Familial osteosarcoma. Journal of the American Medical Association 202: 1055

Roca A N, Smith J L, Jing B S 1970 Osteosarcoma and parosteal osteogenic sarcoma of the maxilla and mandible. American Journal of Clinical Pathology 54: 625–636

Sabanas A O, Dahlin D C, Childs D S, Ivins J C 1956 Postradiation sarcoma of bone. Cancer 9: 528–542

Schwartz D T, Alpert M 1964 The malignant transformation of fibrous dysplasia. American Journal of Medical Sciences 247: 1–20

Skolnik E M, Fornatto E J, Heydemann J 1956 Osteogenic sarcoma of the skull following irradiation. Annals of Otology, Rhinology and Laryngology 65: 915–936

Soloway H B 1966 Radiation-induced neoplasms following curative therapy for retinoblastoma. Cancer 19: 1984–1988

Wolfe J J, Platt W R 1949 Postirradiation osteogenic sarcoma of the nasal bone. Cancer 2: 438–446

Yannopoulos K, Bom A F, Griffiths C O, Crikelair G F 1964 Osteosarcoma arising in fibrous dysplasia of the facial bones. American Journal of Surgery 105: 556–564

Additional references

Coley B L, Stewart F W 1945 Bone sarcoma in Polyostotic fibrous dysplasia. Annals of Surgery 121: 872–881

Curtis M L, Elmore J S, Sotereanos G C 1974 Osteosarcoma of the jaws. Journal of Oral Surgery 32: 125–130

Dodge O G 1965 Tumours of the jaw, odontogenic tissues and
maxillary antrum (excluding Burkitt lymphoma) in
Uganda Africans. Cancer 18: 205–215

Finkelstein J B 1970 Osteosarcoma of the jaw bones.
Radiological Clinics of North America 8: 425–443

Harmon T P, Morton K S 1966 Osteogenic sarcoma in four
siblings. Journal of Bone and Joint Surgery 48B: 493–498

Price C H G 1955 Osteogenic sarcoma: an analysis of age and
sex incidence. British Journal of Cancer 9: 558–574

Steiner G C 1965 Postradiation sarcoma of bone. Cancer 18:
603–612

Zimmerman L E, Ingalls R 1957 Clinical pathologic
conference. American Journal of Ophthalmology 43: 417–
426

22

Miscellaneous mesenchymal tumours and tumour-like lesions

In this chapter are considered a variety of conditions, many of which are essentially non-neoplastic. Some tumours have been included for convenience of discussion relating particularly to their controversial nature.

GIANT CELL LESIONS OF THE NOSE AND SINUSES

Introduction
The existence of tumours or tumour-like lesions characterized by multinucleated giant cells has been recognized for well over a hundred years. The earliest histological description was by Lebert in 1845 but, in retrospect, it is clear that the gross appearances were described long before that date. Thus, Cooper and Travers (1818) illustrated what became known subsequently as 'osteoclastoma' in the upper end of the tibia and it is interesting to note that these authors also referred to tumour-like conditions occurring in the upper and lower jaws of children. Both cranial and extracranial lesions were subsequently correlated with the microscopical picture, dominated in varying degree by the giant cells whose supposed resemblance to the megakaryocytes of the bone marrow prompted Paget (1853) to use the term 'myeloid' tumour in connection with several cranial lesions involving the jaw bones. In 1860, Nélaton published a larger series of lesions of the upper and lower jaws under the title of 'tumeurs à myeloplaxes'. It is noteworthy that nearly all the conditions reported by Paget and Nélaton occurred in young patients, mostly in the second and third decades of life. Paget was of the opinion that these lesions in the jaw were of a benign character and, notwithstanding the subsequent use of the term 'giant cell sarcoma' by many writers, the extracranial lesions tended to be viewed in the same light (Bloodgood, 1910). By this time many of the tumours were recognized as arising in the epiphyses of long bones where their neoplastic nature was generally accepted but, in 1913, Barrie claimed that they should not be regarded as neoplasms but should be classified with inflammatory or granulomatous conditions under the label 'chronic haemorrhagic osteomyelitis'. Although this might seem relevant to the modern concept of craniofacial lesions, the cases on which this author based his view were entirely extracranial and his suggestion was strongly criticized by Stewart (1922) who accepted the neoplastic theory and proposed the term 'osteoclast sarcoma' which later became corrupted to 'osteoclastoma'. In 1924, Coley drew attention to the malignant behaviour of some of these tumours when occurring in long bones and reported metastasis in over ten per cent. Nevertheless, the concept of benign giant cell tumours of bone, particularly in the cranial region, persisted (Wattles, 1937 Peimer, 1954). In 1940, Jaffe, Lichtenstein and Portis drew attention to confusion with other giant cell lesions including hyperparathyroidism, xanthogranuloma and giant cell epulis. They pointed out that the term 'benign' could be misleading since some of the tumours were at least locally aggressive. Out of the continuing controversy there developed the impression that giant cell tumours of the jaws behaved more benignly than those in other parts (Berger, 1947).

A major landmark in the confused history of giant cell lesions was introduced by Jaffe (1953) who proposed the term 'giant cell reparative granuloma' to designate a rare condition involving the jaw bones. He regarded it as non-neoplastic and quite distinct from the giant cell tumour of which he had only seen one case in the skull. Undoubtedly, many of the earlier and even later reports of giant cell tumours of the cranio-facial bones were examples of reparative granuloma, thus accounting for their relatively benign behaviour but reflecting the lack of general agreement on the criteria of distinction. Argument has continued particularly on the issue as to whether the giant cell tumour of long bones occurs at all in the skull. In view of the literary confusion, it was considered more convenient to discuss the giant cell lesions together making points of delineation where ever possible.

Terminology
Many of the earlier labels, mentioned above, have long since been abandoned because their implications are no

longer acceptable and even 'osteoclastoma' finds less favour to-day. The label 'giant cell tumour of bone' should be confined to true neoplasms and only applied to cranial lesions when there is unequivocal identity with those tumours occurring in long bones. The name 'giant cell reparative granuloma of the jawbones' was recommended by Jaffe because it conveyed the more precise idea that the lesion is not a neoplasm in the true sense but represents a local reparative reaction. The lesion has been divided into central and peripheral types, the latter comprising the gingival epulides.

Incidence

Giant cell tumours of bone are not very common in any part of the skeleton. Emley (1971) found less than four per cent amongst nearly 4000 primary bone tumours at the Mayo Clinic. About three quarters of such tumours are located in the long bones, hence the proportion which might involve the walls of paranasal sinuses must be very small indeed. In fact, Bhaskar, Bernier and Godby (1959) denied the existence of such tumours in this region. In a re-evaluation of 66 giant cell lesions of the jaws, Austin, Dahlin and Royer (1959) found two cases which they regarded as genuine tumours in contrast with 64 examples of reparative granuloma. Fu and Perzin (1974) reported four cases of giant cell tumour involving the sinuses, amongst their 256 non-epithelial tumours.

It would seem that the majority of the giant cell lesions involving the cranio-facial bones belong to the reparative granuloma group. Waldron and Shafer (1966) found 32 cases of giant cell reparative granuloma amongst 22,000 oral and para-oral biopsies. In a series of 14 giant cell lesions of the jaws, Hamlin and Lund (1967) found ten reparative granulomas, two giant cell tumours and two 'brown tumours' of hyperparathyroidism. In the I.L.O. material there were two cases of giant cell reparative granuloma reported by Radcliffe and Friedmann (1957).

Clinical features

Attempts have been made to distinguish between true giant cell tumour and reparative granuloma on the basis of age distribution. The latter condition is essentially a disease of the young with a peak age in the second decade (Bhaskar et al, 1959; Austin et al, 1959; Waldron and Shafer, 1966) whereas patients with true giant cell tumours usually show a maximum frequency between the ages of 20 and 40 years (Murphy and Ackerman, 1956; Hutter, Worcester, Francis, Foote and Stewart, 1962; Sissons, 1966). Nevertheless, many reports indicate a considerable overlap; thus one of the four giant cell tumours reported by Fu and Perzin was only 12 years old, whilst four of the reparative granulomas reported by Hamlin and Lund (1967) ranged in age

from 31 to 60 years. The published series of giant cell reparative granuloma show a female predominance.

Whatever their precise nature, these giant cell lesions usually present as painless swellings often producing facial deformity (Fig. 22.1). Proptosis may result from involvement of the orbit. Growth is usually slow, the duration of symptoms being measured in months. The 'soap bubble' pattern of rarefaction in X-ray pictures is not specific.

Anatomical site of origin

In so far as acceptable giant cell tumours have been encountered in the skull, the most commonly reported site has been the maxillary sinus (Austin et al 1959; Friedberg, Eisenstein and Wallner, 1969; Fu and Perzin, 1974). Involvement of the ethmoid and frontal sinuses have been reported by Fu and Perzin (1974) and Hlaváček and Jolna (1974). Emley (1971) reported a giant cell tumour involving the sphenoid sinus and reviewed 13 other cases but it is by no means certain that a number of these were not examples of reparative granuloma.

The giant cell reparative granuloma is more common in the mandible than in the maxilla (Jaffe, 1953). In the 64 cases reported by Austin et al (1959) three involved predominantly the maxillary sinus. In the series reported by Waldron and Shafer (1966) about one third involved the maxilla and two thirds the mandible. Both the cases in the I.L.O. material involved the maxillary sinus.

Gross appearances

Distinction between the various types of giant cell lesion is not always possible to the naked eye. Soft grey tissue may be mottled by vascularity and haemorrhage. A reparative granuloma may have a firmer consistency then the giant cell tumour due to larger amounts of fibrous tissue but haemorrhage may be sufficiently marked in either to mimic the brown tumour of hyperparathyoidism.

Histopathology

The common feature is, of course, the presence of multinucleated giant cells which vary in number and distribution according to the type of lesion but may well be less important than other elements in the microscopical picture. In the true tumour, the giant cells are evenly distributed, the nuclei are regular, round or oval and are often present in very large numbers. The intervening tissue is highly cellular, being composed of mononuclear cells of varying shapes, closely packed with a notable absence of intercellular substance (Fig. 22.2). In the less aggressive tumours the nuclei of the stromal cells show little irregularity and tend to resemble those of the giant cells. In the more malignant types, the proportion of stromal cells is increased relative to the giant cells, with

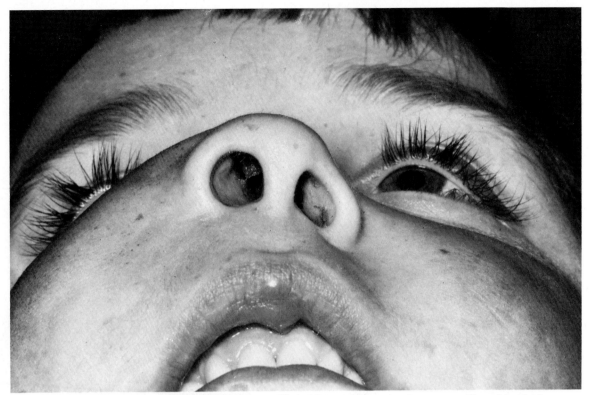

Fig. 22.1 Giant cell reparative granuloma of the maxilla in a 5 year-old boy, showing gross swelling of the cheek.

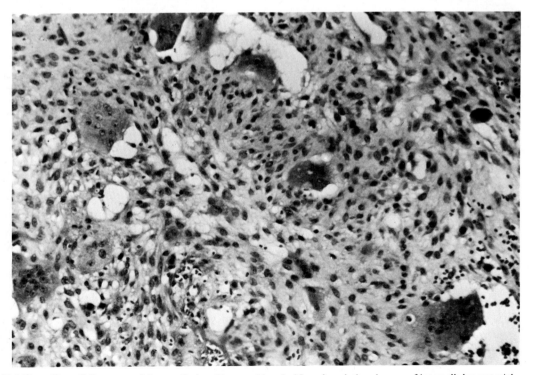

Fig. 22.2 True Giant Cell tumour of the maxilla in a 31 year-old male. Note the relative absence of intercellular material.
M ×224

greater nuclear irregularity and many mitoses. Osteoid or bone formation may be found on the periphery of the lesion where it represents reactive change in the adjacent bone. There may be many vessels lying among the stromal cells and focal haemorrhage is not uncommon.

In the reparative granuloma, the distribution of the giant cells takes the form of irregular aggregates often related to areas of haemorrhage whilst large areas are often devoid of such elements. The stroma contains spindle cells of fibroblastic type and appreciable amounts of collagen are present (Figs. 22.3 & 22.4). Occasional fine trabeculae of bone or osteoid (Fig. 22.5) may be present and deposits of iron pigment are seen as the result of invariable haemorrhage.

Differential diagnostic difficulties may be caused by the so-called 'brown tumour' of hyperparathyroidism (Fig. 22.6), often located in the skull and indistinguishable from reparative granuloma. It is essential in all giant cell lesions involving bone to undertake serum calcium and phosphorus estimations to confirm or exclude this possibility. The microscopical appearances of cherubism may also resemble reparative granuloma and the presence of foam cells may suggest another alternative-xanthogranuloma (Jaffe et al 1940). As has been pointed out by Van Nostrand (1976), any fibro-osseous lesion may contain giant cells. Foci of such cells may be found in

fibrous dysplasia of bone and in osteogenic sarcoma and alkaline phosphatase activity in the stromal cells could be a pointer to either of these conditions.

Small biopsies may be misleading in so far as they are not fully representative and may, at best, indicate the presence of some form of giant cell lesion. The final diagnosis may often require the close consultation of the surgeon, radiologist and pathologist.

The ultrastructure of the extracranial giant cell tumours has been studied by a number of workers, including Hanaoka, Friedman and Mack (1970) and Steiner, Ghosh and Dorfman (1972). The giant cells contain large numbers of mitochondria, sparse rough endoplasmic reticulum and small numbers of lysosome-like bodies, together with many vesicular structures and numerous Golgi complexes. The stromal cells often resemble macrophages though their cytoplasm is less complex than that of the giant cells.

Histochemical studies have shown that the acid phosphatase content of the multinucleated cells of the giant cell tumour is much higher than in the stromal cells (Schajowicz, 1961; Ores, Rosen and Ortiz, 1969).

In the present context, the main histological problem is usually distinction between giant cell tumour and reparative granuloma. Histological criteria have been enumerated by a number of workers (Umiker and

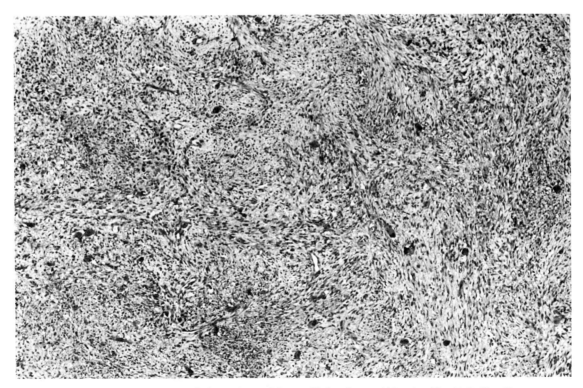

Fig. 22.3 Giant cell reparative granuloma of the maxilla in a 5 year-old boy (see Fig. 22.1). M ×58

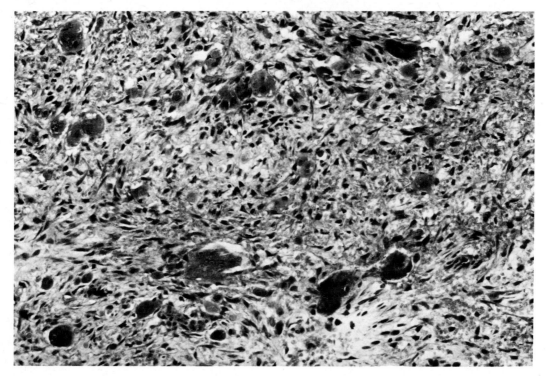

Fig. 22.4 Giant cell reparative granuloma of the maxilla in a 5 year-old boy. Higher magnification of Fig. 22.3. M ×214

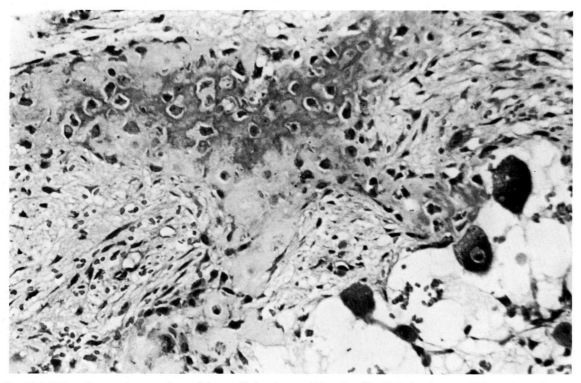

Fig. 22.5 Giant cell reparative granuloma of the maxilla in a 5 year-old boy (see Fig. 22.3) showing osteoid formation and partial calcification. M ×282

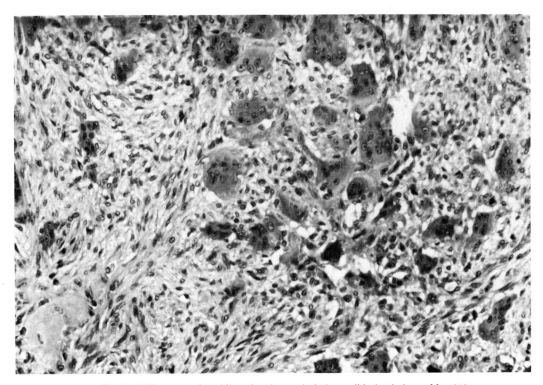

Fig. 22.6 Hyperparathyroidism showing typical giant cell lesion in bone. M × 268

Gerry, 1954; Austin et al., 1959; Hirschl and Katz, 1974). These points of comparison together with other relevant features are summarized in Table (22.1).

Aetiology and pathogenesis

Trauma has been invoked as a causal agent in both giant cell tumour and reparative granuloma. Geschicter and Copeland (1930) found a history of previous injury in between 40 and 50 per cent of 226 cases, including 20 lesions in upper or lower jaws. Although their series must have consisted mainly of true giant cell tumours, there were probably included some examples of reparative granuloma. These authors endeavoured to trace a relationship between bone cysts and giant cell tumours, suggesting that some bone cysts might represent healed tumours. However, Waldron and Shafer (1966) pointed out that traumatic bone cysts are very rare in the maxilla and, contrary to what one might expect, the giant cell reparative granuloma shows a relative high frequency in females.

The prominence of giant cells in these lesions inevitably focussed attention on these elements to which undue emphasis has probably been given and, in the context of giant cell tumours, the stromal cells would appear to be more important (Hanaoka et al, 1970). The close similarity to osteoclasts resulted in the adoption of the term 'osteoclastoma' which persists in the literature.

TABLE 22.1 The differential diagnosis of giant cell tumour and reparative granuloma

Feature	Giant cell tumour	Reparative granuloma
Age	3rd & 4th decades	2nd decade
Behaviour	Variably aggressive May metastasize	Benign. Non-neoplastic
Recurrence	Frequent	Rare
Giant Cells: Number	Many, dominating the picture	Variable, usually less numerous
Distribution	Evenly diffuse	Focal, often related to haemorrhage
Nuclei	Numerous, usually regular. No mitoses	Fewer, regular. No mitoses
Stromal Cells	Variable in shape with fairly abundant cytoplasm	Spindle cells of fibroblastic type
Intercellular substance	Virtually absent	Collagenous
Osteoid	Rare, usually peripheral	Occasionally present
Haemorrhage	Present	Present
Haemosiderin	Present	Present

Geschicter and Copeland (1930) believed that the multinucleated giant cells in the giant cell tumour represented an abnormal proliferation of osteoclasts in relation to new bone formation from cartilage. Jaffe et al (1940) considered that origin was from undifferentiated supporting connective tissue cells in the bone marrow. Another view is that the giant cells are of endothelial origin. This is based on not inconsiderable evidence presented over a long period of time (Stroebe, 1890; Johnson, 1930; Rather, 1951; Hanaoka et al, 1970). There is no doubt that giant cells take part in the lining of vascular spaces but the phenomenon is not peculiar to the giant cell tumour of bone, being observed in other neoplasms of both osseous and non-osseous origin whilst one of the present authors has observed a similar occurrence in the giant cell reparative granuloma. The mechanism of formation has also been disputed. The majority view, based on light and electron microscopical observations and tissue culture studies, is that they are formed by fusion of the mononuclear cells (Stewart, 1922; Aegerter, 1947; Morton, 1956; Hutter et al, 1962; Hanaoka et al, 1970). The assertion of Schajowicz (1961) that the giant cells were formed by repeated amitotic division of nuclei has received little support. The ultra-structural studies of Hanaoka et al (1970) showed not only the fusion of stromal cells to form giant cells but also an intimate relationship between stromal and endothelial cells with the formation of zonula occludens. This could explain the alkaline phosphatase activity in stromal cells reported by Pepler (1958).

Behaviour

The assessment of prognosis is complicated by the difficulties of diagnosis. The observations of Coley (1924) made it quite clear that the giant cell tumour of bone was not necessarily benign and, in 1940, Jaffe et al emphasized this point and divided these tumours into three grades in which particular attention was paid to the stromal cells. Grade 1, the least aggressive, exhibited uniform stromal cells with no significant nuclear irregularity and a virtual absence of intercellular colla-gen. In Grade 2, giant cells were still fairly abundant but nuclear atypism was present in both stromal and giant cells whilst the stroma was less vascular than in the previous grade. Grade 2 tumours showed a tendency to recur with occasional frankly malignant behaviour after several years. Grade 3 was a relatively small group in which stromal cells were more abundant with more marked nuclear irregularity whilst the giant cells tended to be smaller with fewer nuclei. This group was frankly malignant, half of them exhibiting metastasis particu-larly to the lungs. The mitotic activity of the mononu-clear tumour cells has been considered in the grading of giant cell tumours but most pathologists found grading of no real value. Murphy and Ackerman (1956) reported 31 extracranial tumours of which 26 were classified as benign whilst three of the five malignant tumours exhibited metastasis. Hutter et al (1962) reported 76 extracranial tumours of which about 30 per cent were malignant, some undergoing transformation subsequent to initial diagnosis. The antral tumour reported by Austin et al (1959) recurred twice during the first three years after curettage but was without recurrence eight years later following irradiation. Friedberg et al (1969) found that their antral tumour recurred two and a half years after surgery and irradiation but survived a further ten years without recurrence. There are no reports of metastases from cranial tumours of this type.

The natural history of giant cell tumours varies and it is difficult to foretell whether such a tumour might recur after surgical removal. Whether giant cell tumours arising in the skull are necessarily less aggressive than their extracranial counterparts remains an open ques-tion. One of Fu and Perzin's cases survived 18 years without recurrence after excision.

The giant cell reparative granuloma follows a benign course. With adequate removal recurrence is rare. In a follow-up of 45 of their 64 cases, Austin et al (1959) found symptom-free periods ranging from three months to forty four years. The two cases in the I.L.O. material both showed apparent healing following surgery and are known to have been free from recurrence for periods of 11 and 21 years.

BIBLIOGRAPHY

Aegerter E E 1947 Giant cell tumor of bone. American Journal of Pathology 23: 283–297
Austin L T, Dahlin D C, Royer R Q 1959 Giant cell reparative granuloma and related conditions affecting the jaw bones. Oral Surgery, Oral Medicine and Oral Pathology Pathology 12: 1285–1295
Barrie G 1913 Chronic (non-suppurative) haemorrhagic osteomyelitis. Annals of Surgery 57: 244–258
Berger A 1947 Solitary central giant cell tumor of the jaw bones. Journal of Oral Surgery 5: 154–167
Bhaskar S N, Bernier J L, Godby F 1959 Aneurysmal bone cysts and other giant cell lesions of the jaws. Journal of Oral Surgery 17: 30–41
Coley W B 1924 Prognosis in giant cell sarcoma of the long bones. Annals of surgery 79: 321–357

Cooper A P, Travers B 1818 Exostoses in Surgical Essays, 2nd edn. Cox and Sons, London pp 167–224
Emley W E 1971 Giant cell tumor of the sphenoid bone. Archives of Otolaryngology 94: 369–374
Friedberg S A, Eisenstein R, Wallner L J 1969 Giant cell lesions involving the nasal accessory sinuses. Laryngoscope 79: 763–776
Fu Y, Perzin K H 1974 Non-epithelial tumors of the nasal cavity, paranasal sinuses and nasopharynx. II Osseous and Fibro-osseous lesions. Cancer 33: 1289–1305
Geschicter C F, Copeland M M 1930 Tumors of the giant cell group. Archives of Surgery 21: 145–156
Hamlin W B, Lund P K 1967 Giant cell tumors of the mandible and facial bones. Archives of Otolaryngology 86: 658–665

Hanaoka H, Friedman B, Mack R P 1970 Ultrastructure and histogenesis of giant cell tumors of bone. Cancer 25: 1408–1423

Hirschl S, Katz A 1974 Giant cell reparative granuloma outside the jaw bones. Human Pathology 5: 171–181

Hlaváček V, Jolna V H 1974 Giant cell tumours of bone in E.N.T. organs. Acta Otolaryngologica 77: 374–380

Hutter R V P, Worcester J N, Francis K C, Foote F W, Stewart F W 1962 Benign and malignant giant cell tumors of bone. Cancer 15: 653–690

Jaffe H L 1953 Giant cell reparative granuloma, traumatic bone cyst and fibrous (fibro-osseous) dysplasia of the jaw bones. Oral Surgery, Oral Medicine and Oral Pathology 6: 159–175

Jaffe H L, Lichtenstein L, Portis R B 1940 Giant cell tumor of bone. Archives of Pathology 30: 993–1031

Lebert H 1845 Des tumeurs fibroplastiques ou sarcomateuses. Physiologie pathologique, tome 2, pp 120–160. J B Bailière, Paris

Morton J J 1956 Giant cell tumor of bone. Cancer 9: 1012–1026

Murphy W R, Ackerman L V 1956 Benign and malignant giant cell tumors of bone. Cancer 9: 317–339

Nélaton E 1860 Tumeurs benignes des os ou tumeurs à myeloplaxes. A Delahaye, Paris

Ores R, Rosen P, Ortiz J 1969 Localization of acid phosphatase activity in a giant cell tumour of bone. Archives of Pathology 88: 54–57

Paget J 1853 Myeloid tumours. Lecture VIII in Lectures on Surgical Pathology, Vol. 2, pp 212–228 Longmans

Peimer R 1954 Benign giant cell tumors of the skull and the nasal sinuses. Archives of Otolaryngology 60: 186–193

Pepler W J 1958 The histochemistry of giant cell tumours (osteoclastoma and giant cell epulis). Journal of Pathology and Bacteriology 76: 505–510

Radcliffe A, Friedmann I 1957 Reparative giant cell granuloma of the jaw. British Journal of Surgery 45: 50–54

Schajowicz F 1961 Giant cell tumors of bone (osteoclastoma). Journal of bone and joint surgery 43A: 1–29

Sissons H A 1966 Giant cell tumour in Systemic Pathology, (Ed) Symmers W H C 1st edn Longmans 37: p 1417

Steiner G C, Ghosh L, Dorfman H D 1972 Ultrastructure of giant cell tumors of bone. Human Pathology 3: 569–586

Stewart M J 1922 The histogenesis of myeloid sarcoma. Lancet 2: 1106–8

Umiker W, Gerry R G 1954 Pseudo-giant cell tumour (reparative granuloma of the jaws. Oral Surgery, Oral Medicine and Oral Pathology 7: 113–123

Van Nostrand A W P 1976 Pathologic aspects of osseous and fibro-osseous lesions of the maxillary sinus. Otolaryngologic Clinics of North America 9: 35–42

Waldron C A, Shafer W G 1966 The central giant cell reparative granuloma of the jaws. American Journal of Clinical Pathology 45: 437–447

Wattles M 1937 A case of benign giant cell tumor of the ethmoid labyrinth with a review of the literature. Annals of Otology, Rhinology and Laryngology 46: 212–222

FIBROUS DYSPLASIA AND OSSIFYING FIBROMA OF THE NOSE AND SINUSES

Introduction

The term fibrous dysplasia was first introduced by Lichtenstein in 1938 although the condition had been known previously by a variety of other names such as osteitis fibrosa, osteodystrophia fibrosa, fibrous osteoma, ossifying fibroma, unilateral Von Recklinghausen's disease and many others. The last mentioned label indicated the existing confusion with generalized osteitis fibrosa related to parathyroid disease. A number of workers had already recognized an association between multiple bone lesions, skin pigmentation and endocrine dysfunction resulting in sexual precocity in females which became known as Albright's Syndrome (Albright, Butler, Hampton and Smith, 1937). Lichtenstein and Jaffe (1942) reviewed published cases which seemed to fit the pattern of fibrous dysplasia and concluded that about 17 per cent of cases were confined to one bone but, since that time, many more monostotic examples have been recognized, especially in the head region, with the result that they are now regarded as greatly outnumbering the polyostotic lesions (Gross and Montgomery, 1967). It became apparent that a proportion of the cases formerly diagnosed as Leontiasis Ossea were probably examples of fibrous dysplasia of the facial bones (Pugh, 1945; Daves and Yardley, 1957) and it has become common practice to use the expression cranio-facial fibrous dysplasia for those lesions which may involve more than one facial bone but usually have no extra-cranial or extraskeletal manifestations.

Terminology

Although there is general agreement on the use of the label fibrous dysplasia, there is a difference of opinion on whether the term ossifying fibroma represents merely a variant of this condition or whether it is a separate entity. This will be discussed later.

Incidence

The disease is clearly not a common one in the present context but information on its more precise frequency has been misleading owing to confusion in diagnoses. Half the cranio-facial lesions reported by Smith and Zavaleta (1952) were finally classified as osteomas, hence their incidence of fibrous dysplasia should have been 1:20,000 new patients. In the I.L.O. material, the frequency was of the order of 1:60,000 new patients attending for ear, nose or throat conditions. Fu and Perzin (1974) included nine cases of fibrous dysplasia amongst their 256 non-epithelial tumours.

Clinical features

Irrespective of the site of origin, the disease is predominantly one of young subjects. In cranio-facial lesions the majority of patients are under 20 years of age but a smaller number of cases are encountered throughout the remaining decades of life, the oldest recorded example being 81 years (Pound, Pickrell, Huger and Barnes, 1965). The disease undoubtedly occurs more frequently in females, in one series accounting for 70 per cent (Georgiade, Masters, Horton and Pickrell, 1955). I.L.O. cases ranged from 8 to 73 years, four out of seven being female.

The common form of presentation is painless swelling, producing facial deformity, nasal obstruction and proptosis with disturbance of vision. Some cases are asymptomatic, the lesion being identified either as an incidental finding or as a result of malignant transformation (Huvos, Higinbotham and Miller, 1972).

Serum calcium and phosphorus levels are normal in most cases of fibrous dysplasia but alkaline phosphatase activity is often increased, particularly in polyostotic cases and also in some cranio-facial lesions (Williams and Thomas, 1975).

Radiological appearances have been considered in detail by various workers (Fries, 1957; Sherman and Glauser, 1958). They vary according to the composition of the lesion. Where the fibrous element predominates the appearance may be that of an osteolytic lesion, sometimes suggest a cyst. The presence of fine bony trabeculae may impart a 'ground glass' appearance on X-ray. Cranio-facial lesions are said to appear more sclerotic, due partly to increased amounts of bone but also to overlapping of structures. Expansion of the outer table of involved cranial bones is not uncommon.

Anatomical site of origin

Belaval and Schneider (1954) classified fibrous dysplasia in three groups: monostotic (confined to one bone), polyostotic (involving two or more bones) and widely disseminated with extraskeletal manifestations. Schlumberger (1946) reported 67 monostotic lesions amongst which 14 involved the head region. Of cranio-facial lesions, the maxilla is most frequently involved (Georgiade et al, 1955; Zimmerman, Dahlin and Stafne, 1958), followed in order of frequency by the mandible, ethmoidal, frontal and sphenoidal regions. The skull was frequently involved in the disseminated cases reported by Albright et al (1937) and around 20 per cent of patients with the polyostotic type of Albright's syndrome have lesions in the jaws. About 15 per cent of all cases of monostotic fibrous dysplasia occur in the jaws but, although the facial bones may be affected in both types, the monostotic facial lesion does not become polyostotic. In the I.L.O. cases, the distribution was maxillary three, ethmoidal three and frontal one.

Gross appearances

In the more general context, the lesional tissue of fibrous dysplasia is often referred to as firm, rubbery, greyish white tissue but, in cranio-facial lesions, the abnormal tissue is not infrequently described as soft and caseous with a gritty texture due to the presence of bone which may sometimes predominate, imparting to the lesion a harder consistency. Vascularity and haemorrhage account for a patchy reddish-brown colouration.

Histopathology

The microscopical picture is somewhat variable. The basic pattern is one of fibrous displacement of bone in which the background of collagenous tissue shows variable cellularity and density with predominantly slender spindle cells forming bundles or whorls. Oedematous or myxoid areas and even cyst-like spaces may be present. Lichtenstein and Jaffe (1942) regarded the cellular, loosely whorled appearance as the fundamental structure. Within this connective tissue stroma lies immature metaplastic bone. The osseous masses vary greatly in size and shape but often exhibit slender curved trabeculae (Fig. 22.7). Deposition of osteoid around stromal cells and subsequent irregular calcification results in the incarceration of the metaplastic osteoblasts but, characteristically, the trabeculae are not rimmed by these cells as in the common pattern of new bone formation. In this connection, some observers maintain that palisading of trabeculae by osteoblasts does occur in fibrous dysplasia but it is likely that such an event represents reactive change at the periphery of the lesion. The spindle cells in the stroma usually show evidence of marked alkaline phosphatase activity (Changus, 1957; Pepler, 1960). The immature nature of the bony component is indicated by the woven pattern which is readily demonstrated with polarized light (Fig. 22.8). Variable vascularity is found together with areas of haemorrhage, the latter resulting in accumulations of haemosiderin. Osteoclastic resorption is not a feature of the lesion but occasional groups of multinucleated giant cells may be found in relation to vessels or areas of haemorrhage. The presence of areas of hyaline cartilage have been intermittently reported. Occasional groups of foam cells may also be found.

The proportion of fibrous to osseous tissue may vary greatly (Figs. 22.9 and 22.10), a fact which may be reflected in the radiographic appearances. Zimmerman et al (1958) attempted grading of fibrous dysplasia on this basis, ranging from type 1 which was predominantly fibrous to type 4 which was densely ossified. It seems possible that the condition known as non-ossifying fibroma may be a variant at the fibrous end of the spectrum.

Another possible variant, which is still the subject of controversy, is characterized by the presence of small irregular or rounded masses of bone, partially calcified osteoid or cement-like substance embedded in a highly cellular, fibromatoid stroma (Figs 22.11, 22.12 & 22.13).

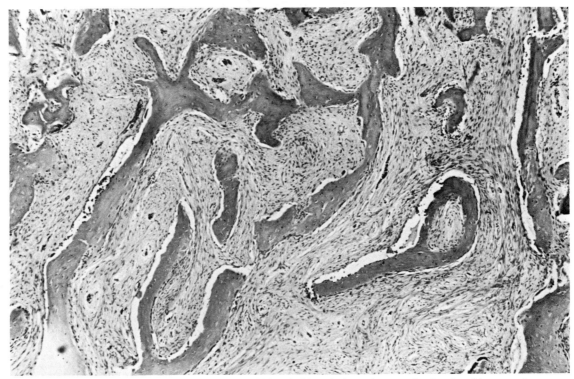

Fig. 22.7 Fibrous dysplasia of the maxilla in a 24 year-old female. Note the irregular curved trabeculae of immature bone embedded in vascular fibrous tissue. M ×58

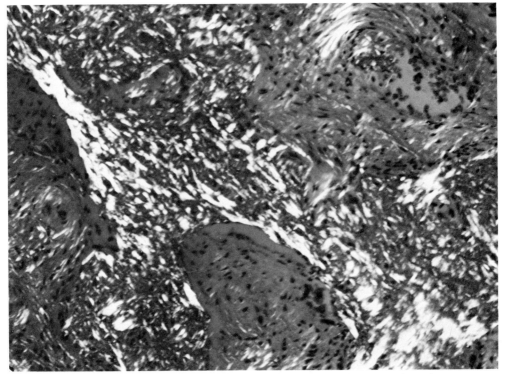

Fig. 22.8 Fibrous dysplasia of the maxilla in a 24 year-old female (see Fig. 22.7). Polarized light shows the woven pattern of bone. M ×54

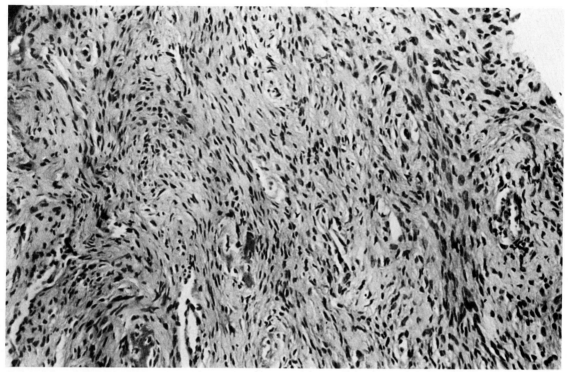

Fig. 22.9 Fibrous dysplasia of the ethmoid region in a 13 year-old girl, showing almost exclusively a fibrous pattern. M ×232

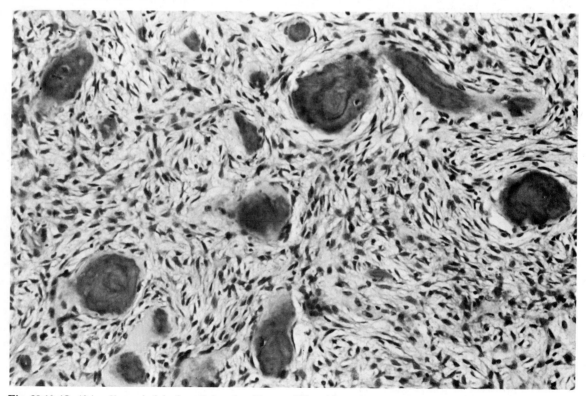

Fig. 22.10 'Ossifying fibroma' of the frontal sinus in a 10 year-old boy. Note spherical bone masses with osteoid formation in a background of spindle celled tissue. M ×225

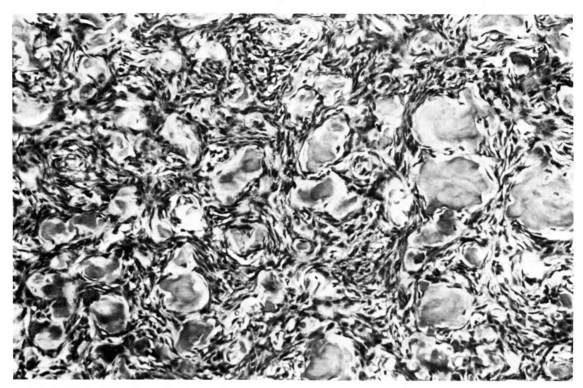

Fig. 22.11 'Ossifying fibroma' of the maxilla in an 8 year-old girl with involvement of the maxillary sinus. M × 232

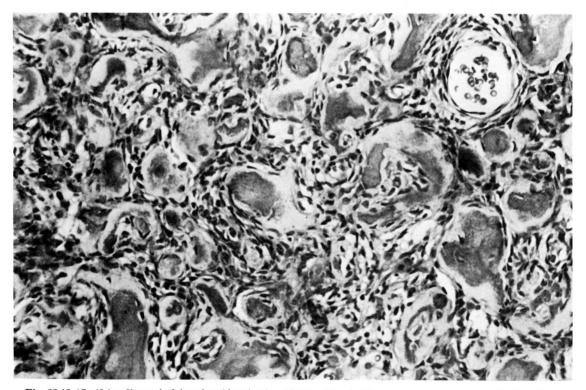

Fig. 22.12 'Ossifying fibroma' of the ethmoid region in a 25 year-old male. Note peripheral zones of osteoid. M × 297

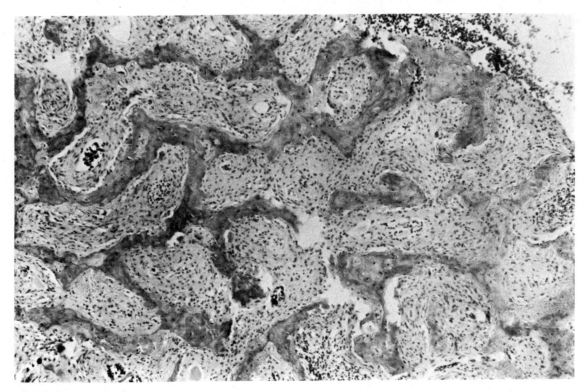

Fig. 22.13 Fibrous dysplasia of the ethmoid region in a 33 year-old female, showing the characteristic curved trabeculae of immature bone. M × 74

This pattern is identified by some observers as 'ossifying fibroma' though there has been much confusion of terminology and interpretation in relation to pathogenesis (q.v.). The psammoma-like masses may lead to confusion with meningioma. The condition has to be distinguished from other fibro-osseous lesions. The fibrous osteoma may bear a superficial resemblance but the trabeculae show a prominence of lamellar structure rather than the woven pattern which characterizes fibrous dysplasia and there may be palisading of osteoblasts. The presence of giant cells may raise the question of other giant cell lesions such as reparative granuloma, cherubism (Jones, 1965) or hyperparathyroidism.

Aetiology and pathogenesis

Although the existence of this condition had been established for more than forty years, there is still no clear understanding of its nature and causation. Against the early background of polyostotic manifestation in young subjects, it was regarded as a developmental defect (Lichtenstein, 1938; Lichtenstein and Jaffe, 1942; Berger and Jaffe, 1953). Reitzik and Lownie (1975) reported familial incidence of cranio-facial fibrous dysplasia but in most cases there is no such evidence.

Schlumberger (1946) did not regard the condition as a hamartoma but suggested that the lesion represented an abnormal response to injury though little support for this view has been forthcoming. The emergence of the monostotic type (including cranio-facial involvement) as the predominating form in a group of lesions with a common histological structure has certainly given grounds for reappraisal. Although a large proportion of monostotic cases have a common age incidence with the polyostotic variety, the occurrence of lesions in older subjects leads one to conclude that the 'perverted activity' of bone forming mesenchyme (Lichtenstein and Jaffe, 1942) is not necessarily a developmental defect. The resemblance to intramembranous ossification has been apparent to many observers and it has been suggested that there is a maturation arrest at the woven bone stage (Reed, 1963). More usually cranio-facial lesions are confined to that region and do not exhibit extraskeletal manifestations. In consequence, some have regarded the monostotic form as distinct from the disseminated variety (Schlumberger, 1946; Smith, 1965).

The occasional presence of a cartilaginous element in the lesion has been variously interpreted. Lichtenstein and Jaffe (1942) regarded it as an integral part of the dysplastic process but others believe it to be part of a reparative process related to callus formation (Harris, Dudley and Barry, 1962).

A particular problem which remains unresolved is the relationship between fibrous dysplasia of the cranio-facial region and the lesion or lesions variously known as ossifying fibroma, fibrous osteoma or fibro-osteoma. The first of these terms was originally used by Mont-gomery (1927) in connection with fibro-osseous lesions of the jaws which appear to have resembled some of the cases subsequently reported by Phemister and Grimson (1937) under the title of fibrous osteoma and by Billing and Ringertz (1946) under the heading fibro-osteoma. Some of these cases were almost certainly examples of fibrous dysplasia. A particular feature noted in some fibro-osseous lesions of the jaws is the presence of small spherular masses composed of calcified material, osteoid, bone or even cementum. Such a pattern was reported by Benjamins (1938) under the title of osteoid fibroma but others have applied the label ossifying fibroma (Klassen and Curtis, 1939; Eden, 1939; Woodruff, 1945). Not-withstanding the fact that the concept of 'ossifying fibroma' was never clearly defined histologically, many workers have accepted this pattern as a variant of fibrous

dysplasia (Lichtenstein, 1938; Mallory, 1942; Schlum-berger, 1946; Mammel, 1948; Daves and Yardley, 1957; Pound et al, 1965). On the other hand, some observers have maintained that 'ossifying fibroma' is a separate entity, even representing a true tumour (Smith and Zavaleta, 1952; Waldron, 1953; Thoma, 1956). Smith and Zavaleta's concept of the ossifying fibroma ranged from a 'young' type, which appeared to resemble the trabeculated form of fibrous dysplasia, to a 'mature' variety exhibiting the spherular pattern seen in figure 22.12.

The trabeculated and spherular patterns are not infrequently coincidental in fibrous dysplasia (Schlum-berger, 1946; Eversole, Sabes and Rovin, 1972) and is demonstrated in Figures 22.13, 22.14 and 22.15 from a case of fibrous dysplasia involving the ethmoid region. It is clear than the distinction between the two histological pictures is, to some extent, arbitrary al-though the spherular pattern is more common in the ossifying fibroma whilst the trabecular structure tends to predominate in fibrous dysplasia. However, a different dimension was introduced into the argument on the basis of radiological appearances (Sherman and Stern-bergh, 1948; Sherman and Glauser, 1958). These

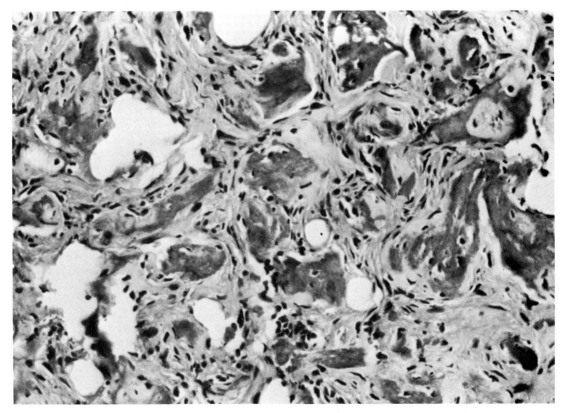

Fig. 22.14 Fibrous dysplasia of the ethmoid region in a 33 year-old female (see Fig. 22.13) showing 'ossifying fibroma' pattern. M × 350

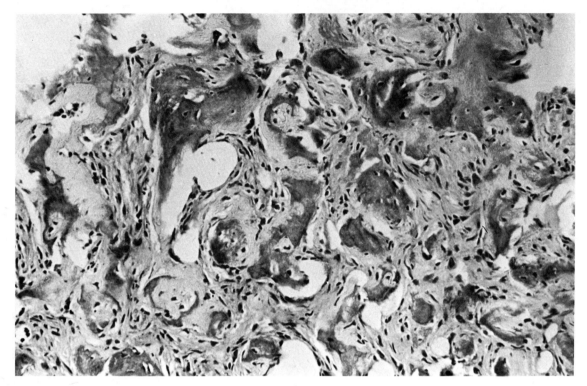

Fig. 22.15 Fibrous dysplasia of the ethmoid region in a 33 year-old female showing another area resembling 'ossifying fibroma'. M × 232

authors have maintained that the ossifying fibroma produces a discrete, predominantly osteolytic lesion with a thin eggshell margin whilst fibrous dysplasia presents a more diffuse infiltrative pattern. Eversole et al (1972) have pointed out the greater tendency to delineation by the ossifying fibroma which may influence the surgical approach to treatment of the lesion.

It is clear that total reliance cannot be placed on the histological pattern alone and that, from a practical point of view there is justification in distinguishing between fibrous dysplasia and ossifying fibroma even though there may be no clear demarcation of pathogenesis (Langdon, Rapidis and Patel, 1976).

Behaviour

Cranio-facial fibrous dysplasia is a slowly growing lesion which exhibits expansile activity, encroaching on the various cavities in the region. Those lesions arising in early life tend to grow more slowly as the patient becomes older and may become quiescent with the cessation of skeletal growth (Reed, 1963). However, there have been reported cases of reactivation by pregnancy (Henry, 1969). 'Recurrence' after local surgery is not uncommon and the evidence for complete healing of these lesions is somewhat tenuous.

Harris et al (1962) reviewed 50 cases of fibrous dysplasia, amongst which were six lesions confined to the cranio-facial bones. Four of these cases were asymptomatic for periods ranging from ten to thirty years after initial treatment but two required further intervention for persistent disease. In the I.L.O. material, five cases were known to have been asymptomatic for seven to seventeen years, two having minor deformity and one dying of old age.

Whilst the natural history of cranio-facial fibrous dysplasia follows this pattern in many cases, there is nevertheless a small risk of malignant transformation. Schwartz and Alpert (1964) reviewed 26 published cases of sarcoma preceded by fibrous dysplasia and added two cases of their own. These authors calculated that the incidence of malignant change was considerably higher than that of spontaneous sarcoma, noting that over one third of the cases involved the cranio-facial region. Furthermore, they found that nearly 40 per cent of all the cases had received irradiation for the primary condition. However, on the basis of a minimum radiation dosage of 3000 r required to induce malignancy, they concluded that less than 20 per cent had developed post-irradiation sarcoma. Most of the non-irradiated cases have developed extracranial sarcomas but Jäger (1962) reported sarcomatous change in the maxilla of a 24 year-old male who had had polyostotic fibrous dysplasia for 18 years but had received no irradiation. Of the twelve cases of sarcomatous change reported by Huvos et al (1972), only one had been irradiated but there were no cases involving the paranasal region. The majority of sarcomas arising in dysplasia are of the osteogenic type, a smaller number develop fibrosarcoma and an occasional chondrosarcoma has been observed.

BIBLIOGRAPHY

Albright F, Butler A M, Hampton A O, Smith P 1937 Symptoms characterized by osteitis fibrosa disseminata, areas of pigmentation and endocrine dysfunction. New England Journal of Medicine 216: 727–746

Belaval G S, Schrieider R W 1954 Fibrous dysplasia of bone. Cleveland Clinical Quarterly 21: 158–168

Benjamins C E 1938 Das Osteoid-Fibrom mit atypischer Verkalkung im Sinus frontalis. Acta Otolaryngologica 26: 26–44

Berger A, Jaffe H L 1953 Fibrous (fibro-osseous) dysplasia of jaw bones. Journal of Oral Surgery 11: 3–17

Billing M L, Ringertz N 1946 Fibro-osteoma. Acta Radiologica 27: 129–152

Changus G W 1957 Osteoblastic hyperplasia of bone. Cancer 13: 1157–1161

Daves M L, Yardley J H 1957 Fibrous dysplasia of bone. American Journal of Medical Sciences 234: 590–606

Eden K C 1939 The benign fibro-osseous tumours of the skull and facial bones. British Journal of Surgery 27: 323–350

Eversole L R, Sabes W R, Rovin S 1972 Fibrous dysplasia: a nosologic problem in the diagnosis of fibro-osseous lesions of the jaws. Journal of Oral Pathology 1: 189–220

Fries J W 1957 Roentgen features of fibrous dysplasia of the skull and facial bones. American Journal of Roentgenology 77: 71–88

Fu Y, Perzin K H 1974 Non-epithelial tumours of the nasal cavity, paranasal sinuses and nasopharynx. Cancer 33: 1275–1305

Georgiade N, Masters F, Horton C, Pickrell K 1955 Ossifying fibromas (fibrous dysplasia) of the facial bones in children and adolescents. Journal of Pedriatrics 46: 36–43

Gross C W, Montgomery W W 1967 Fibrous dysplasia and malignant degeneration. Archives of Otolaryngology 85: 653–657

Harris W H, Dudley H R, Barry R J 1962 The natural history of fibrous dysplasia. Journal of Bone and Joint Surgery 44A: 207–233

Henry A 1969 Monostotic fibrous dysplasia. Journal of Bone and Joint Surgery 51B: 300–306

Huvos A G, Higinbotham N L, Miller T R 1972 Bone sarcomas arising in fibrous dysplasia. Journal of Bone and Joint Surgery 54A: 1047–1056

Jäger M 1962 Osteoidsarkom auf dem Boden einer fibröspolyostotischen Dysplasie (Jaffe-Lichtenstein). Zentralblatt fur allgemeine Pathologie und pathologische Anatomie 103: 291–298

Jones W A 1965 Cherubism. Oral Surgery, Oral Medicine and Oral Pathology 20: 648–653

Klassen K P, Curtis G M 1939 The calcium and phosphorus metabolism in ossifying fibroma of the mandible. Journal of Bone and Joint Surgery 21: 444–450

Langdon J D, Rapidis A D, Patel M F 1976 Ossifying fibroma – one disease of six. British Journal of Oral Surgery 14: 1–11

Lichtenstein L 1938 Polyostotic fibrous dysplasia. Archives of Surgery 36: 874–898

Lichtenstein L, Jaffe H L 1942 Fibrous dysplasia of bone. Archives of Pathology 33: 777–816

Mallory T B 1942 Disease of bone. New England Journal of Medicine 227: 955–960

Mammel C K 1948 Histologic comparisons of localized fibrous dysplasia of bone and ossifying fibroma. Journal of Oral Surgery 6: 27–36

Montgomery A 1927 Ossifying fibromas of the jaw. Archives of Surgery 15: 30–44

Pepler W J 1960 Ossifying fibromas and their relation to fibrous dysplasia and other tumours. Journal of Pathology and Bacteriology 79: 408–412

Phemister D B, Grimson K S 1937 Fibrous osteoma of the jaws. Annals of Surgery 105: 564–583

Pound E, Pickrell K, Huger W, Barnes W 1965 Fibrous dysplasia (ossifying fibroma) of the maxilla. Annals of Surgery 161: 406–410

Pugh D G 1945 Fibrous dysplasia of the skull. Radiology 44: 548–555

Reed R J 1963 Fibrous dysplasia of bone. Archives of Pathology 75: 480–495

Reitzik M, Lownie J F 1975 Familial polyostotic fibrous dysplasia. Oral Surgery, Oral Medicine & Oral Pathology 40: 769–774

Schlumberger H G 1946 Fibrous dysplasia of single bones (monostotic fibrous dysplasia). Military Surgeon 99: 504–527

Schwartz D T, Alpert M 1964 The malignant transformation of fibrous dysplasia. American Journal of Medical Sciences 247: 1–20

Sherman R S, Glauser O J 1958 Radiological identification of fibrous dysplasia of the jaws. Radiology 71: 553–558

Sherman R S, Sternbergh W L A 1948 The roentgen appearance of ossifying fibroma of bone. Radiology 50: 595–609

Smith A G, Zavaleta A 1952 Osteoma, ossifying fibroma and fibrous dysplasia of facial and cranial bones. Archives of Pathology 54: 507–527

Smith J F 1965 Fibrous dysplasia of the jaws. Archives of Otolaryngology 81: 592–603

Thoma K H 1956 Differential diagnosis of fibrous dysplasia and fibro-osseous neoplastic lesions of the jaws and their treatment. Journal of Oral Surgery 14: 185–194

Waldron C A 1953 Ossifying fibroma of the mandible. Oral Surgery, Oral Medicine and Oral Pathology 6: 467–473

Williams D M L, Thomas R S A 1975 Fibrous dysplasia. Journal of Laryngology and Otology 89: 359–374

Woodruff G H 1945 Ossifying fibroma of the ethmoid cells and the frontal sinus. Annals of Otology, Rhinology & Laryngology 54: 582–585

Zimmerman, D C, Dahlin D C, Stafne E C 1958 Fibrous dysplasia of maxilla and mandible. Oral Surgery, Oral Medicine and Oral Pathology 11: 55–68

PAGET'S DISEASE OF THE NOSE AND SINUSES

Introduction

Under the title of 'osteitis deformans', Paget (1877) described what he believed to be an inflammatory disease of bone with polyostotic involvement including the skull but not, apparently, the facial bones. It would appear that the disease has been in existence for a very long time since Wells and Woodhouse (1975) reported the almost total involvement by Paget's disease of an excavated skeleton from an Anglo-Saxon burial ground near Durham. It is of further interest that the subject who, it was estimated, had lived around 950 A.D. showed involvement of the maxillae. Jaffe (1933) noted that the facial bones were rarely involved to the same extent as other parts of the skeleton but occasional severe affliction of the facial region resulted in gross deformity resembling that described under the name of 'leontiasis ossea'.

Incidence

Schmorl (1932) found evidence of Paget's disease in 138 out of 4614 autopsies, an incidence of three per cent in subjects over the age of 40 years. Earlier reports of the frequency of this disease, of the order of 1:10,000 hospital admissions (Novak and Burket, 1944), would appear to have been underestimated. Porretta, Dahlin and Janes (1957), on the basis of radiographic survey, found an incidence of 1:900 registrations of new patients at the Mayo Clinic. There would also appear to be some geographical variation, a higher incidence having been observed in the north west of England (Barker, Clough, Guyer and Gardner, 1977). In the present context, the early impression was that facial bones were not involved, Paget noting apparent normality although the bones in question were not examined in detail. Much later, reports of facial involvement, especially of the maxilla, began to appear (Stafne and Austin, 1938; Glickman, 1943; Novak and Burket, 1944; Rushton, 1948; Yamane and Fleuchaus, 1954; Cooke, 1956).

In the I.L.O. material, four cases of maxillary involvement were encountered between 1948 and 1974 giving an incidence of 1:100,000 patients attending for ear, nose and throat conditions.

Clinical features

The disease is essentially one of older subjects and in the large series studied by Porretta et al (1957) about two thirds of the cases were in the sixth and seventh decades of life. The I.L.O. cases ranged from 64 to 81 years and all were females though wider experience shows a more equable distribution of the sexes.

The common form of presentation is swelling with facial deformity when the maxilla is involved and nasal obstruction results from encroachment on that cavity.

Facial pain or toothache is a common complaint (Cooke, 1956) and not infrequently the patient may present with a badly fitting denture. There may be manifestations of a more generalized form of the disease though only two of the 15 cases reported by Cooke (1956) presented initially with extracranial complaints.

Typical radiographic findings are enlargement of the affected bone which may exhibit 'cotton wool' patches. Another feature in Paget's disease of the jawbones is the presence of hypercementosis around the roots of the teeth (Stafne and Austin, 1938; Rushton, 1948). In most cases, other bones of the skull are also involved and the characteristic thickening of the calvarium clinches the diagnosis. In the absence of gross cranial changes, sharply localized areas of rarefaction may sometimes be observed especially in the frontal region, constituting the condition known as osteoporosis circumscripta which has been shown to be related to Paget's disease (Kasabach and Gutman, 1937).

Serum alkaline phosphatase levels are raised in varying degree according to the extent of the disease. An extraskeletal manifestation is the development of an excessive cardiac output which may put the patient at risk of high output failure.

Anatomical site of origin

This disease involves most frequently the lower half of the skeleton but Schmorl (1932) found the skull to be affected in 28 per cent of cases. Using dental radiographs, Stafne and Austin (1938) found the disease in the maxilla in 20 out of 138 cases of Paget's disease and most showed involvement of other parts of the skull. The case reported by Halazonetis and Darling (1967) involved both maxillae, giving the patient an ape-like appearance. Glickman (1943) reported one case which appeared to affect the maxilla only but the disease is rarely confined to one bone in the head region. The calvarium is commonly affected producing the classical clinical and pathological picture but other parts, such as the temporal bone (Friedmann, 1974) may also be involved.

Gross appearances

The naked eye picture of the diseased bone is characteristically rough and granular, often with a vascular or haemorrhagic and spongy appearance reflecting the presence of sclerotic and lytic areas.

Histopathology

The essential theme in Paget's disease is concomitant resorption and apposition of bone. There is in the early stage of the disease enhanced osteoclastic activity with extensive bone resorption and disorganization followed by re-organization of the bone pattern by means of osteoblastic activity. Both woven and lamellar bone are produced, surrounded by a richly vascular fibrous stroma containing many multinucleated osteoclasts. The typical picture is one of irregular bony trabeculae, often rimmed by osteoblasts with numerous osteoclasts some of which lie in intimate relation with the bone (Figs. 22.16, 22.17 & 22.18). The osteoblastic regeneration and successive waves of resorption lead to a dismantling of the normal structure which is replaced by trabecular bone exhibiting the characteristic mosaic pattern of irregular cement lines (Fig. 22.19). Jaffe (1933) regarded this mosaic pattern as almost pathognomonic of Paget's disease but such an appearance may be produced by any irregular reconstruction of bone, particularly in reactive change related to inflammatory processes.

Aetiology and pathogenesis

The cause of this disease is still not known and Paget's original concept of an inflammatory lesion has not been totally abandoned. There have been a number of isolated reports of familial incidence though the data have been insufficient to establish a clear hereditary pattern. Although the pelvic region and the lower limbs are involved in over 50 per cent of cases, the overall patchy anatomical distribution is inconsistent with endocrine

dysfunction and abnormal biochemical findings are clearly the consequences of the disease process.

Virus particles have been described in the bone of patients with Paget's disease. Rebel, Malkani, Baslé and Bregeon (1976) carried out ultrastructural studies on the osteoclasts in Paget's disease and noted the presence of intranuclear filamentous inclusions. In so far as the inclusion bodies resembled those seen in progressive multifocal leucoencephalopathy (a suspected papova virus infection), the last mentioned writers concluded that the possibility of an external agent in Paget's disease could not be excluded. Smith (1977) suggested that the condition may be either a slowly growing tumour or a virus infection.

The most likely cause could be a disease of connective tissue. Intensive study of collagen, the main extracellular protein of the body, has shown that more than half this material is in the bone matrix on which hydroxyapatite crystals are deposited during mineralization. Different connective tissues contain collagen molecules that are genetically distinct. The collagen fibres are built up from organized chains of cross-linked molecules, each of which is composed of three helical polypeptide (alpha)

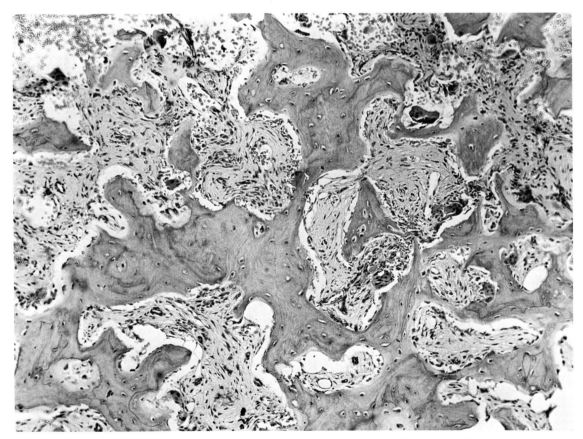

Fig. 22.16 Paget's disease involving a turbinate in a 64 year-old female. M × 130

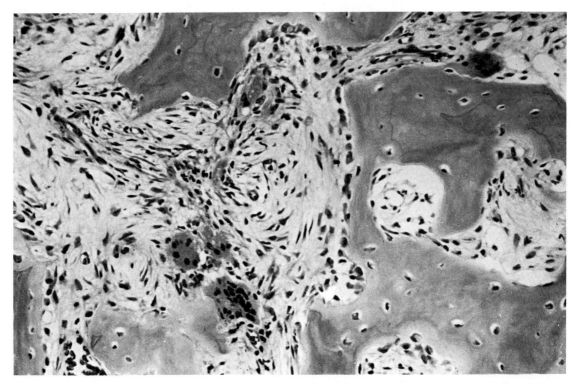

Fig. 22.17 Paget's disease of turbinate in a 64 year-old female. Note osteoclasts and palisading of osteoblasts. M ×232

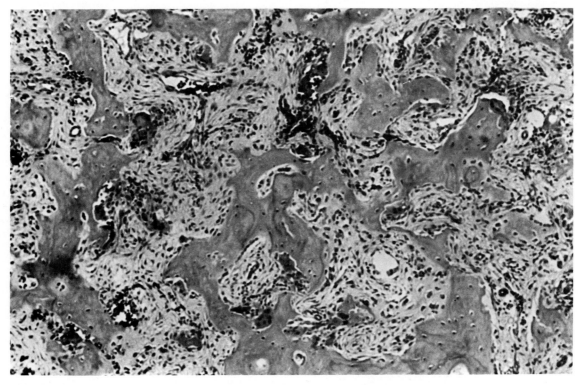

Fig. 22.18 Paget's disease of the maxilla in an 81 year-old female, showing osteoblastic and osteoclastic activity and a highly vascular stroma. M ×93

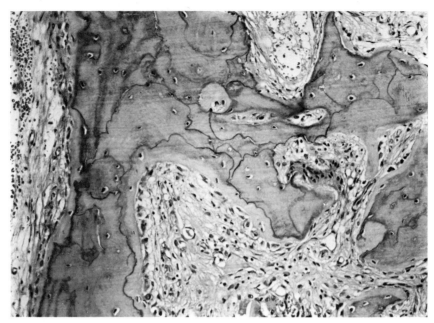

Fig. 22.19 Paget's disease of the maxilla in a 66 year-old female, showing mosaic pattern of cement lines. M × 208

chains wound round each other. These chains are synthesized within the fibroblast or osteoblast and undergo several changes before transfer from the cell. Errors in these synthetic steps may give rise to various disorders. The aminoacids, proline and lysine, are hydroxylated after incorporation in the peptide chain. Hence, they are not re-utilized after breakdown of the chain and consequently hydroxyproline and hydroxylysine are excreted in the urine, thereby providing a readily measured index of collagen turnover.

Hydroxyproline excretion (osteoclastic activity) and serum alkaline phosphatase levels (osteoblastic activity) have been used to follow the course of the disease, particularly in relation to chemotherapy using such agents as mithramycin, glucagon, calcitonin and diphosphonates (Smith 1977). Calcitonin and diphosphonates have been shown to have an inhibitory effect on osteoblastic activity and may relieve pain though the patient may develop antibodies to calcitonin.

Behaviour

Uncomplicated Paget's disease is a slowly progressive condition which, in the craniofacial context, has been alleviated largely by reduction surgery. The long term benefits of the chemotherapeutic approach have yet to be assessed.

This disease predisposes to the development of sarcoma (more usually osteogenic) and, in fact, two of Paget's original five cases had undergone malignant transformation. Such an event has been the subject of widely differing reports as regards its frequency (Freydinger, Duhig and McDonald, 1963). Reported figures have ranged from about one to twelve per cent of all cases of Paget's disease and it has become clear that the discrepancies have resulted from the differing assessments of the true incidence of the primary condition. Porretta et al (1957), who based their evaluation on radiographic skeletal survey, found sarcoma in 16 out of 1753 cases, an incidence of 0.9 per cent. Only ten of their sixteen cases were confirmed by biopsy, six being osteogenic and four fibroblastic but none involved the head region. Osteogenic sarcoma arising in Paget's disease of the maxilla has been reported by Karpawich (1958) and LiVolsi (1977). In the I.L.O. material, there was one case of osteogenic sarcoma of the maxilla in a patient with a ten year history of polyostotic Paget's disease. The patient died within two months of presentation of the tumour, thus underlining the very poor prognosis in Paget's sarcoma.

BIBLIOGRAPHY

Barker D J P, Clough P N L, Guyer P B, Gardner M J 1977 Paget's disease of bone in 14 British towns. British Medical Journal 1: 1181–1183

Cooke B E D 1956 Paget's disease of the jaws: fifteen cases. Annals of the Royal College of Surgeons of England 19: 223–240

Freydinger J E, Duhig J T, McDonald L W 1963 Sarcoma complicating Paget's disease of bone. Archives of Pathology 75: 496–500

Friedmann I 1974 Paget's disease of the temporal bone in Pathology of the ear, 1st edn, Blackwell, London, ch 4, pp 229–233

Glickman I 1943 Paget's disease in the maxilla, mandible and palate. American Journal of Orthodontics and Oral Surgery (Oral surgery section) 29: 591–607

Halazonetis J A, Darling A I 1967 Paget's disease of the maxilla. British Dental Journal 122: 425–429

Jaffe H L 1933 Paget's disease of bone. Archives of Pathology 15: 83–131

Karpawich A J 1958 Paget's disease with osteogenic sarcoma of maxilla. Oral Surgery, Oral Medicine and Oral Pathology 11: 827–834

Kasabach H H, Gutman A B 1937 Osteoporosis circumscripta of the skull and Paget's disease. American Journal of Roentgenology 37: 577–600

LiVolsi V A 1977 Osteogenic sarcoma of the maxilla. Archives of Otolaryngology 103: 485–488

Novak A J, Burket L W 1944 Oral aspects of Paget's disease including case reports and autopsy findings. American Journal of Orthodontics and Oral Surgery (Oral Surgery section) 30: 544–555

Paget J 1877 On a form of chronic inflammation of bones (osteitis deformans). Medico-Chirurgical Transactions 60: 37–64

Porretta C A, Dahlin D C, Janes J M 1957 Sarcoma in Paget's disease of bone. Journal of Bone and Joint Surgery 39A: 1314–1329

Rebel A, Malkani K, Baslé M, Bregeon C 1976 Osteoclast ultrastructure in Paget's disease. Calcified Tissue Reasearch 20: 187–199

Rushton M A 1948 Osteitis deformans affecting the upper jaw and osteoporosis circumscripta of the skull. British Dental Journal 84: 189–192

Schmorl G 1932 Über Osteitis deformans Paget. Virchows Archiv für pathologische Anatomie 283: 694–751

Smith R 1977 Paget's disease of bone, osteogenesis imperfecta and fibrous dysplasia. British Medical Journal 1: 365–367

Stafne E C, Austin L T 1938 A study of dental roentgenograms in cases of Paget's disease (osteitis deformans), osteitis fibrosa cystica and osteoma. Journal of the American Dental Association 25: 1202–1214

Wells C, Woodhouse N 1975 Paget's disease in an anglo-saxon. Medical History 19: 396–400

Yamane G M, Fleuchaus P T 1954 Paget's disease (osteitis deformans). Oral Surgery, Oral Medicine and Oral Pathology 7: 939–947

Additional references

Akin R K, Barton K, Walters P J 1975 Paget's disease of bone. Oral Surgery, Oral Medicine and Oral Pathology 39: 707–712

Hoggins G S, Allan D 1971 Paget's disease of the maxilla. British Journal of Oral Surgery 9: 122–125

Kirshbaum J D 1943 Fibrosarcoma of the skull in Paget's disease. Archives of Pathology 36: 74–79

Lucas R B 1955 The jaws and teeth in Paget's disease of bone. Journal of Clinical Pathology 8: 195–200

Melick R A, Martin R J 1975 Paget's disease in identical twins. Australian and New Zealand Journal of Medicine 5: 564–565

Melick R A, Ebeling P, Hjorth R J 1976 Improvement in paraplegia in vertebral Paget's disease treated with calcitonin. British Medical Journal 1: 627–628

Tubbax J 1974 Osteitis deformans van de maxilla. Acta Stomatologica Belgica 71: 293–308

23

Muscular tumours of the nose and sinuses

RHABDOMYOMATOUS TUMOURS OF THE NOSE AND SINUSES

Introduction
Although skeletal muscle tumours were recognized in the latter half of the nineteenth century (Bard, 1885), it was a long time before their relative frequency was fully appreciated. Distinction between benign and malignant varieties has long been established and, with the exception of the rhabdomyoma of the heart (which some regard as a hamartoma), most of the benign lesions are to be found in the head and neck region though the number reported in the literature is limited. Fu and Perzin (1976) found three such tumours in the naso-pharynx but, so far, no examples of rhabdomyoma have been reported as occurring in the nose and sinuses. The foetal rhabdomyoma described by Dehner, Enzinger and Font (1972) is of questionable neoplastic character but, in any case, has not been encountered in the nose and sinuses.

The term rhabdomyoma was used by earlier writers to include malignant lesions which were also referred to as 'rhabdomyoma sarcomatodes'. The nasal tumours reported by Vail (1908) and Reitter (1921) under the title of rhabdomyoma were unequivocally malignant. In the present context, therefore, we are concerned with rhabdomyosarcoma in its various forms.

Incidence
Increasing recognition of rhabdomyosarcoma has resulted in its acceptance as one of the commonest soft tissue malignant tumours, being second only to fibrosarcoma. Sutow, Sullivan, Ried, Taylor and Griffith (1970) found that rhabdomyosarcoma represented nearly eight per cent of all malignant disease in children and over 13 per cent of malignant tumours in that age range. In the younger patients there is a predilection for the head and neck region, especially the orbit but the nasal and paranasal cavities may be primarily involved. Masson and Soule (1965) found rhabdomyosarcoma in eight per cent of over a thousand sarcomas of the head and neck region and nearly a quarter of these involved

the nose and sinuses. In Nigeria, Williams, Martinson and Alli (1968) found rhabdomyosarcoma in over three per cent of malignant tumours of the upper respiratory tract, most of them arising in the nose and sinuses. Fu and Perzin (1976) found eight nasal or paranasal tumours amongst their 256 non-epithelial tumours of the nose, sinuses and nasopharynx. In the I.L.O. material, there were four cases representing less than 0.3 per cent of all tumours of the nose and sinuses and 1.2 per cent of non-epithelial tumours.

Clinical features
The overall age distribution of rhabdomyosarcoma is very broadly based but with predominance in early life, a fact which is reflected in the pattern encountered in the nose and sinuses. In the literature, those nasal and paranasal tumours in which the age was specified showed a peak distribution in the first decade with a small number of cases between 40 and 70 years. There was a slight excess of males but the difference was probably not significant. There is, hoewever, some degree of correlation between age and the histological type which will be discussed later.

The common form of presentation is swelling with or without pain. The patient may complain of nasal obstruction, discharge or epistaxis and secondary involvement of the orbit results in proptosis and disturbance of vision.

Anatomical site of origin
The nasal cavity is most frequently involved, closely followed by the maxillary sinus but frequently both cavities are found to be affected at the time of presentation. Such tumours arise less frequently in the ethmoid region and one of Fu and Perzin's cases involved the sphenoid sinus. So far, there have been no reports of origin in the frontal sinus. In the I.L.O. material, the nasal cavity was involved in three cases and the maxillary sinus in one.

Gross appearances
Apart from the characteristic polypoid feature of a small group designated the botryoid type, there are no specific

appearances in rhabdomyosarcoma of this region which usually presents a soft greyish white mass of tissue.

Histopathology

As long ago as 1885, Bard subdivided muscular tumours into embryonic and adult forms but the ultimate appreciation of the variegated pattern was inhibited by the reluctance to accept the existence of such tumours in the absence of cross striation. Capell and Montgomery (1937) noted the absence of striation in some tumours which they designated myoblastomas. Stout (1946) emphasized those morphological characteristics, other than cross striation, on which rhabdomyosarcomas may be recognized and in 1958 Horn and Enterline introduced a classification which has been generally accepted. In descending order of common age incidence this comprised pleomorphic, alveolar, embryonal and botryoid types.

The pleomorphic type represents the more classical concept of rhabdomyosarcoma. The malignant rhabdomyoblast may assume various shapes in accordance with its resemblance or otherwise to developing muscle. Small rounded cells, larger ovoid cells, spindle forms, racquet-shaped or straplike cells and multinucleated giant cells make up the polymorphic pattern (Fig. 23.1). Many of the larger cells have an abundant markedly eosinophilic cytoplasm which may be granular or

vacuolated and may show longitudinal striation due to the presence of myofibrils which may be demonstrable with trichrome or P.T.A.H. stains. A smaller number of cells exhibit cross striation (Fig. 23.2 and 23.3). Horn and Enterline (1958) found cross striation in about 60 per cent of their cases in this group. Nuclei show marked irregularity with hyperchromatism and mitoses. This is essentially the adult type of rhabdomyosarcoma and is not often encountered in the nose and sinuses. However, such tumours have been reported in the maxillary sinus by Cooper (1934) and by Pastore, Sahyoua and Mandeville (1950), whilst Williams et al (1968) found one in the nasal cavity of a Nigerian. One primary nasal tumour in the I.L.O. material was of this type (Fig. 23.4).

In 1956, Riopelle and Thériault described a variety of rhabdomyosarcoma under the title 'rhabdomyosarcome alvéolaire'. This variety, which was subsequently well illustrated by Enzinger and Shiraki (1969), is characterized by rounded or polyhedral cells with a moderate amount of eosinophilic cytoplasm forming well defined masses separated by a vascular connective tissue stroma and presenting a superficial resemblance to an epithelial tumour. A looser arrangement of the central cells gives an impression of 'alveoli' lined by one or more compact layers of cells whilst the centre of the 'lumen' is occupied by apparently free cells of greatly varying shape, including multinucleated giant cells and straplike cells

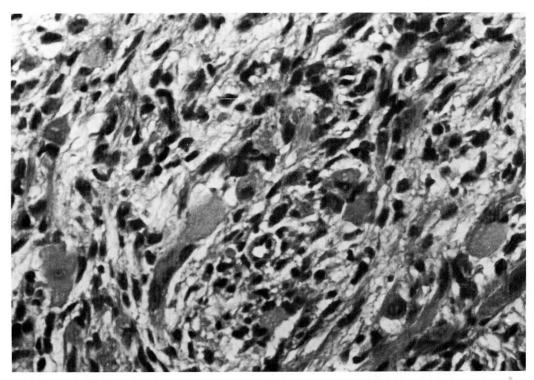

Fig. 23.1 Rhabdomyosarcoma of the nasal cavity in a 16 year-old boy showing a pleomorphic pattern. M × 530

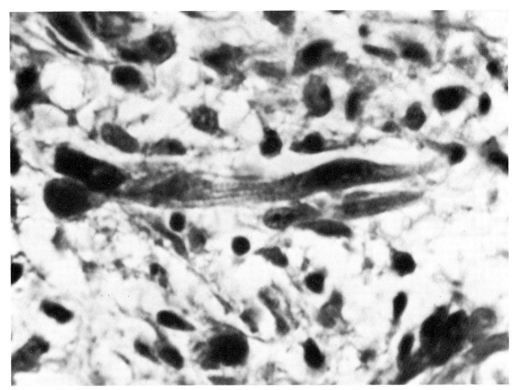

Fig. 23.2 Rhabdomyosarcoma of the nasal cavity in a 16 year-old boy (see Fig. 23.1) showing cross striation. M ×1365

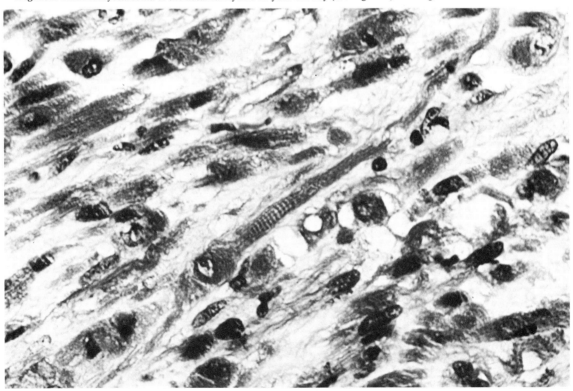

Fig. 23.3 Embryonal rhabdomyosarcoma of the nose in a 44 year-old female, showing cross striation. M ×600

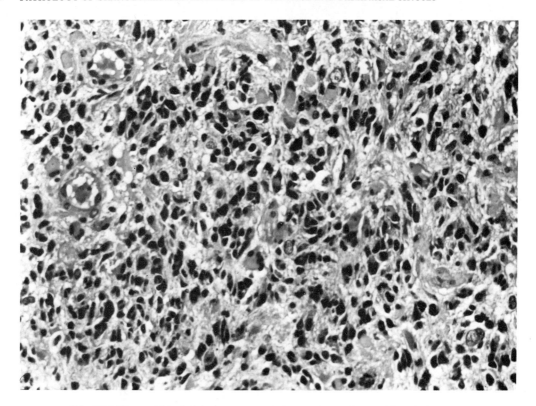

Fig. 23.4 Pleomorphic rhabdomyosarcoma of the nose in a 59 year-old female. M × 325

which sometimes show cross striation. Horn and Enterline (1958) found cross striation in 75 per cent of these tumours. Processes from the peripheral cells appear to blend with the connective tissue stroma. This histological variant occurs largely in adolescents and is encountered mainly in the limbs and trunk but one of the six cases described by Riopelle and Thériault (1956) involved the maxillary sinus. Williams et al (1968) also found one in the antrum whilst Koop and Tewarson (1964) described one such tumour occurring in the nasal cavity. Ethmoidal tumours of the alveolar type have been reported by Dabezies and Naugle (1968) and by Makishima, Iwasaki and Horia (1975).

In 1950, Stobbe and Dargeon drew attention to the existence of an embryonal type of rhabdomyosarcoma in the head and neck region having a resemblance to the sarcoma botryoides in the infantile genital tract. The tumour is composed of largely spindle cells of varying size. Some are long and slender but others may have a moderately abundant eosinophilic cytoplasm and the cell may be expanded in the vicinity of the nucleus, sometimes presenting a tadpole-like appearance. The tumour cells may be very small with darkly stained fusiform nuclei and occasionally an irregular palisading around bizarre shaped vessels may be seen (Fig. 23.5).

The cellular arrangement is usually loose though an interlacing pattern is sometimes present whilst stellate or spider-like cells may help to impart a myxoid appearance. In larger ovoid cells longitudinal and cross striations may be found. Horn and Enterline found cross striation in 30 per cent of their cases but Masson and Soule (1965) could only demonstrate this feature in 15 per cent. This is the more common form of rhabdomyosarcoma, accounting for most of the cases occurring in the first decade of life though such tumours are occasionally encountered in adults as demonstrated by Allen (1960) and one of the present authors' cases. Masson and Soule (1965) found 14 nasal and 7 antral tumours amongst 88 embryonal rhabdomyosarcomas of the head and neck. The two antral tumours reported by Henry and Downs (1968) were also of the embryonal type.

The botryoid variety is essentially a variant of the embryonal type, largely characterized by its grosser appearances. The cellular composition beneath the epithelial covering of the polypoid masses is essentially embryonal in pattern with the same elements of pleomorphism. Horn and Enterline found cross striation in two of their five cases. Antral tumours of the botryoid type have been reported by Horn and Enterline (1958)

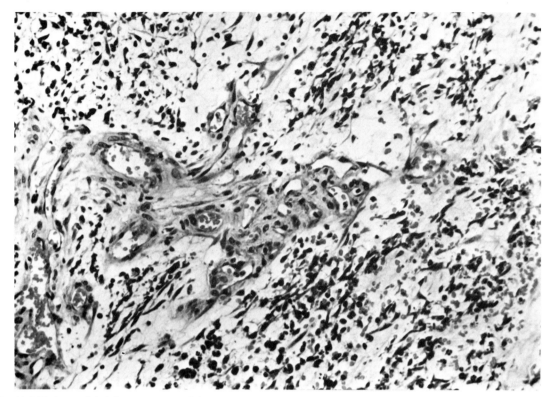

Fig. 23.5 Embryonal rhabdomyosarcoma of the nose in a 4 year-old girl, showing irregular accumulations of tumour cells around bizarre angiomatoid structures. M × 250

and by Koop and Tewarson (1964) whilst one of the I.L.O. cases showed a mixed picture of botryoid, embryonal and even verging on the adult type.

The last mentioned case underlines the fact that overlap of the histological patterns is not uncommon. Furthermore, the variability within the major group of embryonal tumours is emphasized by the classification proposed by Ashton and Morgan (1965) which comprised completely undifferentiated, non-striated and striated embryonal tumours. In the absence of cross striation, the pleomorphic or adult type of rhabdomyosarcoma can often be recognized on a morphological basis but many examples of the embryonal type have been diagnosed merely as undifferentiated sarcoma. The alveolar type has to be distinguished from the alveolar soft part sarcoma though this is rarely encountered in the nasal region. In the absence of cross striation, the projection of cell processes from the periphery of the alveoli into the stroma (Horn and Enterline, 1958) may be a helpful sign.

Ultrastructural studies on rhabdomyosarcomas in the head region have been reported by Kroll, Kuwabara and Howard (1963) and by Friedmann, Harrison, Tucker and Bird (1965). The pattern varies according to the degree of differentiation. In the more primitive cells,

only irregular arrangements of myofilaments are to be seen but in the better differentiated cells the filaments are more organized and show cross striation represented largely by Z-band material (Fig. 23.6). In well differentiated cells there may be recognizable sarcomeres containing A-, H-, I- and Z-bands. The greatly enlarged masses of Z-band material described in the rhabdomyoma (Czernobilsky, Cornog and Enterline, 1968) have not been seen in rhabdomyosarcoma.

Aetiology and pathogenesis

Although rhabdomyosarcoma has been produced experimentally by the injection of nickel sulphide (Friedmann and Bird, 1969) the overall age distribution would not suggest any environmental factor of this nature in the majority of cases. Nevertheless, the possibility of exposure to an external agent in the context of the adult type of tumour cannot be entirely ignored. In a survey of certified deaths from rhabdomyosarcoma in children, Li and Fraumeni (1969) noted the occurrence of soft tissue sarcomas in siblings of five out of 418 cases but this is probably no more than a single predisposing factor.

The fact that nasal and paranasal cavities do not normally contain skeletal muscle posed a problem of derivation of these tumours. The earlier concept of

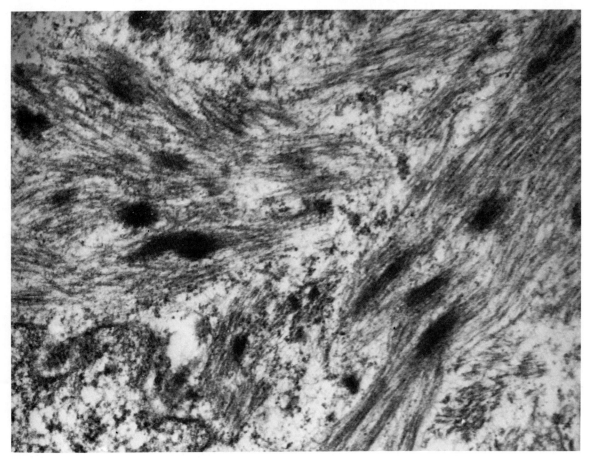

Fig. 23.6 Rhabdomyosarcoma of the nose in a 41 year-old female, showing myofilaments and Z-band material. M × 52 500

origin in ectopic muscular tissue (Vail, 1908) is no longer generally acceptable and the prevailing view (Willis, 1967) is that rhabdomyosarcomas of children and adolescents are derived from embryonic tissue, either from immature prospective muscular tissue or indifferent mesenchymal tissue with a potency for aberrant differentiation into muscle fibres.

Behaviour

Local spread by rhabdomyosarcoma of this region is a common event, as is apparent from the frequency with which both nasal and antral cavities are involved at a relatively early stage and radiological evidence of bone destruction is frequently present (Donaldson, Castro, Wilbur and Jesse, 1973). Recurrence is frequent, often with lymphatic or systemic metastases, lymphnode involvement being more frequent than in other soft tissue sarcomas. Masson and Soule (1965) found metastasis in 37.5 per cent of their head and neck tumours. Fu and Perzin (1976) found metastasis in two thirds of their

cases with cervical lymphnode involvement in 50 per cent. Remote metastases more commonly involved the lungs and the bones.

Millar and Dalager (1974) reviewed 1170 death certificates relating to rhabdomyosarcoma. They found a bimodal pattern showing death peaks at about four and seventeen years which was also reflected in the tumours of the head and neck region, comprising 22 per cent. The infantile peak is clearly related to the embryonal type of tumour but the adolescent peak is not so easily explained except in so far as the alveolar type carries a poor prognosis and may have contributed accordingly. In the general context, Sutow et al (1970) found a five year survival rate of 39 per cent in the embryonal type but only 20 per cent in the alveolar variety. On the other hand, Masson and Soule (1965) recorded a five year survival rate in embryonal rhabdomyosarcoma of the head and neck region of less than six per cent. Fu and Perzin (1976) found a five year survival rate of 21 per cent, most of their tumours being of embryonal type. These authors concluded that prognosis was probably better in peripheral tumours due to greater accessibility to surgery. Three of the I.L.O. cases died after six months, two years and seven years respectively. The shortest survivor was an adolescent with a mixed type of tumour, whilst the other two were pleomorphic varieties in middle-aged adults although the adult type of tumour usually carries a better prognosis in terms of survival (Dito and Batsakis, (1963).

BIBLIOGRAPHY

Allen G W 1960 Embryonal rhabdomyosarcoma of the nose and maxillary sinus. Archives of Otolaryngology 72: 477–478

Ashton N, Morgan G 1965 Embryonal sarcoma embryonal rhabdomyosarcoma of the orbit. Journal of Clinical Pathology 18: 699–714

Bard L 1885 Anatomie pathologique générale des tumeurs. Archives de Physiologie normale et pathologique 5: 247–265

Capell D F, Montgomery G L 1937 On rhabdomyoma and myoblastoma. Journal of Pathology and Bacteriology 44: 517–548

Cooper K G 1934 Plasmacytoma and rhabdomyoma of the paranasal sinuses. Archives of Otolaryngology 20: 329–339

Czernobilsky B, Cornog J L, Enterline H T 1968 Rhabdomyoma. American Journal of Clinical Pathology 49: 782–789

Dabezies O H, Naugle T C 1968 Alveolar rhabdomyosarcoma of paranasal sinuses and orbit. Archives of Ophthalmology 79: 574–577

Dehner L P, Enzinger F M, Font R L 1972 Fetal rhabdomyoma. Cancer 30: 160–166

Dito W R, Batsakis J G 1963 Intraoral, pharyngeal and nasopharyngeal rhabdomyosarcoma. Archives of Otolaryngology 77: 123–128

Donaldson S S, Castro J R, Wilbur J R, Jesse R H 1973 Rhabdomyosarcoma of head and neck in children. Cancer 31: 26–35

Enzinger F M, Shiraki M 1969 Alveolar rhabdomyosarcoma. Cancer 24: 18–31

Friedmann I, Bird E S 1969 Electron microscope investigation of experimental rhabdomyosarcoma. Journal of Pathology 97: 375–382

Friedmann I, Harrison D F N, Tucker W N, Bird E S 1965 Electron microscopy of a rhabdomyosarcoma of the ear. Journal of Clinical Pathology 18: 63–68

Fu Y, Perzin K H 1976 Non-epithelial tumors of the nasal cavity, paranasal sinuses and nasopharynx: V skeletal muscle tumors (rhabdomyoma and rhabdomyosarcoma). Cancer 37: 364–376

Henry F A, Downs J R 1968 Treatment of embryonal rhabdomyosarcoma of the maxilla with combined therapy. Journal of Oral Surgery 26: 316–320

Horn R L, Enterline H T 1958 Rhabdomyosarcoma: a clinico-pathological study and classification of 39 cases. Cancer 11: 181–199

Koop C E, Tewarson I P 1964 Rhabdomyosarcoma of the head and neck in children. Annals of Surgery 160: 95–103

Kroll A J, Kuwabara T, Howard G M 1963 Electron microscopy of rhabdomyosarcoma of the orbit. Investigative Ophthalmology 2: 523–537

Li F P, Fraumeni J P 1969 Rhabdomyosarcoma in children: epidemiologic study and identification of a familial cancer syndrome. Journal of the National Cancer Institute 43: 1365–1373

Makishima K, Iwasaki H, Horia A 1975 Alveolar rhabdomyosarcoma of the ethmoid sinus. Laryngoscope 85: 400–410

Masson J K, Soule E H 1965 Embryonal rhabdomyosarcoma of the head and neck. American Journal of Surgery 110: 585–591

Miller R W, Dalager N A 1974 Fatal rhabdomyosarcoma among children in the United States, 1960–1969. Cancer 34: 1897–1900

Pastore P N, Sahyoua P F, Mandeville F B 1950 Rhabdomyosarcoma of the maxillary antrum. Archives of Otolaryngology 52: 942–947

Reitter G S 1921 Rhabdomyoma of the nose. Journal of the American Medical Association 76: 22–23

Riopelle J C, Thériault J P 1956 Le rhabdomyosarcome alvéolaire. Annales d'Anatomie pathologique 1: 88–111

Stobbe G D, Dargeon H W 1950 Embryonal rhabdomyosarcoma of the head and neck in children and adolescents. Cancer 3: 826–836

Stout A P 1946 Rhabdomyosarcoma of the skeletal muscles. Annals of Surgery 123: 447–472

Sutow W W, Sullivan M P, Ried H L, Taylor H G, Griffith K M 1970 Prognosis in childhood rhabdomyosarcoma. Cancer 25: 1384–1390

Vail D T 1908 Rhabdomyoma of the nose. Laryngoscope 18: 933–942

Williams A O, Martinson F D, Alli A F 1968 Rhabdomyosarcoma of the upper respiratory tract in Ibadan, Nigeria. British Journal of Cancer 22: 12–18

Willis R A 1967 Pathology of tumours, 4th edn. Butterworth, London, ch 48, p 757–771

LEIOMYOMATOUS TUMOURS OF THE NOSE AND SINUSES

Introduction

Smooth muscle tumours have long been recognized in other parts of the body, especially the genito-urinary and alimentary tracts and also in the integument. On the other hand, occurrence in the nose and sinuses is limited and has only been reported within the past quarter of a century. The earliest report was by Dobben (1958) who described a tumour arising in the posterior part of the nose, filling the nasal and nasopharyngeal cavities in a 69 year-old female. Initially regarded as neurofibroma, the diagnosis was subsequently amended to leiomyosarcoma. Subsequent reports of benign and malignant varieties have appeared in the Japanese literature (Kawabe, Kondo and Hosoda, 1969). Only two histological types have, so far, been encountered, namely leiomyoma and leiomyosarcoma, the latter being the more common. The leiomyoblastoma, which is found particularly in the stomach, has not been reported as occurring in the nose and sinuses.

Incidence
Both the benign and malignant varieties are extremely rare in the nasal region. Fu and Perzin (1975) found two leiomyomas and six leiomyosarcomas amongst their 256 non-epithelial tumours of the nose, sinuses and naso-pharynx. Mindell, Calcaterra and Ward (1975) reviewed 31 leiomyosarcomas in the head and neck region of which two tumours involved the antrum and nasal cavity respectively. In a survey of 76 smooth muscle tumours in children, Yannopoulos and Stout (1962) found no examples involving the nose or sinuses.

Clinical features
The two leiomyomas of the nose, mentioned above, occurred in a 60 year-old woman and a 46 year-old man. The one other published case, noted by the same authors, occurred in a 49 year-old female. The age distribution of leiomyosarcoma is broadly based, covering the second to the eighth decade with no significant sex difference.

Fu and Perzin's two leiomyomas presented with multiple polypi and the diagnosis was an incidental histological finding. Leiomyosarcoma may present with nasal obstruction, epistaxis or facial pain. Local invasion may lead to swelling of the cheek or proptosis with disturbance of vision.

Anatomical site of origin
Leiomyoma has, so far, only been reported as occurring in the nasal cavity. Leiomyosarcoma is commonly found in the nose but may also involve the paranasal cavities, as in all the six cases reported by Fu and Perzin. Kawabe et al (1969) published two cases having origin in the maxillary sinus whilst the one case encountered in the I.L.O. material involved the fronto-ethmoidal region.

Gross appearances
Such tumours often present a reddish grey appearance due to a moderate degree of vascularity and cavities may be filled with polypoid masses.

Histopathology
Leiomyomatous tumours form interlacing bundles of spindle cells with fibrillary cytoplasm and elongated, blunt-ended nuclei which, particularly in the benign variety, have been appropriately described as baton-shaped. In the malignant variety, the nuclei tend to be shorter and more irregular and there may also be a tendency to nuclear palisading (Fig. 23.7). Reticulin

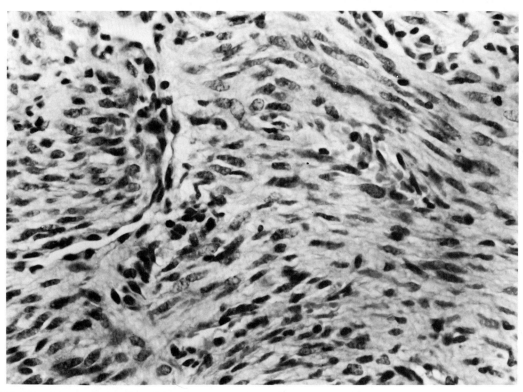

Fig. 23.7 Leiomyosarcoma of the frontal sinus in a 59 year-old female showing nuclear palisading and vascular channels. M × 600

fibres parallel the bundles and surround individual cells. Conventional stains such as phosphotungstic acid haematoxylin and trichrome modifications reveal the presence of 'myofibrils'. According to Stout and Hill (1958), these structures are consistently found in leiomyoma and in the greater proportion of leiomyosarcomas.

In the more general context, the diagnosis of malignancy is based on greater cellularity, cellular and nuclear irregularities and the frequency of mitoses (Ranchod and Kempson, 1977) though none of these features are totally reliable. Necrosis is more likely to be associated with malignancy, whereas myxoid change is more common in benign tumours.

There are often vascular areas and some of the irregular vascular channels may be enveloped by tumour cells, a picture which may sometimes suggest an alternative diagnosis of haemangiopericytoma. The case reported by Pimpinella and Marquit (1965) showed considerable vascularity and was initially diagnosed as 'haemangiofibroma'. Other neoplasms which may enter into the differential diagnosis are fibrosarcoma and neurofibroma or neurofibrosarcoma.

Ultrastructural studies of paranasal leiomyosarcoma have been carried out by Kawabe et al (1969). They observed myofilaments running in the long axis of the cell with aggregation zones as found in normal smooth muscle cells. One point should be emphasized in this context. Filaments in smooth muscle cells are of the order of 50 A in thickness and even the aggregation zones are usually well below the limit of resolution by a light microscope. (Figs. 23.8 and 23.9) It follows, therefore, that the 'myofibrils' demonstrable with time honoured stains must represent a fixation artefact with all its attendant variability.

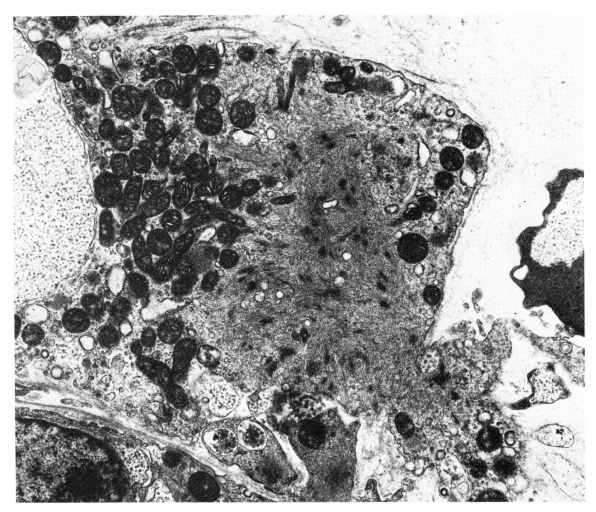

Fig. 23.8 Detail of leiomyoblast containing large mass of myofilaments with dense aggregation zones. Note large groups of mitochondria. M × 18 200. Case as in Fig 23.7

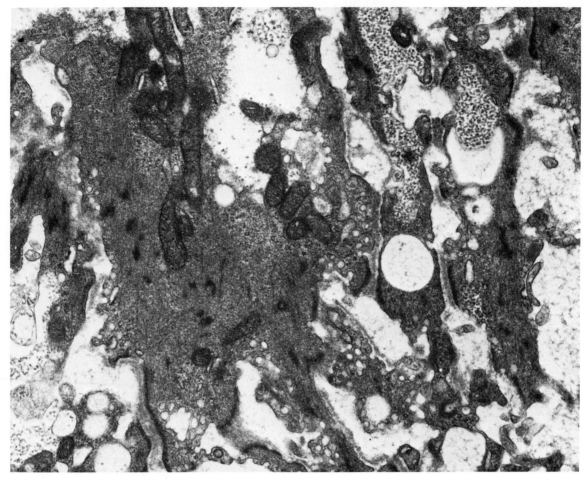

Fig. 23.9 Myofilamentous area with dense aggregation zones. Note pinocytotic vesicles. M × 21 035. Case as in Fig 23.7

Aetiology and pathogenesis

Although one published case had received irradiation 22 years previously for chronic sinusitis, the overall clinical pattern does not indicate any particular aetiological agent. As far as the nose and sinuses are concerned, the only smooth muscle normally present is in the vasculature and some believe that this tissue constitutes the origin of leiomatous tumours though derivation from multipotent mesenchymal cells (Willis, 1967) is at least an equally valid possibility.

Behaviour

The aggressive capability of leiomyosarcoma is manifest in its tendency to local invasion and remote spread. All the six cases reported by Fu and Perzin (1975) involved more than one cavity. Dropkin, Tang and Williams

(1976) reported a tumour in the nasal cavity which recurred five years later, involving the maxillary sinus. Jakobiec, Mitchell, Chauhan and Iwamoto (1978) described secondary invasion of the orbit from a primary leiomyosarcoma of the maxillary sinus.

Systemic metastasis commonly involves the lungs. In both the antral cases reported by Kawabe et al (1969) there was metastatic spread to cervical lymphnodes.

Few cases have been reported as surviving as long as five years. The nasal tumour of Pimpinella and Marquit (1965) recurred after nine and fourteen years. The naso-antral lesion of Dropkin et al (1976) had survived seven years with one recurrence. Three out of Fu and Perzin's cases died of their disease in less than four years. The I.L.O. case died from an unrelated cause fourteen years after local surgery followed by irradiation for an early recurrence.

BIBLIOGRAPHY

Dobben G D 1958 Leiomyosarcoma of the nasopharynx. Archives of Otolaryngology 68: 211–213

Dropkin L R, Tang C K, Williams J R 1976 Leiomyosarcoma of the nasal cavity and paranasal sinuses. Annals of Otology. Rhinology and Laryngology 85: 399–403

Fu Y, Perzin K H 1975 Non-epithelial tumours of the nasal cavity, paranasal sinuses and nasopharynx: IV smooth muscle tumors (leiomyoma, leiomyosarcoma). Cancer 35: 1300–1308

Jakobiec F A, Mitchell J P, Chauhan P M, Iwamoto T 1978 Mesectodermal leiomyosarcoma of the antrum and orbit. American Journal of Ophthalmology 85: 51–57

Kawabe Y, Kondo T, Hosoda S 1969 Two cases of leiomyosarcoma of the maxillary sinus. Archives of Otolaryngology 90: 492–495

Mindell R S, Calcaterra T C, Ward P H 1975 Leiomyosarcoma of the head and neck. Laryngoscope 85: 904–910

Pimpinella R J, Marquit B 1965 Leiomyosarcoma of nose, nasopharynx and paranasal sinuses. Annals of Otology, Rhinology and Laryngology 74: 623–630

Ranchod M, Kempson R L 1977 Smooth muscle tumors of the gastrointestinal tract and peritoneum. Cancer 39: 255–262

Stout A P, Hill W T 1958 Leiomyosarcoma of the superficial soft tissues. Cancer 11: 844–854

Yannopoulos K, Stout A P 1962 Smooth muscle tumors in children. Cancer 15: 958–971

Willis R A 1967 Pathology of tumours, 4th edn. Butterworth, London, ch 47: 747–756

24

Metastatic tumours of the nose and sinuses

METASTATIC TUMOURS OF THE NOSE AND SINUSES

The relative rarity of metastases in a region where primary tumours are more likely to occur inevitably leads to initial oversight, not only clinically but also from a histopathological point of view since certain metastatic tumours may resemble primary neoplasms in the region. Secondary tumours in the nasal or paranasal region are uncommon. In a review of metastatic carcinoma, Abrams, Spiro and Goldstein (1950) found none in the nose and sinuses, nor were any noted in reports of metastatic tumours in the jaws (Castigliano and Rominger, 1954; Cash, Royer and Dahlin, 1961; Clausen and Poulsen, 1963; McDaniel, Luna and Stimson, 1971). Nevertheless, there have been numerous solitary reports of metastatic tumours in the region.

In a review by the present authors (Friedmann and Osborn, 1965), it was noted that nearly 50 per cent of secondary tumours in the Ear, Nose and Throat region involved the nose and sinuses and of these nearly 80 per cent were derived from primary renal carcinoma. Flocks and Boatman (1973) reported a random selection of metastases from 100 renal carcinomas occurring in the head and neck region and referred to one case involving the nasal cavity which they regarded as unusual. In the I.L.O. material there have been five metastatic tumours in the nose and sinuses, representing less than 0.5 per cent of all tumours in the region and approximately 1.5 per cent of all malignant tumours. Four out of the five cases had primary renal carcinoma.

Metastases from renal carcinoma may present a variety of histological problems. The papillary adenomatoid structure (Fig. 24.1) has sometimes led to an erroneous diagnosis of 'papillary cystadenoma' (Friedmann and Osborn, 1965); the clear cell structure (Fig. 24.2) may be confused with a variant of acinic cell tumours of mucosal or salivary glands (see Fig. 14.19) whilst an occasional angiomatoid pattern may be mistaken for a haemangioma (Barmwater, 1931). The marked vascularity of these secondary tumours may often result in presentation with profound epistaxis

(Eneroth, Martensson and Thulin, 1961). It should be emphasized that primary renal carcinoma may remain occult until the patient presents with a metastasis (Biendara, 1951; Harrison, Doey and Osborn, 1964) but, on the other hand, a nasal secondary tumour may appear after the primary neoplasm has been removed (Achar, 1955; Edwards, 1964).

Secondary tumours from the alimentary tract are very uncommon in the nose and sinuses. Castigliano and Rominger (1954) found eight alimentary carcinomas which had metasized to the jaws but the sinuses were not involved. Garrett (1959) reported a secondary tumour in the antro-ethmoidal region from a gastric carcinoma. The possibility of confusion with primary adenocarcinoma in the naso-ethmoidal region has to be borne in mind.

The breast and bronchus are more common sites of primary tumours producing metastases in the jaws but, again, involvement of the nose and sinuses is rare. Garrett (1959) found one case each of mammary and bronchial carcinoma metastasizing in the nose. Ungerecht (1950) reported a paranasal metastasis from a mammary carcinoma whilst Reuter (1960) published a case of secondary carcinoma in the nose arising from a primary in the lung.

Occasional cases of metastasis from the genital tract have been reported. Garrett (1959) published two cases of seminoma of the testicle which produced secondary tumours in the nose and antrum respectively. The present authors (Friedmann and Osborn, 1965) previously reported a metastasis in the frontal sinus from a leiomyosarcoma of the uterus (Fig. 24.3). More recently, there have been several reports of metastatic choriocarcinoma in the nose and sinuses (Subramanyam and Lal, 1970; Salimi, 1977; Mukherjee, 1978).

Castigliano and Rominger (1954) noted a high incidence (26 per cent) of metastases in the jaws from carcinoma of the thyroid gland. Involvement of the sinuses did not occur in their series but one of the present authors encountered a case of secondary carcinoma of the thyroid in the nasal cavity (Figs. 24.4 & 24.5).

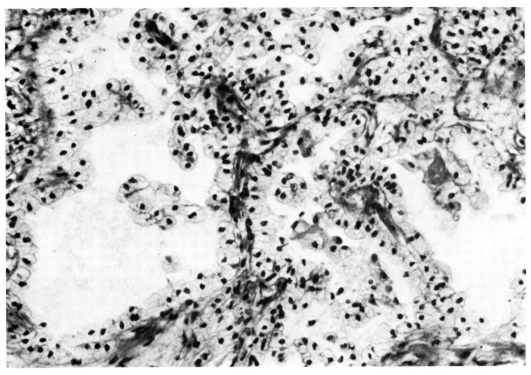

Fig. 24.1 Metastatic renal carcinoma in the maxillary sinus of a 63 year-old male, showing the 'papillary cystadenoma' pattern. M × 335

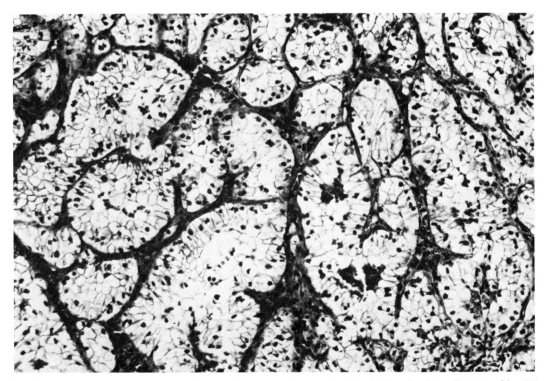

Fig. 24.2 Metastatic renal carcinoma in the frontal sinus of a 49 year-old male, showing the clear cell pattern. M × 268

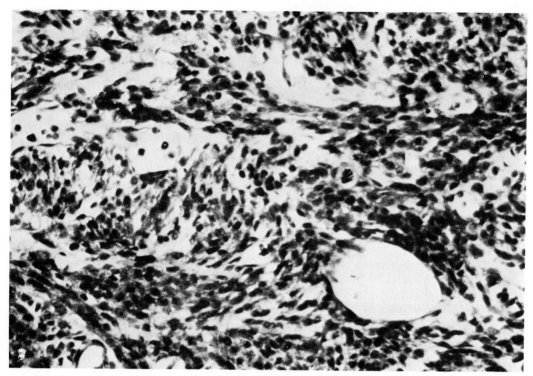

Fig. 24.3 Metastatic leiomyosarcoma of the uterus in the frontal sinus of a 56 year-old female. M ×335

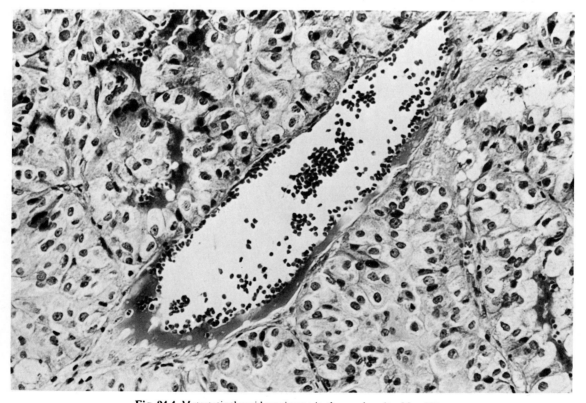

Fig. 24.4 Metastatic thyroid carcinoma in the nasal cavity. M ×525

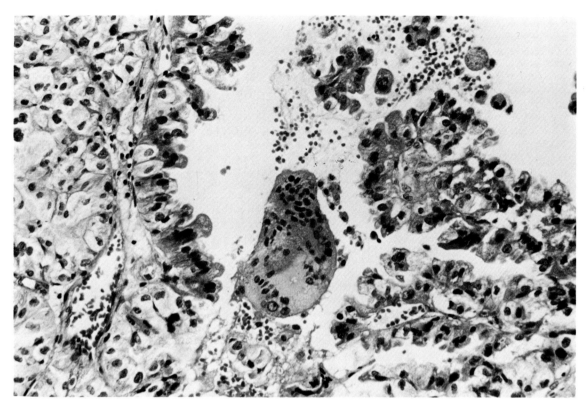

Fig. 24.5 Metastatic thyroid carcinoma in the nasal cavity. M × 525

BIBLIOGRAPHY

Abrams H L, Spiro R, Goldstein N 1950 Metastases in carcinoma. Cancer 3: 74–85

Achar M V R 1955 Metastatic hypernephroma occurring in the nasal septum. Archives of Otolaryngology 62: 644–648

Barmwater K 1931 Endothelioma cavi nasi. Zentralblatt für Hals-, Nasen- und Ohrenheilkunde 17: 42

Biendara E 1951 Zur Klinik der Hypernephrommetastasen im Nasen-nebenhöhlengebiet. Zeitschrift für Laryngologie und Rhinologie 30: 313–317

Cash C D, Royer R Q, Dahlin D C 1961 Metastatic tumors of the jaws. Oral Surgery, Oral Medicine and Oral Pathology 14: 897–905

Castigliano S G, Rominger C J 1954 Metastatic malignancy of the jaws. American Journal of Surgery 87: 496–507

Clausen F, Poulsen H 1963 Metastatic carcinoma of the jaws. Acta Pathologica et Microbiologica Scandinavica 57: 361–374

Edwards W G 1964 Epistaxis from metastatic renal carcinoma. Journal of Laryngology and Otology 78: 96–102

Eneroth C M, Martensson G, Thulin A 1961 Profuse epistaxis in hypernephroma metastasis. Acta Otolaryngologica 53: 546–550

Flocks R H, Boatman D L 1973 Incidence of head and neck metastases from genito-urinary neoplasms. Laryngoscope 83: 1527–1539

Friedmann I, Osborn D A 1965 Metastatic tumours in the ear, nose and throat region. Journal of Laryngology and Otology 79: 576–591

Garrett M J 1959 Metastatic tumours of the paranasal sinuses simulating primary growths. Journal of the Faculty of Radiologists (London) 10: 151–155

Harrison M S, Doey W D, Osborn D A 1964 Intranasal metastasis from renal carcinoma. Journal of Laryngology and Otology 78: 103–107

McDaniel R K, Luna M A, Stimson P G 1971 Metastatic tumor in the jaws. Oral Surgery, Oral Medicine and Oral Pathology 31: 380–386

Mukherjee D K 1978 Choriocarcinoma of the nose. Annals of Otology, Rhinology and Laryngology 87: 257–259

Reuter G 1960 Metastasis to the frame of the nose of a lung tumor. Krebsarzt 15: 61–63

Salimi R 1977 Metastatic choriocarcinoma of the nasal mucosa. Journal of Surgical Oncology 9: 301–305

Subramanyam C, Lal M 1970 Unusual presentation of chorion epithelioma malignum. Medical Journal of Malaya 24: 306–307

Ungerecht K 1950 Spätmetastase eines Mamma-Carcinoms. Zentralblatt für Hals-, Nasen- und Ohrenheilkunde 40: 130

Additional reference
Ferlito A, Recher G, Polidorf F 1979 Nasal metastases from primary cancer of the kidney. Journal of Laryngology 93: 1115–1120

Index